Hospital Care of the Recovering NICU Infant

Hospital Care of the Recovering NICU Infant

Edited by

M. Douglas Jones, Jr., M.D.
Professor and Chairman of Pediatrics
University of Colorado Health Sciences Center
Denver, Colorado

Christine A. Gleason, M.D.
Associate Professor of Pediatrics
Director, Eudowood Neonatal Pulmonary Division
The Johns Hopkins University School of Medicine
Baltimore, Maryland

Susan U. Lipstein, M.S., C.H.A., PA-C
Assistant in Pediatrics
The Johns Hopkins University School of Medicine
Baltimore, Maryland

WILLIAMS & WILKINS
BALTIMORE • HONG KONG • LONDON • MUNICH
PHILADELPHIA • SAN FRANCISCO • SYDNEY • TOKYO

Editor: Laurel Craven
Associate Editor: Victoria M. Vaughn
Copy Editor: Clifford L. Malanowski, Jr.
Designer: Wilma Rosenberger
Illustration Planner: Lorraine Wrzosek
Production Coordinator: Adèle Boyd
Cover Designer: Wilma Rosenberger

Williams & Wilkins
428 East Preston Street
Baltimore, Maryland 21202, USA

Accurate indications, adverse reactions, and dosage schedules for drugs are provided in this book, but it is possible that they may change. The reader is urged to review the package information data of the manufacturers of the medications mentioned.

Printed in the United States of America

Library of Congress Cataloging-in-Publication Data

Hospital care of the recovering NICU infant / edited by M. Douglas Jones, Jr., Christine A. Gleason, Susan U. Lipstein.
p. cm.
Includes index.
ISBN 0-683-04476-1
1. Neonatal intensive care. I. Jones, M. Douglas. II. Gleason, Christine A. III. Lipstein, Susan U.
[DNLM: 1. Infant, Newborn, Diseases. 2. Intensive Care, Neonatal.]
RJ253.5.H67 1991
618.92'01—dc20
DNLM/DLC
for Library of Congress 90-13158
CIP

90 91 92 93 94
1 2 3 4 5 6 7 8 9 10

To our teachers

Lula O. Lubchenco, Roberta A. Ballard, and Henry K. Silver

To our spouses

Ann, Erik, and Steven

With love and appreciation

Foreword

This book, Hospital Care of the Recovering NICU Infant, very nicely fills the void created by other textbooks that deal primarily with the acutely ill newborn.

Most physicians can be conveniently divided into two groups—"firemen" and "farmers." This book should appeal to the farmers in neonatology. A farmer is the physician who plays the crucial role in seeing that the infant survivors of the intensive care units grow and develop optimally.

Frank A. Oski, M.D.

Preface

The sick newborn is initially cared for in a Neonatal Intensive Care Unit (NICU) but recovers in either a less intensive, separate section of the NICU, a NICU step-down unit, a level II nursery, or even a nursery for fullterm newborns. Many are transferred back to referring hospitals for as long as several months prior to discharge. Although these recovering infants are often called "feeders and growers," as if little else were happening, they are not yet healthy and require special knowledge and care throughout the remainder of their hospitalization.

Medical care issues in the step-down nursery are not always covered in standard texts, or if they are, they are discussed with the critically ill infant in mind. We have attempted to describe the pathophysiology and management of the medical conditions encountered most frequently in recovering infants as well as to address the often complicated psychosocial and neurodevelopmental issues of the step-down nursery. Our goal is to take some of the mystery out of caring for these infants.

Because these infants usually recover outside of a NICU, they are often cared for by caretakers other than those specializing in neonatology. It is for these physicians, physician extenders, nurses, social workers, and other personnel that this book is primarily intended.

M. Douglas Jones, Jr., M.D.
Christine A. Gleason, M.D.
Susan U. Lipstein, M.S., C.H.A., PA-C

The editors gratefully acknowledge the excellent secretarial assistance provided by Karen Lingerman.

Contributors

Marilee C. Allen, M.D.
Associate Professor of Pediatrics
The Johns Hopkins University School of Medicine
The Kennedy Institute for Handicapped Children
Baltimore, Maryland

Bernard A. Cohen, M.D.
Assistant Professor of Pediatrics & Dermatology
University of Pittsburgh School of Medicine
Director of Pediatric Dermatology
Children's Hospital of Pittsburgh
Pittsburgh, Pennsylvania

Pamela Kimzey Donohue, M.S., C.H.A., PA-C
Assistant in Pediatrics
The Johns Hopkins University School of Medicine
Baltimore, Maryland

Jacob K. Felix, M.D.
Director, Division of Neonatology
Sinai Hospital
Baltimore, Maryland

Estelle B. Gauda, M.D.
Assistant Professor of Pediatrics
The Johns Hopkins University School of Medicine
Baltimore, Maryland

Emily Germain-Lee, M.D.
Fellow, Division of Endocrinology
The Johns Hopkins University School of Medicine
Baltimore, Maryland

Christine A. Gleason, M.D.
Associate Professor of Pediatrics
Director, Eudowood Neonatal Pulmonary Division
The Johns Hopkins University School of Medicine
Baltimore, Maryland

Janet E. Graeber, M.D.
Assistant Professor of Pediatrics
West Virginia University Hospital
Morgantown, West Virginia

Bonnie B. Hudak, M.D.
Assistant Professor of Pediatrics
SUNY School of Medicine at Buffalo
Buffalo, New York

Mark L. Hudak, M.D.
Associate Professor of Pediatrics
SUNY School of Medicine at Buffalo
Buffalo, New York

M. Douglas Jones, Jr., M.D.
Professor and Chairman of Pediatrics
The University of Colorado Health Sciences Center
Denver, Colorado

Susan U. Lipstein, M.S., C.H.A., PA-C
Assistant in Pediatrics
The Johns Hopkins University School of Medicine
Baltimore, Maryland

John F. Modlin, M.D.
Assistant Professor of Pediatrics
The Johns Hopkins University School of Medicine
Baltimore, Maryland

Leslie P. Plotnick, M.D.
Associate Professor of Pediatrics
The Johns Hopkins University School of Medicine
Baltimore, Maryland

Phoebe Rostov, M.S.W., L.C.S.W.
The Children's Guild
Baltimore, Maryland

L.R. Scherer, III, M.D.
Assistant Professor of Pediatric Surgery
The Johns Hopkins University School of Medicine
Baltimore, Maryland

Kenneth G. Zahka, M.D.
Associate Professor of Pediatrics
Director, Division of Pediatric Cardiology
Rainbow Babies and Childrens Hospital
Cleveland, Ohio

Contents

Foreword — *vii*
Preface — *ix*
Acknowledgment — *xi*
Contributors — *xiii*

1 Nutrition — 1
Mark L. Hudak

2 Apnea and Bradycardia — 33
Estelle B. Gauda

3 Postnatal Anemia — 49
M. Douglas Jones, Jr.

4 The Cardiovascular System — 61
Kenneth G. Zahka

5 Temperature Regulation — 79
Christine A. Gleason

6 Infectious Disease — 85
John F. Modlin

7 Chronic Lung Disease — 103
Susan U. Lipstein and Bonnie B. Hudak

8 Retinopathy of Prematurity — 125
Janet E. Graeber

9 Neurodevelopmental Outcome and Interventions — 133
Marilee C. Allen

10 Assessment of Risk for Developmental Disability — 149
Marilee C. Allen

11 The Thyroid — 161
Emily L. Germain-Lee and Leslie P. Plotnick

12 Screening for Hearing Loss 177
Jacob K. Felix

13 Surgical Management 187
L. R. Scherer, III

14 Dermatology 197
Bernard A. Cohen

15 Discharge Planning 219
Pamela Kimzey Donohue and Christine A. Gleason

16 The Family's Perspective 227
Phoebe Rostov

Appendices 239
A. Laboratory Values 239
B. Growth Parameters 240
C. Miscellaneous 243
Index 247

1

Nutrition

Mark L. Hudak

The cumulative effect of evolutionary advances in infant nutrition unquestionably surpasses that of many of the more dramatic advances in the technology of neonatal intensive care. Progress will continue as new therapies decrease the severity of acute lung disease and allow neonatologists to devote more attention to nutritional issues. Moreover, the recent extension of the "limits of viability" to the 23 to 24 week fetus has brought new and complex challenges to nutritional management. The success with which these are met will be an important determinant of long-term outcome.

What are the appropriate nutritional objectives for the management of the premature infant? For over a decade, the American Academy of Pediatrics Committee on Nutrition has advocated achievement of a "postnatal growth that approximates the in utero growth of a normal fetus at the same postconceptional age." With time, the agenda has become increasingly sophisticated. The initial aim was to achieve intrauterine weight gain, but as specific nutritional deficiencies were recognized in infants with adequate weight gain, strategies refocused on duplicating fetal accretion rates for specific nutrients. More recently, it has been recognized that the preterm infant fed a typical premature formula stores macronutrients (protein and lipid) in different proportions than the fetal counterpart. However, modifications of diet can mimic fetal macronutrient accretion rates, and some investigators have suggested such regimens might further improve outcome. Other investigators argue that, because birth results in profound environmental changes that necessitate adaptive responses, the preterm infant may be better served by growth that does not precisely reproduce fetal patterns. At present, whether "maintenance of an extrauterine fetus" or "accelerated development" is the better nutritional strategy awaits the results of randomized trials. As MacLean has noted, "Perhaps the most appropriate goal of nutritional management is to do whatever possible during the short-term care . . . to produce a long-term outcome that is compatible with both normal physical development and, especially, normal mental development."

This chapter is organized into two sections. The first section presents selected basic nutritional information and summarizes the nutritional requirements and recommendations. The second section outlines some practical aspects of nutritional management.

Nutritional Requirements of the Preterm Infant

FETAL GROWTH

Reproduction of fetal growth has become the de facto standard of successful nutrition in the premature infant. Most of fetal growth occurs between 28 and 40 weeks as weight increases at a rate of 1 to 2% per day (Fig. 1.1). The proportion of total body and extracellular water decreases; intracellular water increases coincident with cellular hyperplasia and hypertrophy. Of the macronutrients, protein and lipid content increase fourfold and tenfold,

Figure 1.1. Smoothed curve values for fetal and postnatal growth of absolute weight in grams, growth velocity in grams per day, and incremental growth rate by percent increase in body weight per day between 8 weeks fetal life and 6 months postnatal life. Growth during the third trimester averages between 1.5 and 2% of body weight per day. (Reprinted with permission from Usher RH, McLean FH. Normal fetal growth and the significance of fetal growth retardation. In: Davis JA, Dobbing J, eds. Scientific foundation of pediatrics. Philadelphia: Saunders, 1974.)

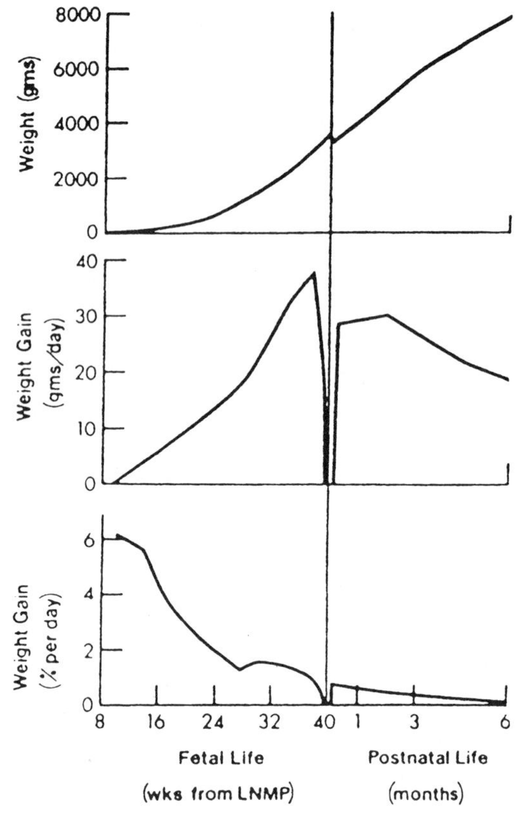

Table 1.1. Body Composition of the Reference Fetus[a]

Gestational Age (weeks)	Body Weight (grams)	Per 100 g Body Weight: Water (grams)	Protein (grams)	Lipid (grams)
24	690	88.6	8.8	0.1
28	1160	84.6	9.6	3.3
32	1830	80.7	10.6	6.3
36	2690	77.3	11.4	8.7
40	3450	74.0	12.0	11.2

[a]Reprinted with permission from Ziegler EF et al. Body composition of the reference fetus. Growth 1976;40:329–341.

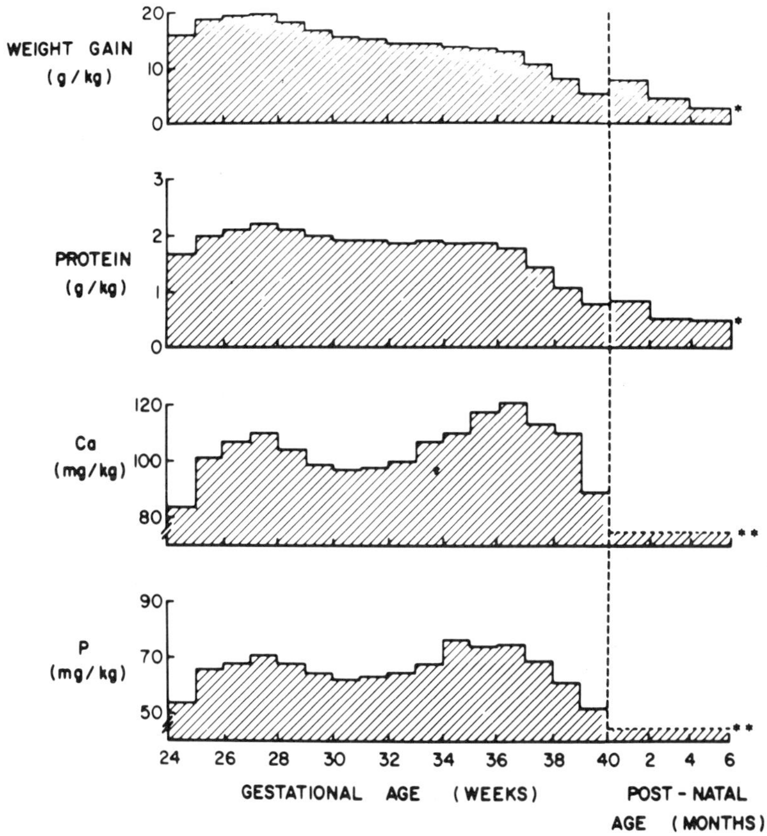

Figure 1.2. Daily weight gain and accretion rates of protein, calcium, and phosphorus during gestation and during the first 6 postnatal months. (Reprinted with permission from Okamoto E, Heird WC. Feeding the low-birth-weight infant. Pediatric Annals 1981;10:440.)

respectively (together they comprise 23% of body weight at term), thereby outpacing the rate of weight gain (Table 1.1). Carbohydrate stores also increase, but they comprise only 1% of body weight at term. Fetal skeletal maturation results in a fourfold rise in calcium and phosphorus stores. Fetal rates of accretion of protein (g/kg/day), calcium (mg/kg/day) and phosphorus (mg/kg/day) as derived from the reference fetus data of Ziegler are depicted as a function of gestational age in Figure 1.2.

FETAL ENERGY REQUIREMENTS

Energy requirements are the sum of energy expended for metabolism and energy stored in new tissue. Metabolism supports maintenance of existing tissue as well as the cost of synthesizing new tissue. Human fetal oxidative metabolism ranges from 5 to 8 ml of O_2/kg/min. Because consumption of 1 liter of oxygen corresponds to an energy consumption of approximately 7 kcal (this figure varies depending on the exact proportion of metabolic substrates), the human fetus consumes 35 to 56 kcal/kg/day.

Energy stored in new tissue can be calculated from changes in fetal body composition. Figure 1.3 demonstrates the protein, fat, and total energy (kcal/kg/day) stored during growth

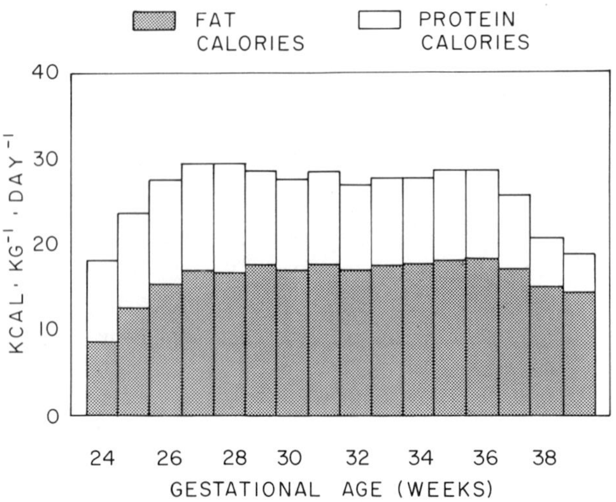

Figure 1.3. Fat, protein, and total energy stores (kcal/kg/day) in the fetus between 24 and 39 weeks gestation based on data from Ziegler.

vs. gestational age as derived from analysis of the data in Table 1.1 (assuming caloric values of 5.65 and 9.25 kcal/g of tissue stored as protein and fat, respectively, and negligible storage of carbohydrate). These data suggest that, during the third trimester, energy stored in new tissue during growth is fairly constant at approximately 30 kcal/kg/day and declines only after the 37th week of gestation. Sparks et al., using a different set of body composition data that reflected increased lipid deposition, calculated a slightly greater stored energy component (Fig. 1.4).

Taking into account both sets of data, total fetal energy requirements are on the order of 50 to 85 kcal/kg/day at 28 weeks and 56 to 98 kcal/kg/day at 38 weeks. Postnatally, cold stress, increased physical activity, and in the enterally fed infant, fecal nutrient loss increase energy requirements.

ENERGY REQUIREMENTS OF THE PRETERM INFANT

Clinicians often aim to provide 120 kcal/kg/day as "full calories." This is based on the usual breakdown of energy balance of the growing premature infant as shown in Table 1.2. Before we examine the individual components of energy balance in more detail, however, it must be noted that 120 kcal/kg/day is at best a guideline. In practice, the energy intake required to achieve the intrauterine growth rate of 1 to 2% of body weight per day varies among infants and over time in the same infant. Some premature infants (generally 1200 to 1800 grams) will grow at a rate greater than 2% of body weight per day on fewer than 120 kcal/kg/day; infants with chronic lung disease may require more than 120 kcal/kg/day to grow. In a healthy infant mature enough to nipple all feedings, appetite safely determines energy intake. Many premature infants may demand ad lib feedings in excess of 120 kcal/kg/day. Growth rates of 2 to 3% of body weight per day may result. This "catch-up" growth in part compensates for the lag time before consistent postnatal weight gain is achieved (up to several weeks in the smallest infants). Once attained, this growth spurt may persist for weeks to months as an infant attempts to achieve his or her genetic growth potential.

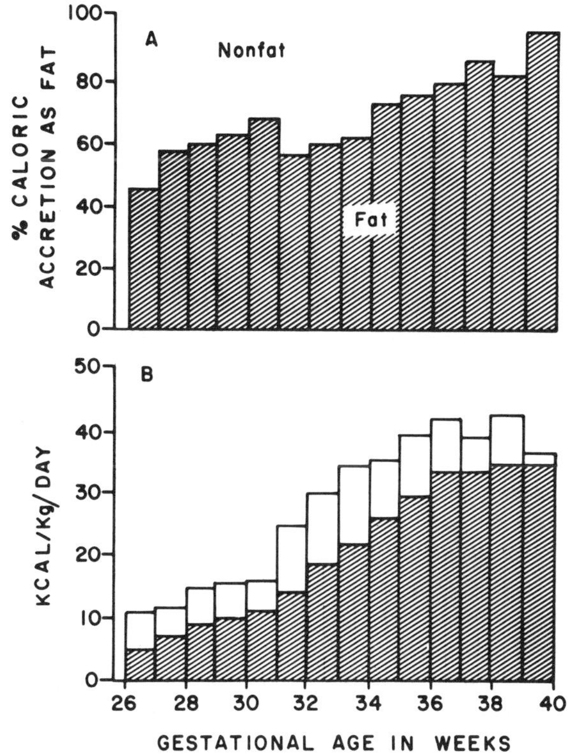

Figure 1.4. Lipid accretion as percentage of caloric accretion (Panel A) and in absolute terms, obtained by multiplying the daily increase in fat weight by 9.5 kcal/g and the increase in nonfat dry weight by 4.5 kcal/g (Panel B), for each week of gestation from 27 weeks to term. (Reprinted with permission from Sparks JW, Girard JR, Battaglia FC. An estimate of the caloric requirements of the human fetus. Biol Neonate Basel, Switzerland: S. Karger AG, 1980;38:113.)

Table 1.2. Energy Requirements of the Preterm Infant

Category	Energy Requirement (kcal/kg/day)
Basal metabolic rate	50
Intermittent physical activity	15
Intermittent cold stress	10
Thermic effect of food	8
Fecal caloric excretion	12
Growth	25
Total	120

Components of Energy Requirement

Several recent studies have investigated energy balance in the healthy, growing premature infant. Estimates of the basal metabolic rate (BMR) in premature infants between 1000 and 2000 grams range from 35 to 50 kcal/kg/day. Estimates of the BMR in full-term infants are slightly higher (43 to 60 kcal/kg/day). In both premature and term infants, brain metabolism accounts for 60 to 70% of the BMR. Diseases (e.g., infection), chronic hypoxia, thermal stress, and certain drugs (e.g., inotropic agents) may increase basal metabolic requirements.

Physical activity accounts for a relatively small part of energy needs. Estimates range from 3 kcal/kg/day in the sedentary, nongrowing infant to about 15 kcal/kg/day in the active, growing infant. In a term newborn, vigorous crying will transiently increase metabolism by 50%.

Extra energy needs for thermoregulation are incurred whenever an infant is cared for outside a thermoneutral environment. Thermoregulatory requirements increase in proportion to the decrease (or increase) in environmental temperature outside the zone of thermoneutrality. Even normal care may decrease isolette temperature and result in transient cold stress.

Diet-induced thermogenesis (DIT) (also known as the thermic effect of food or specific dynamic action) is due to the energy costs of synthesizing absorbed nutrients into fat, protein, and carbohydrate stores. Chessex et al. found that metabolism increased by 0.67 kcal/kg/day for each gram of weight gain. Thus, a weight gain of 15 g/kg/day was associated with an approximate 10 kcal/kg/day increase in resting metabolic expenditure.

Energy requirements for growth depend on the composition of weight gain. For example, Reichman et al. compared growth and macronutrient storage in infants fed approximately 110 and 150 kcal/kg/day of preterm breast milk and SMA formula, respectively. Despite the difference in caloric intakes, weight gain was equivalent. New body tissue was leaner (same proportion of protein but lower percentage of fat) and more closely resembled fetal macronutrient accretion in infants fed their own mother's milk (Fig. 1.5). As a result, infants fed their own mother's milk required 3.09 kcal/g of weight gain vs. 4.26 kcal/g in formula-fed infants. Results of a large number of studies can be summarized as follows: if protein needs are met, dietary energy in excess of that required for full protein utilization is stored as body fat.

PROTEIN

Protein is perhaps the single most important nutrient for the growing infant. In contrast to carbohydrate and fat, the body has no mechanisms for storing protein and cannot synthesize it without dietary essential amino acids. In the infant, protein is required both for maintenance (replenishment of fixed losses via fecal, dermal, and urinary routes) and for growth.

Protein is well-absorbed even by very premature infants. Net protein absorption rates average 83% and 87%, respectively, for breast and formula-fed infants. The premature infant is as capable as the term infant in the ability to absorb protein but is at a disadvantage with respect to both the synthetic and degradative aspects of amino acid metabolism. Due to immature enzyme systems, certain amino acids that are nonessential to adults are "semi-essential" in the newborn. Tyrosine is considered to be semi-essential because phenylalanine hydroxylase activity, which converts phenylalanine to tyrosine, is decreased in the preterm infant. Similarly, the sulfur amino acids cysteine and taurine (metabolites of methionine) are semi-essential because of immaturity of the hepatic enzymes cystathionase and sulphinic acid decarboxylase, respectively. In addition, the preterm infant has a limited capacity to catabolize excess amino acids; intake of excessive or poor quality protein places the infant at risk for acidosis, azotemia, hyperammonemia, and abnormal elevations of plasma amino acids. For these reasons, the difference between an inadequate and a toxic intake is much narrower for protein than for other nutrients.

The goals of protein nutrition are threefold: to supply a quantity and quality of protein sufficient to support fetal nitrogen retention rates; to achieve a normal plasma amino acid profile; and to avoid metabolic complications (e.g., acidosis, azotemia, hyperammonemia).

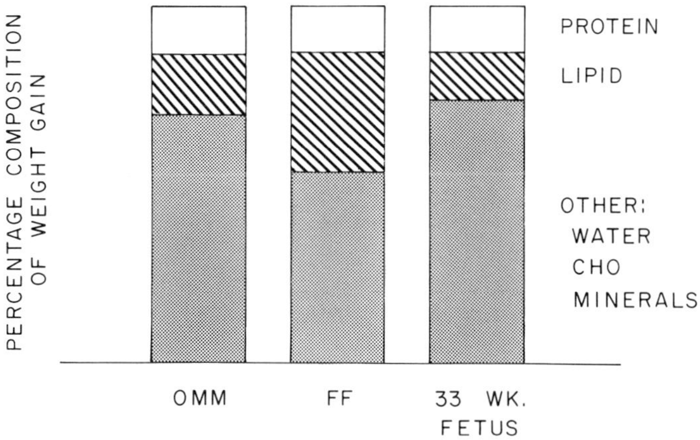

Figure 1.5. Composition of new weight gain at a postconceptional age of approximately 33 weeks in infants fed their own mother's milk (OMM) or formula (FF) and in the 33 week reference fetus. Formula-fed infants had greater proportion of lipid; composition of new weight gain in breast-fed infants more closely resembled that of the fetus. (Modified from Reichman B, Chessex P, Verellen G, Putet G, et al. Dietary composition and macronutrient storage in preterm infants. Pediatrics 1983;72:322, and Ziegler EE, O'Donnell AM, Nelson SE, Fomon SJ. Body composition of the reference fetus. Growth 1976;40:329.)

Quantity of Protein

In a 1 kg fetus, protein accrues at a rate of 2.32 g/kg/day. Dermal and urinary protein losses of 0.85 g/kg/day and a net protein absorption rate of 87% in the 1 kg newborn infant suggest that the protein requirement is at least 3.64 g/kg/day [(2.32 + 0.85)/0.87]. The requirement for a 1.5 kg infant calculated in this way is somewhat less (3.2 g/kg/day) due to a lower in utero protein accretion rate (2.0 g/kg/day) and reduced rate of dermal and urinary protein loss.

Heird and colleagues have clarified the protein requirement of the premature infant by evaluating the growth and metabolic responses of infants fed formulas that differed both in the proportions and in the absolute amounts of energy and protein. Infants with mean birth weights and gestational ages of 1450 grams and 31 weeks, respectively, were fed one of three formulas (protein [g/kg/day]:energy [cal/kg/day] ratios of 2.24:115, 3.6:115, and 3.5:149). Results are summarized in Table 1.3. Several conclusions are important. First, a protein intake of 2.25 g/kg/day supported weight gain but not protein retention at the intrauterine rate. The higher protein intake of 3.6 g/kg/day resulted in greater rates of weight gain and protein retention without metabolic complications. Second, an increase in the energy intake in infants who received 3.6 g protein/kg/day increased the rate of weight gain but did not improve protein retention. Increased weight gain was associated with increased fat deposition but not with increased lean body mass. Third, when all data were considered together, energy intake (whether provided by fat or carbohydrate) above that required for full protein utilization was stored as fat.

Heird and co-workers repeated this study using formulas that provided slightly different ratios of protein:energy intakes (2.8:119, 3.8:120, and 3.9:142). Infants fed the lower protein intake gained weight and retained protein at close to intrauterine rates without sustaining metabolic complications. Infants fed the higher protein intake exhibited greater

Table 1.3. Comparison of Nutritional Outcomes in Premature Infants Fed Three Formulas with Differing Proportions of Energy and Protein[a]

Formula Number	Energy (kcal/kg/day)	Protein (g/kg/day)
1	115	2.24
2	115	3.6
3	149	3.5
Nutritional outcomes		
Weight		1 < 2 < 3
Length, Head Circumference, Nitrogen Retention, BUN, Albumin		1 < 2 = 3
Fat Stored, Skinfold Thickness, Energy Expenditure, Energy Stored		1 = 2 < 3

[a]Modified from Kashyap S et al. Effects of varying protein and energy intakes on growth and metabolic response in low birth weight infants. J Pediatr 1986;108:955–963 and Schulze KF et al. Energy expenditure, energy balance, and composition of weight gain in low birth weight infants fed diets of different protein and energy content. J Pediatr 1987;110:753–759.

weight gain and nitrogen retention but developed metabolic abnormalities (elevated BUN and plasma amino acid levels), irrespective of energy intake.

In summary, these studies demonstrated that, although 3.5 to 3.6 g/kg/day of protein was completely utilized on an energy intake of 115 kcal/kg/day, a slightly higher intake of 3.8 to 3.9 g/kg/day was not completely utilized on an energy intake of 120 to 142 kcal/kg/day. In both studies, greater energy intakes increased fat deposition but not lean body mass.

To meet the three goals of protein nutrition stated above, it can be recommended that premature infants with birth weights between 900 and 1750 grams receive 3.0 g protein per 100 kcal/kg/day. This intake is provided by Similac Special Care formula, approximated by Premature Enfamil and SMA Premie formulas, and rarely met by premature human milk. Breast milk protein supplementation by breast milk fortifiers will meet this recommendation. As infants approach discharge, protein requirements for growth decrease and allow successful transition to standard formulas with lower protein concentrations.

The optimal protein intake of premature infants with birth weights less than 1000 grams has not adequately been studied. These infants may require more than 3.0 g protein per 100 kcal/kg/day to achieve intrauterine rates of nitrogen retention; however, it is not clear that such protein intakes could be tolerated without metabolic complications.

LIPID

Four major classes of lipid are needed: fatty acids, glycerides, phospholipids, and steroids. Lipids are especially important for growth and development during the third trimester of fetal life when lipid increases from 0.1% to from 11 to 15% of body weight. Functions of the various classes of lipids are shown in Table 1.4.

Fatty Acids

Biologically important fatty acids are unbranched, monocarboxylic acids that generally contain an even number (range, 2 to 24) of carbon atoms. Linoleic (18:2) and linolenic (18:3) acids are termed essential fatty acids because animals, unlike plants, cannot synthesize these compounds from precursors. They are especially important for brain development, cell proliferation, myelination, and retinal function.

Table 1.4. Functions of Lipid Classes

Fatty acids	Major lipid energy source
Glycerides	Storage form of fatty acids
Phospholipids	Cell membrane structure and function
	Precursors of prostaglandins; Major component of surfactant
Sterols	Cell membrane and lipoprotein structure and function
	Precursor of bile salts and adrenal and sex hormones
	Storage and transport of fatty acids

Glycerides

Glycerides are the esterification products of fatty acids and glycerol. Triglycerides comprise 98% of the lipid content and 40 to 50% of the energy content in breast milk and infant formulas. Lipid is stored in fat cells as triglycerides. After hydrolysis of triglycerides, energy is derived from oxidation of the fatty acid moieties. Fat storage is virtually without limit due to lack of feedback regulation.

Phospholipids and Sterols

Phospholipids are phosphorus-containing lipids. This lipid class includes derivatives of glycerol-3-phosphate (e.g., membrane and surfactant phospholipids). Arachidonic acid, the precursor of prostaglandins, is derived from the action of phospholipases on the fatty acid sidechains of certain membrane phospholipids. The sterol class of lipids includes cholesterol, adrenocortical and sex hormones, and bile acids.

Dietary Lipids

The sources of fat in different infant formulas are listed in Table 1.5. Table 1.6 compares the fatty acid composition of these fat sources. The combinations of vegetable fats and medium-chain triglycerides that are used in current infant formulas have been chosen to accomplish two clinical goals: to facilitate fatty acid absorption and to insure essential fatty acid sufficiency. The long-chain unsaturated fatty acids that predominate in vegetable fats are more easily absorbed than the saturated fatty acids that comprise the majority of animal fat (e.g., cow's milk). Similarly, absorption of the fatty acids released by hydrolysis of medium-chain triglycerides occurs rapidly because the process does not require solubilization and hydrolysis by intraduodenal bile salts, which may be deficient in premature infants. Furthermore, medium-chain fatty acids are absorbed directly into portal venous blood and are not (as are long-chain fatty acids) repackaged as chylomicrons for secretion into the lacteals.

The ratio of saturated to unsaturated fatty acids is approximately 2:3 in both preterm and term breast milk; however, concentrations of medium- and long-chain saturated fatty acids in preterm breast milk are increased and decreased, respectively, compared to term breast milk. For this reason, preterm infants may digest the fat in their own mother's milk more efficiently than the fat in pooled (term) breast milk. Breast milk contains C20 and C22 fatty acids (important for synthesis of neural tissue) that are not present in infant formulas. This may be of benefit to the preterm infant in whom the synthetic mechanisms for these fatty acids from linoleic and linolenic acid precursors are relatively immature.

Table 1.5. Sources of Fat in Infant Formulas

Cow's milk	Butterfat
Term formulas	
Similac 20, Isomil	Coconut and soy oils
Enfamil 20, Prosobee	Coconut and soy oils
SMA 20, Nursoy	Oleo, coconut, safflower, and soy oils
Preterm formulas	
Similac Special Care and Premature Enfamil	Medium-chain triglycerides (40 to 50%); coconut and soy oils
Premie SMA	Medium-chain triglycerides (10%); oleo, coconut, safflower, and soy oils
Pregestimil	Medium-chain triglycerides; corn and safflower oils

Table 1.6. Fatty Acid Composition (%) of Fat Sources in Infant Formulas[a]

Fatty Acids		Butterfat (Cow milk)	Coconut Oil	Soy Oil	Olive Oil	Safflower Oil	Corn Oil
Saturated							
Butyric	4:0	3.6					
Caproic	6:0	0.9	0.8				
Caprylic	8:0	0.8	5.4				
Capric	10:0	2.5	8.4				
Lauric	12:0	3.3	45.4	0.2			
Myrisitic	14:0	10.4	18.0	0.1	Trace		1.4
Palmitic	16:0	32.0	10.5	9.8	6.9	6.8	10.2
Stearic	18:0	14.5	2.3	2.4	2.3		3.0
	20:0		0.4	0.9	0.1		
Unsaturated							
Palmitoleic	16:1	2.7		0.4			1.5
Oleic	18:1	23.4	7.5	28.9	84.4	18.6	49.6
Linoleic	18:2	3.5	Trace	30.7	4.6	70.1	34.3
Linolenic	18:3	0.8		6.5		3.4	
Other		5.2	1.3	0.1	1.7	1.1	

[a]Adapted from Hamosh M. Fat needs for term and preterm infants. In: Tsang RC, Nichols BL, eds. Nutrition during infancy. Philadelphia: Hanley and Belfus, 1988.

Human milk fat has absorptive advantages compared to vegetable fats. First, the fatty acid composition in human milk favors absorption. Second, bile-salt stimulated lipase (recently shown to be identical to pancreatic cholesteryl esterase) is secreted in breast milk and becomes active in the small intestine at alkaline pH. It completely hydrolyzes medium- and long-chain triglycerides into glycerol and free fatty acids. This enzyme remains active even after breast milk is refrigerated.

It is recommended that total fat intake comprise 30 to 50% of calories. Intake of linoleic and linolenic acids should exceed 3.0 and 0.5% of total calories, respectively. These basic requirements are met or exceeded by human milk and premature infant formulas.

CARBOHYDRATE

Carbohydrate is an important energy source in the newborn infant. Carbohydrate stores at birth comprise about 1% (34 g) of body weight. Carbohydrate is stored in liver and skeletal and cardiac muscle as glycogen and is present as components of nucleic acids, mucopolysaccharides, glycoproteins, glycolipids, connective and collagenous tissue, and some hormones and enzymes.

Carbohydrate is provided in breast milk as the disaccharide lactose. Premature formulas supply carbohydrates as either lactose or nonbranched glucose polymers or both. Lactose accounts for 42% of the calories in breast milk. Similarly, infant formulas provide 41 to 44% of calories as carbohydrate.

Lactose is hydrolyzed into glucose and galactose by lactase, a brush border enzyme concentrated at the tips of the small intestinal villi. Lactase activity is detectable by 24 weeks of fetal life. Enzymatic activity is maximal in the midjejunum and decreases proximally and distally.

Glucose polymers are hydrolyzed by a combination of salivary amylase and intestinal maltase and glucoamylase; pancreatic amylase is not secreted in significant amounts before a month of age. Maltase and glucoamylase activity are present by the third trimester. These enzymes are concentrated in the crypts of the intestinal villi and are more resistant than lactase to villous atrophy from starvation and enteritis.

Glucose and galactose monosaccharides are absorbed by a sodium-linked, ATP-dependent active transport mechanism. Absorption is limited by intestinal surface area and transit time.

Healthy preterm and term infants are capable of digesting lactose. However, lactose malabsorption may occur due to congenital or acquired lactase deficiency (e.g., any of the causes of villous atrophy), congenital or acquired short bowel syndrome, decreased intestinal transit times, or excessive lactose intake. A small degree of lactose malabsorption is common and produces no clinical symptoms due to the capacity of colonic bacteria to ferment lactose. Excessive lactose malabsorption may cause proliferation of pathogenic intestinal flora and/or lead to intestinal distention and diarrhea. Signs of lactose malabsorption include the presence of reducing substances in stool, low fecal pH (<5), and acidosis. Because premature infants are at risk for lactose malabsorption, premature infant formulas are prepared with a 50:50 mixture of lactose and glucose polymers. Replacement of lactose with glucose polymers provides the additional benefit of reducing osmolality.

Under steady state conditions, systemic glucose consumption is about 5 mg/kg/min. Assuming complete lactose absorption, this rate can be fully fueled by providing about 70 cal/kg/day of breast milk or formula. Similarly, in the exclusively parenterally fed infant, approximately 70 ml/kg/day of 10% dextrose water is adequate. Cerebral metabolism accounts for the major portion of glucose consumption and is proportionately greater in the preterm infant.

No specific dietary requirement for carbohydrate has been established. In practice, however, sufficient carbohydrate should be provided to avoid hypo- and hyperglycemia. For this reason, it is recommended that 40 to 45% of full calories be supplied as carbohydrate.

MINERAL AND VITAMIN REQUIREMENTS

Water, Sodium Chloride, and Potassium

This section will consider salt requirements only in the healthy or growing premature infant. Recommendations are summarized in Table 1.7. The reader is referred to other sources for a discussion of fluid and electrolyte management in infants with significant derangements of salt and water homeostasis.

Table 1.7. Recommendations for Sodium and Potassium Intakes

Birth weight (grams)	Sodium (mEq/kg/day)	Potassium (mEq/kg/day)
> 2500	1.2 to 2.0	2.0
1500 to 2500	1.5 to 3.0[a]	2.0
< 1500		
1 to 3 weeks	2.0 to 4.0[a]	2.5
> 3 weeks	2.0 to 3.0	2.5

[a]Sodium requirement may be much higher (4 to 10 mEq/kg/day), depending on renal function. Sodium supplementation should be weaned according to serum sodium.

In a nongrowing, healthy adult, water and sodium chloride balance is zero. Normal renal function and intact regulatory mechanisms guarantee homeostasis over a wide range of intakes. However, provision of salt and water to premature infants must take into account other factors such as growth requirements, immature renal function, variable insensible water loss, and the effects of commonly used pharmacological agents (e.g., diuretics).

Water intake is determined by the amount necessary to make milk or formula isoosmolar. When adequate calories are provided, water intake greatly exceeds insensible losses. Thus, urine output averages 4 to 6 ml/kg/hr, and urine osmolality is low.

Term infants grow normally on 1.2 to 1.4 mEq Na/kg/day. This amount is supplied in 120 kcal/kg/day of mature breast milk or formula. Higher sodium intakes of 3 to 5 mEq/kg/day are also well tolerated. Indeed, "maintenance intravenous fluids" for infants less than 10 kg are commonly written as 100 ml/kg/day of 10% dextrose with 35 mEq/liter NaCl and provide 3.5 mEq Na/kg/day. Chloride is also essential. This fact was underlined a decade ago when infants fed a formula providing less than 0.5 mEq of chloride/kg/day developed severe metabolic alkalosis and failed to thrive.

Premature infants with birth weights above 1500 grams will generally thrive on sodium and chloride intakes of 1.5 mEq/kg/day. Hyponatremia (Na < 130 mEq/liter) occasionally develops in more immature infants and in infants with ileostomies. Such infants may require sodium chloride supplementation (3 to 10 mEq/kg/day). Infants recovering from chronic lung disease on diuretic therapy must also be observed for hyponatremia and/or hypochloremic, hypokalemic metabolic alkalosis and supplemented with sodium chloride and/or potassium chloride as necessary.

The very low birth weight (VLBW) infant (birth weight < 1500 grams) has a narrower tolerance range for salt and water intake primarily due to higher insensible water losses and less mature renal function (i.e., a higher renal fractional excretion of sodium). "Late hyponatremia" with diminished growth has been observed between the 2nd and the 6th week of life in infants with birth weights < 1000 grams who receive < 1.5 mEq Na/kg/day. This has been attributed to sodium chloride deficiency as a result of increased obligatory sodium excretion by an immature kidney and increased sodium incorporation into bone during rapid growth. Elevated plasma and urinary ADH and aldosterone levels support a functional sodium chloride deficiency.

After the first few days of life, the optimal intake of sodium chloride in the VLBW infant can be inferred to be between 1.5 and 5.0 mEq/kg/day. Intakes of 1.2 to 1.5 mEq/kg/day (with adequate protein and energy intake) in the first weeks of life have been associated with slow growth, decreased retention of potassium and nitrogen, abnormal levels of vasoactive hormones, and an increased incidence of hyponatremia and hyperkalemia compared to intakes of 2.2 to 5.0 mEq/kg/day. Elevated atrial natriuretic peptide on an intake of 4 to 5 mEq/kg/day suggests salt and water overload. On the basis of these findings, it seems prudent to provide VLBW infants with 2 to 4 mEq/kg/day until they reach a weight of 1500 grams and then wean toward 1.5 mEq/kg/day. Premature infant formulas (e.g., Similac Special Care, Premature Enfamil, and Premie SMA) provide 2.4 mEq/kg/120 kcal and meet these recommendations. Adjustments in salt intake can be made based on weekly measurements of the serum sodium concentration. Greater amounts of sodium chloride are frequently necessary if urinary or intestinal losses of sodium are high (e.g., as in infants on diuretic therapy or in infants following intestinal resection, respectively).

Potassium accrues at rates of 1 mEq/kg/day in the VLBW infant growing at 15 g/kg/day and at half that rate in the term infant growing at 7 g/kg/day. To cover losses, an extra 1.5 mEq/kg/day is recommended (Table 1.7). In the premature infant, diuretic and sodium bicarbonate, penicillin, or ticarcillin therapy may deplete total body potassium and cause hypokalemia (serum K $<$ 3.5 mEq/liter) that requires supplementation.

Hyperkalemia is uncommon in the recovering patient. Unexpected hyperkalemia in a previously stable patient is usually due to a medication error.

Calcium and Phosphorus

Providing calcium and phosphorus in quantities sufficient to avoid abnormalities of bone growth and development is one of the great challenges in the management of the very premature infant. Deficiency of these minerals can produce a spectrum of bone disease, ranging from mild osteopenia to severe rickets with pathological fractures. To avert bone demineralization, it is necessary to replenish obligatory fecal and urinary losses of these minerals even in the absence of skeletal growth. This is particularly crucial in the very low birth weight infant, who may not demonstrate consistent growth until several weeks of life. Growth adds enormously to mineral requirements. At the fetal rate of growth (a daily weight gain of 1.5% of body weight), retention of calcium and phosphourus should replicate fetal accretion rates of approximately 125 and 75 mg/kg/day, respectively. Higher (or lower) growth rates require commensurately greater (or less) mineral retention to achieve normal bone mineralization as assessed by bone radiographs or photon absorptiometry (see Fig. 1.6).

ABSORPTION AND EXCRETION OF CALCIUM AND PHOSPHORUS

Enteral absorption of calcium occurs by passive diffusion in the jejunum and ileum and by a process of active transport in the duodenum and jejunum that is dependent on vitamin D and a calcium binding protein. In the premature infant, passive diffusion predominates. The net rate of calcium absorption depends on the diet. For example, true calcium absorption is greater from term or preterm human milk (80 to 90%) than from infant formulas (30 to 80%). Calcium absorption tends to increase with postconceptional age. Net calcium retention is always less than net calcium absorption because of obligatory urinary calcium excretion.

Phosphorus is absorbed separately from calcium, both by passive diffusion and by a vitamin D mediated active transport mechanism in the jejunum and ileum. The capacity to absorb phosphorus also increases with postconceptional age. Phosphorus absorption depends on dietary composition and varies with the prevailing need for phosphorus. Absorption is inhibited by phytates in soy formula and by aluminum and magnesium containing antacids.

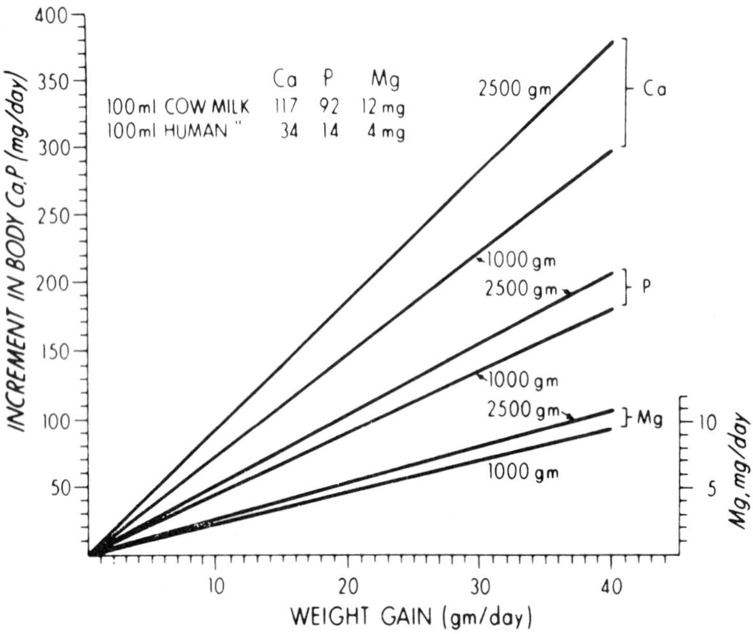

Figure 1.6. Increments in body calcium, phosphorus, and magnesium content as functions of body weight and weight gain, as derived from analyses of human fetuses. (Reprinted with permission from Committee on Nutrition of the American Academy of Pediatrics. Pediatric nutrition handbook. Elk Grove Village, IL: American Academy of Pediatrics, 1985.)

Normally, approximately 98% of the calcium that is filtered at the glomerulus is reabsorbed. Urinary calcium excretion is increased by sodium and glucose loads and by all diuretics (lasix > lasix + thiazide > thiazide + aldactone). Urinary loss of calcium delivered by parenteral nutrition is also increased. The percentage of filtered phosphorus that is reabsorbed is more variable and can range from 85 to 95%.

RECOMMENDATIONS FOR ENTERAL INTAKES OF CALCIUM, PHOSPHORUS, AND VITAMIN D

In term infants, human milk is assumed to provide the requirement for calcium and phosphorus. Human milk contains approximately 50 and 25 mg/kg/120 kcal of calcium and phosphorus, respectively. This, even with very efficient absorption and retention, will be insufficient for small infants (See Fig. 1.2). The concentrations of calcium and phosphorus in standard formulas are higher (75 to 90 and 50 to 70 mg/kg/120 kcal, respectively) to allow for less efficient absorption and retention.

Although intrauterine rates of calcium and phosphorus accretion cannot be met by pooled term human milk, preterm human milk, or standard formulas, fortification of preterm human milk with protein and minerals will support fetal accumulation rates. The composition of one commonly used fortifier is shown in Table 1.8. The use of premature formulas that contain 200 to 220 and 100 to 110 mg/kg/120 kcal of calcium and phosphorus, respectively, will allow attainment of intrauterine rates of mineral retention. The amount of calcium and phosphorus that should be provided to promote normal bone mineralization can be estimated from body weight and growth rate (Fig. 1.6). For example, a 1000 gram infant growing at

10 g/day should retain 75 and 42 mg, respectively, of calcium and phosphorus. Assuming net mineral retention rates of 65%, the required intakes of calcium and phosphorus are 115 and 65 mg, respectively.

The requirement for vitamin D in the premature infant is not known; currently, provision of 400 to 800 IU/day is recommended. Infants on full feedings of preterm human milk and most infants on premature formulas should receive 400 IU/day of supplemental vitamin D.

RECOMMENDATIONS FOR PARENTERAL INTAKES OF CALCIUM, PHOSPHORUS, AND VITAMIN D

Parenteral nutrition solutions should routinely contain calcium, phosphorus, and vitamin D. Until several years ago, precipitation of calcium phosphate crystals in parenteral solutions severely curtailed provision of intravenous calcium and phosphorus. One of the advantages of amino acid solutions formulated specifically for the neonate is that they permit solubilization of greater concentrations of minerals. For example, with Trophamine (McGaw Laboratories) one may add calcium and phosphorus in proportion to the concentrations of amino acids as listed in Table 1.9. Higher concentrations of calcium and phosphorus (600 and 465 mg/liter, respectively) have been used when indicated. Vitamin D should be added to provide 400 IU/day.

RECOGNITION AND TREATMENT OF CALCIUM AND PHOSPHORUS DEFICIENCIES

Inadequate retention of calcium and/or phosphorus is suggested by one or more of the following: osteopenia or rickets; pathological fractures; hypophosphatemia (serum phosphate < 5 mg/dl); elevated concentrations of serum alkaline phosphatase (> 500 IU/liter). Hypocalcemia is generally not observed until severe depletion of total body calcium occurs or unless one or more of the regulatory mechanisms controlling serum calcium fails (e.g., coexisting vitamin D deficiency). Radiological rickets will not be evident until bone growth begins. A very high serum alkaline phosphatase level (> 700 IU/liter) is a useful predictor that radiographical rickets will develop with growth in an unsupplemented infant.

Table 1.8. Composition of Enfamil Human Milk Fortifier (EHMF)

Nutrient	Amount (in four packets)[a]
Kilocalories	14.0
Protein (g)	0.7
Fat (g)	0.04
Carbohydrate (g)	2.7
Minerals	
Sodium (mEq)	0.3
Potassium (mEq)	0.4
Chloride (mEq)	0.5
Calcium (mg)	60
Phosphorus (mg)	33
Magnesium (mg)	4
Trace elements	
Zinc (mcg)	800
Copper (mcg)	40

[a]EHMF is mixed with breast milk in the ratio of four packets to 100 ml of breast milk. This results in a caloric density and concentrations of protein, minerals, and trace elements similar to Premature Enfamil 24 formula.

Table 1.9. Guidelines for Calcium and Phosphorus Concentrations in Trophamine Amino Acid Solution

Percent Amino Acids	Calcium (mg/liter)	Phosphorus (mg/liter)
0.8	300	200
0.8 to 1.4	400	267
1.5 to 1.9	500	333
≥ 2.0	600	400

Occasionally, very low birth weight infants show chemical and/or radiographical evidence of calcium and/or phosphorus deficiency despite full enteral feedings. These infants almost always have a history of significant medical complications such as chronic lung disease or necrotizing enterocolitis. Phosphorus should be supplemented initially with potassium phosphate solution (approximately 20 mg P per 1 mEq of K) beginning at 20 to 25 mg/kg/day. This will lower the calcium:phosphorus intake ratio below the 2:1 ratio delivered by the premature formulas, but it may be more appropriate. Although bones accrue calcium and phosphorus in a 2:1 ratio, the fetal accretion ratio is lower (1.4 to 1.7:1) and reflects the combined mineral needs of soft tissue and bone. Supplementation with calcium and phosphorus is also indicated if serum calcium and phosphorus are normal but serum alkaline phosphatase is increasing and osteopenia is worsening. Calcium carbonate or lactate salts are preferred because feeding intolerance and/or diarrhea sometimes complicate administration of calcium gluconate or glubionate.

Vitamin D doses above 400 IU/day have not been demonstrated to improve calcium or phosphorus retention. However, many clinicians choose to supply an additional 400 IU of vitamin D during feeding as part of a multivitamin preparation. This practice is without known side effects. However, very high doses of vitamin D increase bone reabsorption and may aggravate osteopenia or rickets.

Iron

For a discussion of iron requirements in the premature infant, see Chapter 3.

Trace Elements

Elements that comprise less than 0.01% of body weight are defined as trace elements. Some of the essential trace elements play an important role in metabolism, generally as fixed structural components or as activating cofactors of enzyme systems. To date, nine essential trace elements have been identified; zinc, copper, iodine, fluorine, selenium, chromium, manganese, molybdenum, and cobalt. Clinical deficiency states have been recognized in human infants for four of these; zinc, copper, iodine, and fluorine.

ZINC AND COPPER

In the fetus between 26 and 40 weeks, zinc accrues at a rate of 250 mcg/kg/day, and total body zinc increases fourfold. Similarly, copper stores increase sixfold as copper accumulates at a rate of 50 mcg/kg/day.

After birth, zinc is absorbed primarily by the ileum, and copper is absorbed in the stomach and proximal small intestine. The bioavailability of zinc and copper is greatly influenced by diet. Absorption of zinc and copper from enteral feedings ranks as follows:

preterm human milk > zinc and copper-fortified preterm human milk > term formula > preterm formula. The greater bioavailability of zinc in human milk compared to infant formulas or cow's milk has been attributed in part to the presence in human milk of citrate, which may facilitate mucosal cell uptake of zinc via its function as a zinc binding ligand. In the premature infant, absorption of zinc and copper increases as a function of postconceptional age.

The optimal accretion rates for zinc and copper in the premature infant are unknown. Achievement of intrauterine accretion rates may be unnecessary because significant amounts of these elements are stored in the fetal liver and released after birth.

Recommendation for Zinc and Copper Intakes

Currently, the American Academy of Pediatrics recommends enteral zinc and copper intakes of 600 and 108 mcg/kg/day, respectively. On 120 kcal/kg/day, these intakes are achieved with preterm human milk and most term and preterm infant formulas. Concentrations of these trace elements are deliberately greater in premature formulas than in human milk to compensate for decreased bioavailability. Recommended intakes of zinc and copper in the exclusively parenterally fed infant are lower (300 and 20 mcg/kg/day, respectively).

Zinc and Copper Deficiency States

Zinc and copper deficiencies have been described in infants with prolonged inadequate dietary intake or with conditions that interfere with adequate absorption (e.g., ileostomy).

The signs and symptoms of zinc deficiency are a characteristic dermatitis involving the periorificial, acral, and perineal areas, diarrhea, poor growth, delayed wound healing, decreased cell-mediated immunity, and hypoalbuminemia. An inherited defect in zinc absorption, acrodermatitis enteropathica (See Chapter 14), may manifest later in infancy with the additional signs of alopecia, delayed sexual maturation, and hypogeusia. Because of the excellent bioavailability of zinc in breast milk, this syndrome does not develop in the breast-fed infant until after weaning. It is successfully treated by providing oral zinc supplements (1 to 2 mg/kg/day).

Copper deficiency presents with pallor, failure to thrive, diarrhea, edema, lethargy, hypotonia, seborrheic dermatitis, hepatosplenomegaly, osteoporosis, sideroblastic anemia, and neutropenia. It is easily treated by provision of a supplement.

OTHER TRACE ELEMENTS

Iodine is essential for normal thyroid function. The recommended intake of 6 mcg/kg/day is based on the iodine content of breast milk and is met by all current term and premature infant formulas. Selenium deficiency has been reported to cause cardiomyopathy. Adequate selenium is present in breast milk and formula. Parenterally fed infants should receive 2 to 3 mcg selenium/kg/day.

Vitamins

The recommended daily allowances (RDAs) of vitamins as suggested by Dr. Reginald Tsang and the American Academy of Pediatrics are listed in Table 1.10. The table also shows the volume (ml/day) of fortified preterm breast milk and selected infant formulas required to meet these recommendations.

Table 1.10. Vitamin Requirements

Recommended Intake[a]		PE[c] 20	SSC 20	Premie SMA 20	Preterm human milk with EHMF	Pregestimil 20	Poly-vi-sol 1 ml	Vi-Daylin 1 ml
		Volume of Formula to Supply Recommendation[b] (ml)						
Vitamin A	1400 IU	173	304	438	170	560	1500	1500
Vitamin D	400 IU	182	396	784	182	784	400	400
Vitamin E								
Weeks 2–4	25 IU	806	926	1667	658	1000	5	5
>Week 4	5 IU	161	185	333	131	200		
Vitamin K	5 μg/kg	55/kg	60/kg	71/kg	45/kg	40/kg		
Vitamin B_1 (Thiamin)	250 μg/100 kcal	Yes	Yes	No	Yes	No	500	500
Vitamin B_2 (Riboflavin)	335 μg/100 kcal	Yes	Yes	No	Yes	No	600	600
Vitamin B_6	250 μg/100 kcal	Yes	Yes	No	Yes	No	400	400
Vitamin B_{12}	0.15 μg/100 kcal	Yes	Yes	Yes	Yes	Yes	2	1.5
Niacin	4 mg/100 kcal	Yes	Yes	No	Yes	No	8	8
Folic acid	50 μg/day	217	200	500	192	472		
Vitamin C	60 mg/day	260	240	857	214	768	35	35
		Volume (ml) Needed to Meet Requirements for All Vitamins						
		260[d]	396[d]	857[d]	214	784[d]		

[a]Compiled by Jeanne Cox from Tsang RC. Vitamin and mineral requirements in premature infants. New York: Marcel Dekker, 1985 and Committee on Nutrition of the American Academy of Pediatrics. Nutritional needs of low birth weight infants. Pediatrics 1985; 75:976–986.
[b]Assuming Vitamin E supplementation with 12.5 IU b.i.d.
[c]PE, Premature Enfamil; SSC, Similac Special Care; EHMF, Enfamil Human Milk Fortifier
[d]Volumes of 24 kcal formula to provide recommended intakes: PE 24, 216 ml; SSC 24, 330 ml; Premie SMA 24, 714 ml; Pregestimil 24, 653 ml.

Prescription of vitamin supplements should take into account the type and volume of enteral feeding. For instance, an intake of 150 mg/kg/day of premature Enfamil 24 or fortified preterm human milk in a 1.5 kg infant supplies the RDA for all vitamins. On the other hand, a 1.0 kg infant taking 100 ml/day of Similac Special Care requires vitamin supplements to meet the RDA for all vitamins. Supplementation must take into account the osmolality of multivitamin preparations, which can exceed 10,000 mosm/liter. Addition of 1 ml of a multivitamin preparation to 30 ml of formula nearly doubles the osmolality. Oral vitamin supplementation may be started when an infant tolerates 60 to 70 kcal/kg/day of enteral feedings or when parenteral nutrition is discontinued. Doses of 0.5 ml/day (0.25 ml b.i.d.) and 1 ml/day (0.5 ml b.i.d.) seem reasonable for infants less than and greater than 1250 grams, respectively.

RDAs for several vitamins are based upon the average quantity of vitamin consumed by a healthy, breast-fed term neonate. For example, the RDA of vitamin A is derived as the product of the concentration of vitamin A in term breast milk (2230 IU/liter) and the volume of breast milk consumed by a term neonate (3.5 kg × 180 ml/kg = 630 ml), or approximately 1400 IU. However, the vitamin requirements of premature infants are not necessarily equivalent to these RDAs. Several factors may increase vitamin requirements of the premature infant. These include lower body stores at birth, increased utilization, and decreased intestinal absorption of vitamins. A recent report that early intramuscular vitamin A supplementation in infants with acute lung disease decreased the incidence and severity of chronic lung disease has highlighted this point.

Practical Considerations in Feeding the Preterm Infant

A host of factors complicates enteral delivery of nutrients to even the healthy preterm infant. Factors related to immature neurophysiological functions are easily circumvented, but there are no quick fixes for immature gastrointestinal function (delayed gastric emptying, diminished peristalsis, decreased digestive and absorptive capabilities) and metabolism. Complications of prematurity (acute and chronic respiratory disease, patent ductus arteriosus, apnea and bradycardia, sepsis, necrotizing enterocolitis) add to the actual and perceived difficulty of establishing adequate enteral nutrition. The net result is that, on average, the length of time required to achieve full enteral feedings increases as gestational age decreases. For example, in 1987, infants cared for in the Columbia University NICU with birth weights between 900 and 1750 grams tolerated full enteral feeds (120 kcal/kg/day) and regained birth weight by 2 to 3 weeks of age. Thereafter, weight gain in excess of the intrauterine rate (catch-up growth) allowed discharge at a weight greater than the 10th percentile. In contrast, infants with birth weights less than 1000 grams did not regain birth weight or tolerate full enteral feeds until 5 to 6 weeks of life. In the latter infants, catch-up growth had not occurred by a postconceptional age of 40 weeks; these infants remained below the 10th percentile in weight.

Optimal nutritional management of premature infants with birth weights below 1500 grams and/or gestational ages less than 30 weeks is best achieved with a combination of parenteral and enteral feeding regimens until enteral feeding is well established. Parenteral supplementation of amino acids and lipid can be discontinued when enteral feedings of 60 to 70 kcal/kg/day are tolerated. The following discussion is limited to the practical aspects of the management of enteral feeding of the premature infant and will include the following topics:

1. Initiation of enteral feedings;
2. Choosing breast milk or formula;
3. Methods of enteral feeding;
4. Advancing enteral feedings;
5. Concentration of feedings;

6. Monitoring feeding tolerance;
7. Nutritional assessment; and
8. Discharge recommendations.

INITIATION OF ENTERAL FEEDINGS

Over the past 50 years, the timing of the first enteral feeding in the premature infant has swung through two cycles of the pendulum. Before World War II, clinicians commonly began milk feedings within the first several hours of life. By the 1940s, however, it was advocated that feedings be delayed 3 to 4 or more days after birth to minimize aspiration pneumonia and to facilitate the resolution of peripheral edema. In the 1960s, early institution of feedings was recommended as concerns surfaced about the effect of even short periods of starvation on neurodevelopment. The introduction of parenteral nutrition in the 1970s, coupled with the linkage of necrotizing enterocolitis to enteral feeding, led to a reemergence of the practice of delaying oral feedings. A survey conducted in 1983 revealed that, in 80% of tertiary care nurseries, infants with birth weights less than 1000 grams received no enteral feedings during the first week of life.

Although the optimal time to begin oral feedings in the extremely low birth weight infant is still controversial, several lines of evidence suggest that the early institution of hypocaloric enteral feedings may be beneficial. First, prolonged enteral fasting in experimental animals adversely affects gastrointestinal structure and function even if adequate calories and nutrients are provided parenterally. Second, recent clinical trials have demonstrated beneficial, but not detrimental, effects of early feeding in sick premature neonates. Two controlled trials were unable to demonstrate that early feeding increases the incidence of necrotizing enterocolitis. Indeed, in the first trial, Ostertag and associates found that the incidence of NEC was greater in infants fasted for 2 weeks compared to infants with shorter fasts. Their follow-up study showed that two groups of high-risk infants differing only in the timing of initial feeding (day 1 vs. day 7) had equivalent rates of NEC.

Other investigators have reported that a regimen of hypocaloric feeds (5 to 8 kcal/kg/day) begun on day 2 to 7 and continued for 7 to 10 days (in conjunction with parenteral nutrition) improved feeding tolerance, decreased the time to full feedings, and reduced the incidence of indirect hyperbilirubinemia, cholestatic jaundice, and metabolic bone disease compared to an isocaloric prescription of parenteral nutrition and enteral fasting through day 9 to 17. Infants on early hypocaloric feedings also had improved oral glucose tolerance compared to fasted infants, perhaps in part related to the earlier induction of gastrointestinal hormones.

In summary, there is no consensus regarding the optimal time to begin enteral feeds in the premature infant. Decisions tend to be individualized and depend on the birth weight, maturity, and clinical condition of each infant. Confirmation by additional controlled trials that early institution of hypocaloric enteral feedings is both safe and beneficial should have an important impact on clinical practice.

CHOOSING BREAST MILK OR FORMULA

Is breast milk best? That the mother's breast milk initially provides the best nourishment for a term infant is a key operational axiom of nutritional science. On the basis of this assumption, term formulas (Similac, Enfamil, SMA) have been modeled after mature breast milk. Current formulas indeed have excellent nutritional quality. Breast milk, however, has several potentially important immunological advantages compared to formula

Table 1.11. Components of Breast Milk and Immunological Function

Protein	
Casein subunit	Potentially enhances growth of *Lactobacillus bifidus*
Whey proteins	
Lactoferrin	Inhibits coliform, fungal growth by binding iron Bactericidal in combination with secretory IgA (SIgA) Anti-inflammatory properties Comprises 20% of breast milk protein (only trace amounts present in cow's milk)
Lysozyme	Bactericidal vs. coliforms in conjunction with SIgA Anti-inflammatory agent
Secretory IgA	Inhibits adherence and proliferation of bacteria at epithelial surfaces Confers "environmental specificity" to breast milk because IgA antibodies derived from entero- and bronchomammary pathways reflect antigenic and microorganism exposure of mother Comprises 90% of IgA and 10% of total protein in breast milk (but only 0.1% of cow's milk protein) Concentration probably increased in preterm vs. term breast milk
Carbohydrate	
Oligosaccharides	Analogus in structure to bacterial receptors, potentially inhibit binding of bacteria to cell surfaces Promote growth of *Lactobacillus bifidus* Comprise 15 to 20% of total carbohydrate in breast milk
Lymphocytes	Secrete immunoglobulins

because of its unique protein, carbohydrate, and cellular components (Table 1.11). Whenever possible, infants should be fed fresh breast milk. Immune factors related to cellular elements are lost with freezing or refrigeration of breast milk; cellular and immunoglobulin-related properties are destroyed during the process of heat sterilization. Finally, breast feeding may provide important but difficult to quantitate psychological benefits.

Breast feeding of the premature infant is more controversial. It is clear, however, that the special nutritional needs of the preterm infant are not met by unsupplemented, pooled, banked term human milk. Preterm infants fed term milk are likely to develop deficiencies of energy, protein, salt, and minerals.

The composition of preterm breast milk, however, differs substantially from term human milk and, in some ways, more closely approximates the nutritional requirements of the premature infant. Preterm breast milk, in general, has higher concentrations of energy, protein, salt, magnesium, and IgA but lower concentrations of calcium and phosphorus than term human milk. Like term breast milk, the nutritional composition of preterm milk is subject to considerable individual variability and also changes after birth as a function of the duration of lactation. For example, changes in protein concentration for both term and preterm breast milk are summarized in Table 1.12. One can calculate that, at usual volumes, unsupplemented preterm breast milk will not meet the protein needs of the premature infant after 4 weeks of lactation.

Despite some controversy, the literature tends to support the practice of initiating feeding of the preterm infant with his or her own mother's milk. By the time an infant can tolerate full volumes, it is essential to supplement preterm breast milk (<32 weeks gestation) with protein, salt, minerals, and trace elements. Otherwise, hyponatremia will occur at 4 to 5 weeks, hypoproteinemia at 8 to 12 weeks, and rickets at 4 to 5 months of age.

Table 1.12. Changes in Protein Concentration of Breast Milk with Respect to Duration of Lactation[a]

	Average Protein Concentration (g/dl)	
Days Postpartum	**Preterm Breast Milk**	**Term Breast Milk**
3	2.83	2.24
7	2.25	1.88
14	1.97	1.60
28	1.65	1.38
Mature	—	0.8

[a]Values obtained by averaging results of the following studies:
Gross SJ, et al. J Pediatr 1980;96:641.
Atkinson SA, et al. Am J Clin Nutr 1980;33:811.
Gross SJ, et al. Pediatrics 1981;68:490
Lemons JA, et al. Pediatr Res 1982;16:113.
Anderson DM, et al. Am J Clin Nutr 1983;37:810.

Supplementation with a human milk fortifier such as Enfamil HMF (Table 1.8) is recommended (see Concentrations of Feedings below).

Preterm Infant Formulas

As MacLean has pointed out (Ross Seminars), preterm infant formulas have been designed specifically to meet the nutritional requirements of infants with birth weights of 1200 to 1500 grams. Nonetheless, these formulas by necessity are often fed to very low birth weight infants (<1000 grams). It is possible that future research will demonstrate that selective nutritional modifications of current premature formulas may enhance the growth of the more immature infant.

The current premature formulas include Premature Enfamil, Similac Special Care, and Premie SMA. Use of one of these formulas is recommended if mother's breast milk is not available. These formulas are similar in many ways, but differences do exist. Unfortunately, no comparative studies have been reported to guide the clinician's choice of formula.

Unlike term formulas, preterm formulas have been designed to facilitate digestion and absorption of nutrients as much as to supply nutrients specific to breast milk:

1. Protein in preterm formulas is whey-predominant. Presumably, this results in enhanced digestion because, unlike casein proteins, whey proteins are soluble in gastric fluid. However, much of the whey protein is β-lactoglobulin, a protein present in only small amounts in human milk. Protein concentration is higher in preterm than in term formulas.
2. Carbohydrate is provided by an approximate 1:1 mix of lactose and glucose polymers. Theoretically, the latter are more easily digested and absorbed by a preterm infant.
3. The fat composition of preterm formulas differs from term formulas in that a variable proportion of medium-chain triglycerides is added. In reasonable amounts, medium-chain triglycerides are better absorbed than long-chain fatty acids. Medium-chain triglycerides may also improve retention of nitrogen and calcium.
4. Preterm formulas are supplemented with salt and with calcium and phosphorus to meet increased requirements of preterm infants for these nutrients.

METHODS OF ENTERAL FEEDING

Gavage Feeding

Infants with a postconceptional age less than 32 weeks usually receive all enteral feedings by gavage due to immaturity and/or incoordination of gag, suck, swallow, and breathing mechanisms. These neurophysiological functions are generally mature enough by a postconceptional age of 32 to 35 weeks to allow a safe trial of nipple feeding. Other candidates for gavage feeding include neurologically abnormal infants (secondary to asphyxia or to a congenital anomaly) and infants with an excessively high respiratory rate. In addition, larger infants (>34 weeks) recovering from acute illnesses such as respiratory distress syndrome often require gavage feedings well beyond a postconceptional age of 35 weeks secondary to easy fatigability with nipple feedings. A judgment of when to begin and how aggressively to advance nipple feedings in the individual infant is best made in consultation with an experienced nurse. Many premature infants are able to coordinate sucking, swallowing, and breathing before the strength of their suck reflex matures. These infants often do well with a "premie" nipple that decreases the resistance of milk flow.

Gavage feedings may be delivered either by intermittent bolus or by continuous infusion via tubes placed orally or nasally directly into the stomach or transpylorically into the duodenum or jejunum. Guidelines for placing and changing feeding tubes and for delivering gavage feedings are summarized in Table 1.13. Nasal tubes can be more easily secured than oral tubes. However, they carry the disadvantage of obstructing the nasal airway, which is a particular practical problem in an infant receiving supplemental oxygen by nasal cannula; they are also irritating and cause increased nasal secretions. The theoretical advantages of transpyloric feedings (averting feeding problems secondary to delayed gastric emptying and/or gastroesophageal reflux and aspiration) are outweighed by the practical difficulties of placing and securing transpyloric catheters. In addition, complications of transpyloric feeding have been reported, including impaired fat absorption, diarrhea, abdominal distention, pyloric incompetence, alterations of intestinal flora, and intestinal perforation. Finally, there is no persuasive evidence that transpyloric feedings confer any nutritional advantage compared to gastric feedings.

CONTINUOUS VS. INTERMITTENT GAVAGE FEEDING

In the larger premature infant (e.g., birth weight > 1000 to 1250 grams), most clinicians initiate intermittent bolus feedings. For smaller premature infants, some clinicians advocate continuous feedings while others promote a bolus feeding regimen with equal vigor. For selected infants, continuous feedings may increase the rate of weight gain compared to isocaloric intermittent feedings. On the other hand, continuous feedings are technically more complicated (Table 1.13) and tolerance of continuous feedings are more difficult to monitor than bolus feedings. The advantages and disadvantages of each method are summarized in Table 1.14. In the individual infant, it is best to maintain a flexible approach. Some infants who do not tolerate continuous feedings respond well to bolus feedings; conversely, other infants who fail intermittent feedings thrive on continuous enteral infusions.

In order to administer continuous feeding of formula, a volume of formula greater than or equal to a 4 hour aliquot plus the dead space of extension tubing is drawn up into a syringe and attached to an infusion pump set at the prescribed rate. The aliquot is refreshed every 4 hours. Continuous feedings of breast milk are feasible, but precautions must be employed to prevent loss of fat in the delivery system. Separation of cream in nonhomogenized breast milk and adherence of lipid to tubing and cassettes mandates use of microinfusion pumps without cassettes and with minimal dead space in the length of plastic tubing. These precautions have been shown to result in a minimal (<4%) loss of fat and minimal time-related variations in nutrient composition. For both formula and breast feedings, the extension tubing is changed every 8 to 12 hours to minimize bacterial colo-

Table 1.13. Guidelines for Gavage Feedings

Catheter material	Polyethylene or silastic with radiopaque strips (Never use polyvinylchloride catheters; these catheters stiffen with exposure to gastric contents and result in an unacceptably high incidence of esophageal and gastric perforation)
Catheter size	5 F ($<$ 1300 grams) 8 F ($\geq$ 1300 grams)
Orogastric catheter	
Indications	Intermittent bolus gavage feedings Continuous feedings in absence of endotracheal tube or presence of nasal CPAP
Placement	Measure from mouth to earlobe to xiphoid process + 1 cm; secure with clear tape Auscultate stomach during injection of 2 to 3 ml air
Advantages	Does not interfere with nasal respiration
Disadvantages	More difficult to secure than nasogastric tube
Nasogastric catheter	
Indications	Continuous feedings in presence of endotracheal tube
Placement	Measure from nares around ear to xiphoid + 1 cm; secure with clear tape on cheek and at nose Ausculate stomach during injection of 2 to 3 ml air
Advantages	Easier to secure
Disadvantages	Interferes with nasal respiration May increase nasal secretions
Changing of catheters	
Intermittent bolus feedings	Change q12hr to minimize bacterial colonization
Continuous feedings	Change q24hr
Delivery of feedings	
Intermittent bolus method	Prescribed volume of feeding measured into a syringe Syringe (without plunger) connected to feeding tube and suspended above infant's head Feeding allowed to flow by gravity into the stomach Indwelling tube clamped after full feeding delivered, and infant is positioned in prone or right side down position to encourage gastric emptying Catheter pinched on withdrawal for changing
Continuous infusion method	For most premature formulas, a volume of greater than or equal to a 4 hour aliquot plus dead space of extension tubing is drawn up into a syringe and attached to an infusion pump set at the prescribed rate. Aliquot refreshed every 4 hours. Continuous feedings of breast milk are feasible if precautions are used. Separation of cream in nonhomogenized breast milk and adherence of lipid to tubing and cassettes mandates use of microinfusion pumps without cassettes and minimal dead space extension tubing as well as more frequent (q 2 to 3 hr) changes of aliquot. These precautions have been shown to result in minimal ($<$4%) loss of fat and minimal time variation in nutrient composition. Teleologically, a minor time variation in nutrient composition is reasonable considering the changes that occur in the lipid concentration of milk secreted during a single breast feeding. For both formula and breast feedings, the extension tubing is changed every 8 to 12 hours to minimize bacterial colonization

Table 1.14. Comparison of Bolus and Continuous Gavage Feedings

Bolus feeding
Minimizes risk of tube dislodgement and aspiration
Simplifies monitoring of feeding tolerance
Alters pulmonary mechanics through postconceptional age 35 weeks (decreases tidal volume, minute ventilation, and dynamic compliance; increases total lung resistance)
Produces cyclical variation of plasma levels of gastrointestinal hormones (e.g., insulin, gastrin, gastrointestinal inhibitory peptide)
Continuous feeding
Complicates monitoring of feeding tolerance
Minimizes change in pulmonary mechanics
Improves weight gain in 1000 to 1249 gram infants compared to isocaloric bolus feedings
Maximizes percentage delivery of prescribed enteral feedings
Minimizes gastric distention
Minimizes disturbance of the infant
Decreases frequency of apnea and bradycardia
Establishes steady-state plasma levels of gastrointestinal hormones

nization. The schedule of continuous enteral feedings depends on the predilection of the individual caretaker and ranges from 24 hours on to 3 hours on and 1 hour off. There is no reason a priori why any one schedule is preferable. In the extremely low birth weight infant, we generally attempt conversion from continuous to bolus feedings when the infant is growing well on full enteral calories and weighs between 1000 to 1250 grams. "Off" time is slowly lengthened by gradually increasing the hourly volume rate of feedings. Once an infant tolerates an aliquot infused over 1 hour, bolus feedings are begun.

Candidates for continuous enteral feedings include very immature infants, infants with symptomatic gastroesophageal reflux (GER), infants with acquired or congenital short bowel syndrome, and infants with significant chronic lung disease. Continuous feedings may decrease GER or at least the more overt symptoms of GER. Constant infusion of feedings is the preferred method in infants with short bowel syndrome because, with the limited digestive and absorptive capabilities of the gut, they are more likely to tolerate the lower steady-state amounts of luminal substrate than the higher peak surges associated with isocaloric bolus feedings. A combination of nipple feedings during the day supplemented by continuous feedings at night has improved weight gain and other nutritional indicators in selected older infants with chronic lung disease.

Gastrostomy

Gastrostomy placement should be considered in a term-equivalent infant if it is expected that continuous feedings will be required for an indefinite period of time (See Chapter 13).

ADVANCING ENTERAL FEEDINGS

Postnatal adaptations in gastric capacity, digestive and absorptive functions, and intestinal motility require prudent advancement of enteral feedings in the premature infant. Too rapid advancement of feedings may overwhelm the adaptive capabilities of the gastrointestinal tract and cause feeding intolerance (abdominal distention, ileus, gastric aspirates with or without vomiting) indistinguishable from early necrotizing enterocolitis (NEC).

In a frequently cited paper, Brown and Sweet proposed that extreme caution in increasing feedings might prevent necrotizing enterocolitis. For example, in the 1000 gram birth weight infant, they recommended a gradual increase to full enteral calories over a 2 week period. Their recommendations must be considered with the caveat that it is difficult to interpret a retrospective review of an uncontrolled intervention for an epidemic disease. One controlled study reported no difference in the incidence of necrotizing enterocolitis as a function of rate of increase in feedings. However, this study cannot justify aggressive feeding of the very low birth weight infant because the maximum rate of advancement studied (20 ml/kg/day) was quite conservative. More recent data from the Case Western University NICU tend to support the supposition that advancing feedings more than 25 to 35 ml/kg/day increases the risk of NEC.

"Cookbook" recommendations for advancing the rate and concentration of enteral feedings as a function of birth weight are needlessly complex. The clinician need only choose (*a*) the daily caloric increment (kcal/kg/day) and (*b*) the initial concentration of enteral substrate (i.e., full strength vs. dilute formula). The general rule is that the time (and patience) required to advance enteral feedings is inversely proportional to the immaturity and degree of illness of the infant. Clinicians differ as to whether they begin with full strength or dilute formula and how rapidly they advance volume and concentration. However, advancement to 100 kcal/kg/day over 5 to 7 days is usually successful in the stable infant with a gestational age between 29 to 32 weeks. A 23 to 24 week infant may require 10 to 14 days or longer to tolerate the same enteral intake. These cautious regimens do not guarantee that NEC will not develop. However, prudent daily increments probably minimize feeding intolerance and pratically result in earlier establishment of full feedings.

In the full-term infant, it is common to begin with a test feeding of sterile water because, if the infant is neurologically abnormal or has esophageal atresia, aspiration of water is more benign than aspiration of dextrose water or formula. In the gavage-fed preterm infant in whom esophageal patency has been verified, this practice has no rationale. Alternatively, many clinicians prefer to initiate feedings of preterm infants with half-strength (10 kcal/oz; 0.33 kcal/ml) or even more dilute solutions of formula or breast milk. The linkage between hyperosmolar feedings and NEC appears to have motivated this practice, with the additional leap of faith that, if isosmolar are safer than hyperosmolar feedings, then hypoosmolar feedings are safer still. It is usually forgotten that the association between hyperosmolar feedings and NEC was established for a "superosmolar" (>700 mosm/liter) elemental formula. Current, full-strength premature formulas are already slightly hypoosmolar (240 to 268 mosm/liter), and there is no evidence that dilution of these formulas will alter the incidence of NEC. One study, however, has suggested that moderately premature infants (mean birth weight 1225 grams) reached full enteral calories earlier and had a lower incidence of gastric residuals if advanced to full volume on half-strength rather than full-strength feedings. These results must be confirmed in order to recommend routine use of diluted feedings. At present, the choice between diluted or full-strength feedings is best left to the individual practitioner.

One word of caution is necessary if diluted formulas are used. When the concentration is increased, the volume of feedings may need to be decreased to avoid an excessive daily caloric increment. For example, an abrupt change from half-strength to full-strength formula at a volume of 120 ml/kg/day results in a substantial caloric increment (40 kcal/kg/day) that many infants will not tolerate. For this reason, it is safer to increase caloric density at lower enteral volumes and avoid sudden larger alterations in caloric intake.

Advancing Feedings in the Chronically NPO Infant

Feeding an infant who has been chronically starved presents special challenges. Such infants generally fall into two categories: premature infants in whom feedings were withheld for an extended period of time due to extreme illness or instability; and infants who have undergone intestinal resection. For such infants, it often requires courage to initiate feedings in the face of traditional taboos. Chronic disuse of the gastrointestinal tract predictably leads to an ileus with diminished or absent bowel sounds and bilious aspirates. Moreover, small volumes of feedings may result in even larger volumes of gastric residuals or in significant abdominal distention. In most cases, perseverance with feedings eventually induces the necessary adaptations of intestinal motility and of digestive and absorptive capabilities. Feedings with breast milk or elemental formulas are probably more likely to succeed than those with more complex formulas. Continuous rather than bolus feedings may also enhance success. A trial of metoclopramide may be worthwhile if delayed gastric emptying is a significant component of feeding intolerance.

Changing the Frequency of Feedings

Once an infant is growing on full enteral calories by bolus gavage or nipple feedings, the interval between feedings must eventually be increased in preparation for discharge. In many nurseries, the volume of the feeding determines the interval between feedings. For example, feedings may be changed to q3hr intervals at a volume of 15 to 20 ml q2hr, and to q4hr intervals at a volume of 35 to 40 ml q3hr. When the feeding interval is changed, the volume should be increased gradually over several feedings.

CONCENTRATION OF FEEDINGS

The need to restrict fluid intake sometimes requires increasing the concentration of feedings. The need to supply more than 120 kcal/kg/day is not per se a reason to concentrate feedings; however, many infants with caloric requirements greater than 120 kcal/kg/day also require fluid restriction (e.g., infants with chronic lung disease).

Feedings can be "concentrated" in several ways: by prescribing a ready-mixed formula (24 or 27 kcal/oz); by adding supplements to breast milk or to ready-mixed formulas; or by changing the proportion of powder to water in formulas prepared from powder. These methods affect nutrient deliveries differently; therefore, the clinician must carefully consider the macro- and micronutrient requirements of each infant before prescribing energy concentration of feedings.

The initial step in concentrating feedings is to increase caloric density from 20 to 24 kcal/oz. Formulations of Similac Special Care and Enfamil Premature formulas containing 24 kcal/oz are across-the-board concentrations of the 20 kcal/oz preparations that change neither the proportion of macro- and micronutrients nor the quantity of nutrients per 100 kcal. On the other hand, 24 kcal/oz "premie" SMA contains less protein, calcium, phosphorus, salt, and vitamins and more fat and carbohydrate per 100 kcal than its 20 kcal/oz counterpart. All three 24 kcal/oz premature formulas are isosmolar to breast milk. For preterm breast milk, a human milk fortifier may be used (Table 1.8). One packet of fortifier per 25 ml of breast milk increases caloric density from 20 to approximately 24 kcal/oz. This method of fortification provides additional protein, salt, calcium, phosphorus, zinc, and copper that may be deficient in preterm breast milk relative to the infant's needs.

Table 1.15. Useful Parameters in the Assessment of Feeding Tolerance

Serial measurement of abdominal girth
Abdominal examination (assess for visible or palpable loops of bowel; auscultate bowel sounds)
Gastric residuals (volume; assess composition: yellow gastric secretions, formula, bile, gross blood)
Stooling pattern (composition and frequency)
Systemic signs (lethargy, apnea and bradycardia)
Hemoccult testing of gastric residuals, stool
Stool reducing substances

Fortification can also be achieved by mixing equal volumes of breast milk and Similac Natural Care human milk fortifier (identical to 24 kcal/oz Similac Special Care except for a 16% increase in calcium and phosphorus). However, this method increases caloric density by only 10% (to 22 kcal/oz).

Energy concentration above 24 kcal/oz is occasionally necessary and is most easily accomplished by adding carbohydrate and/or fat supplements to the feedings. Protein supplements (e.g., Casec powder) should ordinarily not be added to premature formulas. Carbohydrate can be added as Polycose liquid, a solution of glucose polymers with caloric density of 2 kcal/ml, or as Polycose powder (3.8 kcal/g). Lipid can be added as medium-chain triglycerides (7.7 kcal/ml). This method of energy concentration reduces the delivery of other nutrients per 100 kcal. For example, raising caloric density from 24 to 27 kcal/oz with MCT oil reduces the amount of protein and minerals delivered per 100 kcal by approximately 9%. Excessive supplementation may result in diarrhea. It is helpful to have a nutritionist assist with the preparation of formulas with caloric concentrations above 24 kcal/oz.

MONITORING FEEDING TOLERANCE

Assessment of feeding tolerance is an important aspect of the care of the premature infant (Table 1.15). A sudden increase in abdominal girth (> 1 to 2 cm) may be the first indication of feeding intolerance. This may be due to excessive volume or substrate load or may be an early sign of NEC. Other explanations include constipation (common in very premature infants), aerophagia, or in an intubated infant, malposition of the endotracheal tube. A physical examination often helps determine the etiology. Abdominal distention with visible and/or palpable loops of bowel, even in the absence of other signs of feeding intolerance, should be managed conservatively. Occasionally, an infant will develop repetitive but benign "loopy" episodes that may signify only a need for a glycerine suppository. Diminution or disappearance of bowel sounds, development of abdominal tenderness or guarding, or abdominal wall erythema usually indicates significant pathology.

Gastric residuals should be assessed before each bolus gavage feeding and at least every 4 hours during continuous feedings. The normal volume of gastric residual depends on the type and concentration of enteral substrate and the schedule of feeding. The time required for gastric emptying is greater for formula than for breast milk and for concentrated compared to dilute formulas. Infants on a bolus schedule usually have no more than 1 to 2 ml gastric residuals of formula 2 to 3 hours after a feeding. As a rule of thumb, normal residual volumes on continuous feedings should be no more than the sum of the hourly infusion volume and the dead space of the feeding catheter.

Stools may be watery or increased in frequency secondary to overfeeding, bacterial or viral enteritis, or NEC. In each case, the concentration of reducing substances in stool may rise; this indicates increasing lactose malabsorption. Occult blood in the stool may be due to catheter-induced gastritis or perineal excoriation; however, it may also result from an incarcerated inguinal hernia or NEC. Streaks of blood are most frequently due to rectal or anal fissures. Frank blood in the stool is always abnormal.

NUTRITIONAL ASSESSMENT

The simplest and most important way to monitor the nutritional status of the preterm infant is to plot growth parameters and caloric intakes over time. An accurate weight should be charted daily, and length and head circumference should be noted weekly. Serial measurements of triceps skinfold thickness, if determined by an experienced nutritionist, give some information about the composition of weight gain.

The following laboratory measurements should be monitored weekly: electrolytes, serum urea nitrogen, and blood sugar; total protein and albumin; calcium, phosphorus, and alkaline phosphatase; and hemoglobin/hematocrit.

DISCHARGE RECOMMENDATIONS

Most infants can be discharged on an ad lib feeding schedule. Except in a neurologically impaired infant, it is rarely necessary to schedule feedings. Similarly, most infants who have reached 35 to 37 weeks postconception can be discharged on standard formulas with iron. This is fortunate because special formulas are often difficult to obtain. They are more expensive, and there is a greater likelihood that an error will be made in their preparation. They are sometimes necessary in infants with severe chronic lung disease or congestive heart failure who require fluid restriction and in an infant with persistent hypophosphatemia and an elevated serum alkaline phosphatase who requires supplemental phosphorus and calcium.

SUGGESTED READINGS

General

Committee on Nutrition of the American Academy of Pediatrics. Nutritional needs of low-birth-weight infants. Pediatrics 1985;75:976–986.

Committee on Nutrition of the American Academy of Pediatrics. Pediatric nutrition handbook. Elk Grove Village, IL: American Academy of Pediatrics, 1985.

Cowett RM, Hay WW Jr, eds. The micropremie: the next frontier. Report of the 99th Ross Conference on Pediatric Research. Columbus, OH: Ross Laboratories, 1990.

Grand RJ, Sutphen JL, Dietz WH, eds. Pediatric nutrition: theory and practice. Stoneham, MA: Butterworths, 1987.

Tsang RC, ed. Vitamin and mineral requirements in preterm infants. New York: Marcel Dekker, 1985.

Tsang RC, Nichols BL, eds. Nutrition during infancy. Philadelphia: Hanley and Belfus, 1988.

Uauy R, ed. Current concepts in newborn nutrition: nutrition beyond growth. Seminars in Perinatology 1989;13(2).

Fetal Growth and Energy Requirements

Okamoto E, Heird WC. Feeding the low birth-weight infant. Ped Ann 1981;10:440–445.

Sparks JW, Girard JR, Battaglia FC. An estimate of the caloric requirement of the human fetus. Biol Neonate 1980;38:113–119.

Usher RH, McLean FH. Normal fetal growth and the significance of fetal growth retardation. In: Davis JA, Dobbing J, eds. Scientific foundations of pediatrics, Philadelphia: Saunders, 1974.

Ziegler EE, O'Donnell AM, Nelson SE, Fomon SJ. Body composition of the reference fetus. Growth 1976;40:329–341.

Energy Requirements

Chessex P, Reichman BL, Verellen GJE, et al. Influence of postnatal age, energy intake, and weight gain on energy metabolism in the very low-birth-weight infant. J Pediatr 1981;99:761–766.

Freymond D, Schutz Y, Decombez J, et al. Energy balance, physical activity, and thermogenic effect of feeding in preterm infant. Pediatr Res 1986;20:638–645.

Putet G, Senterre J, Rigo J, Salle B. Nutrient balance, energy utilization, and composition of weight gain in very low-birth-weight infants fed pooled human milk or a preterm formula. J Pediatr 1984;105:79–85.

Reichman B, Chessex P, Putet G, et al. Diet, fat accretion, and growth in premature infant. N Engl J Med 1981;305:1495–1500.

Reichman BL, Chessex P, Putet G, et al. Partition of energy metabolism and energy cost of growth in the very low-birth-weight infant. Pediatrics 1982;69:446–451.

Reichman B, Chessex P, Verellen G, et al. Dietary composition and macronutrient storage in preterm infants. Pediatrics 1983;72:322–328.

Sauer PJJ, Dane JH, Visser HKA. Longitudinal studies on metabolic rate, heat loss, and energy cost of growth in low birth weight infants. Pediatr Res 1984;18:254–259.

Whyte RK, Campbell D, Stanhope R, et al. Energy balance in low birth weight infants fed formula of high or low medium-chain triglyceride content. J Pediatr 1986;108:964–971.

Whyte RK, Haslam R, Vlainic C, et al. Energy balance and nitrogen balance in growing low birthweight infants fed human milk or formula. Pediatr Res 1983;17:891–898.

Protein

Kashyap S, Forsyth M, Zucker C, et al. Effects of varying protein and energy intakes on growth and metabolic response in low birth weight infants. J Pediatr 1986;108:955–963.

Kashyap S, Okamoto E, Kanaya S, et al. Protein quality in feeding low birth weight infants: a comparison of whey-predominant versus casein-predominant formulas. Pediatrics 1987;79:748–755.

Kashyap S, Schulze KF, Forsyth M, et al. Growth, nutrient retention, and metabolic response in low birth weight infants fed varying intakes of protein and energy. J Pediatr 1988;113:713–721.

Pencharz PB, Steffee WP, Cochran W, et al. Protein metabolism in human neonates: nitrogen balance studies, estimated obligatory loss of nitrogen and whole-body nitrogen turnover. Clin Sci Mol Med 1977;52:485–498.

Raiha NCR, Heinonen K, Rassin DK, Gaull GE. Milk protein quantity and quality in low-birthweight infants: I. Metabolic responses and effects on growth. Pediatrics 1976;57:659–674.

Schulze KF, Stefanski M, Masterson J, et al. Energy expenditure, energy balance, and composition of weight gain in low birth weight infants fed diets of different protein and energy content. J Pediatr 1987;110:753–759.

Calcium and Phosphorus

Abrams SA, Schanler RJ, Garza C. Bone mineralization in former very low birth weight infants fed either human milk or commercial formula. J Pediatr 1988;112:956–960.

Ehrenkranz RA. Mineral needs of the very-low-birthweight infant. Sem Perinatol 1989;13:142–159.

Evans JR, Allen AC, Stinson DA, et al. Effect of high-dose vitamin D supplementation on radiographically detectable bone disease of very low birth weight infants. J Pediatr 1989;115:779–786.

Greer FR, McCormick A. Improved bone mineralization and growth in premature infants fed fortified own mother's milk. J Pediatr 1988;112:961–969.

Gross SJ. Bone mineralization in preterm infants fed human milk with and without mineral supplementation. J Pediatr 1987;111:450–458.

Laing IA, Glass EJ, Hendry GMA, et al. Rickets of prematurity: calcium and phosphorus supplementation. J Pediatr 1985;106:265–268.

Rowe JC, Goetz CA, Carey DE, Horak E. Achievement of in utero retention of calcium and phosphorus accompanied by high calcium excretion in very low birth weight infants fed a fortified formula. J Pediatr 1987;110:581–585.

Schanler RJ, Abrams SA, Garza C. Mineral balance studies in very low birth weight infants fed human milk. J Pediatr 1988;113:230–238.

Schanler RJ, Garza C. Improved mineral balance in very low birth weight infants fed fortified human milk. J Pediatr 1988;112:452–456.

VITAMINS

Shenai JP, Kennedy KA, Chytil F, Stahlman MT. Clinical trial of vitamin A supplementation in infants susceptible to bronchopulmonary dysplasia. J Pediatr 1987;111:269–277.

CLINICAL ISSUES IN THE FEEDING OF THE PRETERM INFANT

Aynsley-Green A. Hormones and postnatal adaptation to enteral nutrition. J Pediatr Gastroenterol Nutr 1983;2:418–427.

Aynsley-Green A. Metabolic and endocrine interrelations in the human fetus and neonate. Am J Clin Nutr 1985;41:399–417.

Book LS, Herbst JJ, Atherton SO, et al. Necrotizing enterocolitis in low-birth-weight infants fed an elemental formula. J Pediatr 1975;87:602–605.

Book LS, Herbst JJ, Jung AL. Comparison of fast- and slow-feeding rate schedules to the development of necrotizing enterocolitis. J Pediatr 1976;89:463–466.

Brown EG, Sweet AY. Preventing necrotizing enterocolitis in neonates. JAMA 1978;240:2452–2454.

Churella HR, Bachhuber WL, MacLean WC. Survey: methods of feeding low-birth-weight infants. Pediatrics 1985;76:243–249.

Currao WJ, Cox C, Shapiro DL. Diluted formula for beginning the feeding of premature infants. ADJC 1988;142:730 731.

Dunn L, Hulman S, Weiner J, Kliegman R. Beneficial effects of early hypocaloric enteral feeding on neonatal gastrointestinal function: preliminary report of a randomized trial. J Pediatr 1988;112:622–629.

Heldt GP. The effect of gavage feeding on the mechanics of the lung, chest wall, and diaphragm of preterm infants. Pediatr Res 1988;24:55–58.

LaGamma EF, Ostertag SG, Birerbaum H. Delayed feeding fails to prevent necrotizing enterocolitis. AJDC 1985;139:385–389.

Levine GM, Deren JJ, Steiger E, Zinno R. Sole of oral intake in maintenance of gut mass and disaccharide activity. Gastroenterology 1974;67:975–982.

Lucas A, Bloom F, Aynsley-Green A. Gut hormones and minimal enteral feeding. Acta Paediatr Scand 1986;75:719–723.

Ostertag SG, LaGamma EF, Reisen CE, Ferrentino FL. Early enteral feeding does not affect the incidence of necrotizing enterocolitis. Pediatrics 1986;77:275–280.

Ross Laboratories. Using concentrated formulas and caloric supplements to meet special infant feeding needs. Columbus, OH: Ross Laboratories, 1987.

Schanler RJ. Human milk for preterm infants: nutritional and immune factors. Sem Perinatol 1989;13:69–77.

Siegel M, Lebenthal E, Krantz B. Effect of caloric density on gastric emptying in premature infants. J Pediatr 1984;104:118–122.

Slagle TA, Gross SJ. Effect of early low-volume enteral substrate on subsequent feeding tolerance in very low birth weight infants. J Pediatr 1988;113:526–531.

Toce SS, Keenan WJ, Homan SM. Enteral feeding in very-low-birth-weight infants: a comparison of two nasogastric methods. AJDC 1987;141:439–444.

2

Apnea and Bradycardia

Estelle B. Gauda

INTRODUCTION

The ability to breathe without mechanical ventilation is one of the greatest challenges facing the infant who is born prematurely. Unstable ventilation characterized by apnea and periodic breathing is the normal ventilatory pattern for many otherwise stable premature infants because the mechanisms that control breathing are still quite immature. However, it is generally accepted that frequent and prolonged apnea associated with hypoxemia and bradycardia is not optimal for brain and other organ development. Medical interventions are thus recommended to decrease or prevent the occurrence of prolonged apnea in premature infants.

To better understand the basis for the recommendations that will be made, this chapter will (*a*) briefly review those mechanisms that may account for the unstable breathing patterns observed in premature infants; (*b*) outline and discuss those illnesses and conditions that are associated with apnea; (*c*) recommend when an infant should be treated, what treatment modality should be employed, and the duration of treatment; (*d*) discuss who should be monitored and for how long; (*e*) recommend what additional evaluations should be done; (*f*) suggest discharge planning for the infant who still has apnea; and lastly, (*g*) discuss the associated risk of Apparent Life-Threatening Events (ALTE) and Sudden Infant Death Syndrome (SIDS) with prematurity.

DEFINITION

Apnea is simply defined as the cessation of airflow. Because short respiratory pauses are normal, more specific definitions are given to select out those infants who might be at risk for adverse outcome. For clarity and consistency, the following definitions have been extracted from the National Institutes of Health Consensus Development Conference on Infantile Apnea, Sept. 29 to Oct. 1, 1986.

Pathological Apnea. A respiratory pause is abnormal if it is prolonged (≥20 seconds) or associated with hypotonia, bradycardia, cyanosis, or abrupt, marked pallor.

Periodic Breathing. A breathing pattern in which there are three or more central respiratory pauses of greater than 3 seconds duration with less than 20 seconds of respiration between pauses. Periodic breathing can be a normal event.

Apnea of Prematurity. Periodic breathing with pathological apnea in premature infants (≤37 weeks gestation). Apnea of prematurity usually ceases by 37 weeks gestation, but it may persist for several weeks postterm.

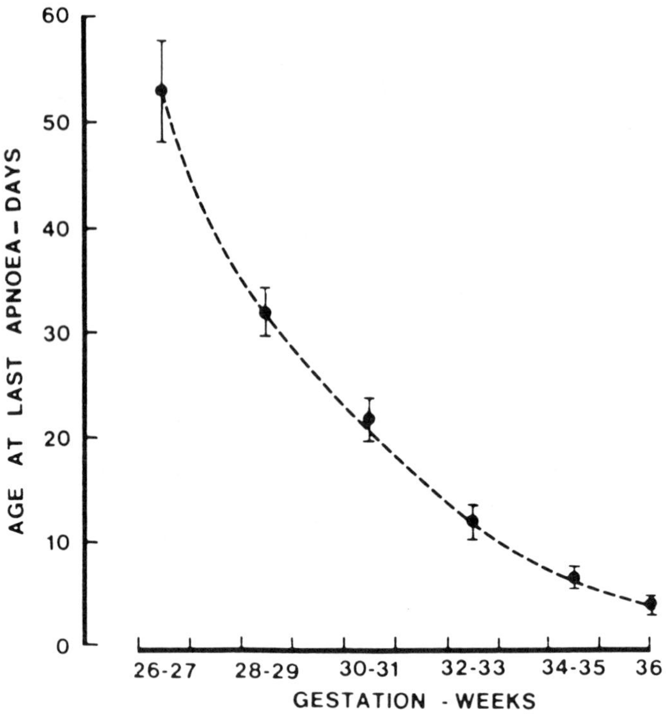

Figure 2.1. Postnatal age when last apnea was detected vs. gestational age at birth in 231 preterm babies with recurrent apnea of greater than 20 sec duration. The mean postnatal age of the last apnea detected decreased with increasing gestational age. Data points are mean ± S.E.M. (Reprinted with permission from Henderson-Smart DJ. The effect of gestational age on the incidence and duration of recurrent apnoea in newborn babies. Aust Pediatr J 1981;17:273–276.)

Symptomatic Premature Infants. Preterm infants who continue to have pathological apnea at the time when they otherwise would be ready for discharge.

Asymptomatic Premature Infants. Preterm infants who either never had apnea of prematurity or whose apnea of prematurity has resolved.

INCIDENCE

Periodic breathing occurs in 95% of premature infants and 30% of term infants. In premature infants, the frequency of periodic breathing and apnea is inversely related to gestational and postnatal age. Periodic breathing is usually considered a benign, unstable breathing pattern because, unlike prolonged apnea, it is *not* associated with significant hypoxia or bradycardia.

In contrast to periodic breathing, pathological apnea, by definition, can be associated with cyanosis and bradycardia. Pathological or prolonged apnea occurs in virtually all infants <28 weeks postconception; in 50% of infants between 30 and 32 weeks; and in <7% of infants at 34 to 35 weeks. As expected, the duration of apnea decreases with postconceptional age. The postnatal age at which the last apneic episode may be detected decreases exponentially with increasing postconceptional age (Fig. 2.1). Thus, the gestational age of the infant predicts the frequency of apnea and the postnatal age at which apnea might resolve. As a rule of thumb, apnea of prematurity should resolve when the

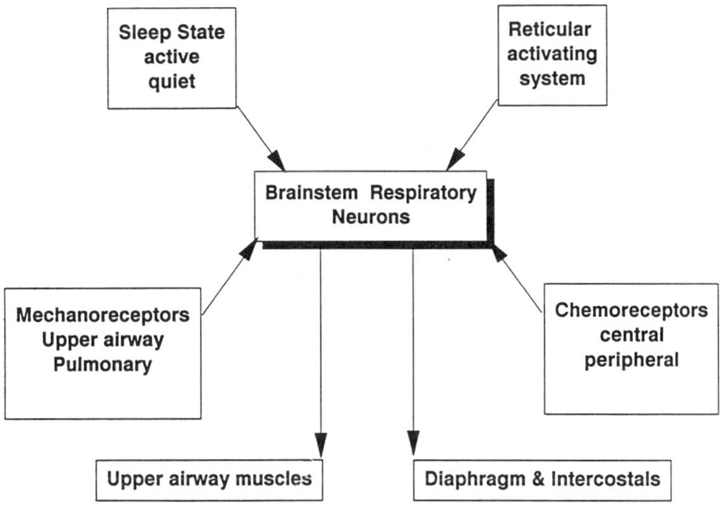

Figure 2.2. Schematic illustration of the modulators of breathing.

infant reaches 34 to 37 weeks postconception. This becomes helpful when predicting who needs treatment, the duration of treatment, and when more extensive evaluations should be done.

PATHOGENESIS

Stable ventilation results from a complex integration of afferent inputs from (*a*) peripheral and central chemoreceptors, (*b*) the reticular activating system, (*c*) the cortex, and (*d*) upper airway and pulmonary mechanoreceptors. All of these are integrated by the central respiratory controller located in the brainstem (Fig. 2.2). Perturbations of any one or all of these afferent inputs or dysfunctional processing in the brainstem can result in unstable breathing patterns. Alterations of efferent output to the muscles of respiration (upper airway muscles, diaphragm, and intercostals) may also lead to unstable ventilation. The relevance to apnea of prematurity is discussed below.

Brainstem Immaturity

Implicit in the definition of apnea of prematurity is the fact that immaturity is the major predisposing factor for the development of apnea and periodic breathing. In studies of neonatal animals, there is histological evidence of incomplete synaptic connections and dendritic projections of the brainstem respiratory neurons. The physiological consequence of this has been suggested from clinical studies by Henderson-Smart et al. Using auditory evoked potentials in premature infants with and without apnea, they have shown that the latency of the auditory evoked response decreases with increasing postconceptional and postnatal age. In addition, at any given postconceptional age, infants with longer latencies had more apnea. With maturation, the frequency of apnea decreased, and latency times shortened. Maturity is thus associated with improved myelination of synaptic connections in the brainstem and more stable ventilatory patterns.

Airway Obstruction Associated with Apnea of Prematurity

As previously mentioned, apnea is defined as the cessation of airflow. However, lack of airflow may be secondary to either diaphragmatic arrest or airway obstruction. Therefore, three types of apnea are observed in premature infants: (*a*) *Central apnea*—no diaphragmatic activity; (*b*) *Obstructive apnea*—upper airway obstruction with continuous diaphragmatic activity; and (*c*) *Mixed apnea*—a combination of upper airway obstruction preceded or followed by central apnea. Originally, it was thought that premature infants had only central apneas. This is not the case. Studies that have simultaneously measured both airflow and diaphragmatic activity have demonstrated that upper airway obstruction is frequent. Thus, central and mixed apneas probably occur in equal frequencies (40 to 45%), with 10 to 15% of apnea being purely obstructive. Any form of apnea may predominate in any given infant. Of particular interest is the fact that infants with predominately obstructive apnea frequently are neurologically abnormal.

The site of airway obstruction is thought to be pharyngeal, as in adults with obstructive sleep-apnea syndrome. Therefore, upper airway muscles that dilate the pharynx are important in maintaining, preventing, or reestablishing upper airway patency in premature infants. Because of this, mechanisms that modulate upper airway muscles are equally as important as those that modulate diaphragmatic activity.

Effect of Sleep State on Apnea

Premature infants are particularly prone to apnea during sleep, and they are asleep 80% of the time. Of the following sleep states: (*a*) *active sleep*—rapid eye movement, REM; (*b*) *quiet sleep*—nonREM, slow wave sleep; and (*c*) *indeterminant sleep*, apnea is more common during active and indeterminant sleep. The premature infant is again at a disadvantage because the percent of time spent in active and indeterminant sleep is inversely related to gestational age.

Modulation of Accessory Muscles of Respiration During Sleep

The phasic activity of accessory muscles of respiration (upper airway and intercostal muscles) are inhibited during sleep. Inhibition of the muscles that dilate the pharynx predisposes the upper airway to collapse. Noninvasive electromyographical measurements in preterm infants have shown infrequent, inspiratory-related genioglossus muscle (a pharyngeal dilator) activity during sleep unless the airway becomes occluded or breathing is stimulated by CO_2. Diminished or absent activity of pharyngeal dilating muscles may predispose the infant to develop upper airway obstruction during sleep. Both baseline tone of pharyngeal dilators as well as their activation to reestablish patency after airway collapse are also essential for effective ventilation.

The intercostal muscles stabilize the chest and contribute to maintenance of lung volume. Inhibition of the intercostal muscles during active sleep further destabilizes the already very compliant chest wall in premature infants. This is important because distortion of the chest wall may promote reflex shortening of inspiration via the intercostal-phrenic reflex. In addition, destabilization of the chest wall further reduces lung volume, resulting in oxygen desaturation.

Ventilatory Responses to Hypoxia and Hypercapnia

The adult ventilatory response to hypoxia is a sustained increase in ventilation. In contrast, when infants are exposed to low O_2 tensions, their ventilation initially increases, but this increase in ventilation is not sustained (Fig. 2.3). This hypoxic ventilatory depression is a function of postconceptional age.

The ventilatory response to CO_2 in infants is similar to that of adults; with increasing CO_2, there is a linear increase in ventilation. However, the slope of the CO_2 response curve is less steep in premature infants than it is in term infants. The reduction is even greater in premature infants who also have apnea. Hypoxia may further reduce the ventilatory response to CO_2 in infants.

CLINICAL PRESENTATION

In infants without respiratory distress syndrome (RDS), apnea of prematurity usually starts within the first week of life. The infant appears otherwise well and is usually thriving. The onset of apnea may be later in infants with RDS and coincident with the resolution of lung disease. There are many physiological and pathological conditions that are associated with and exacerbate apnea in premature infants; some of these are discussed below. In addition, there may be a spectrum of the severity of the apnea in any one infant. Many of

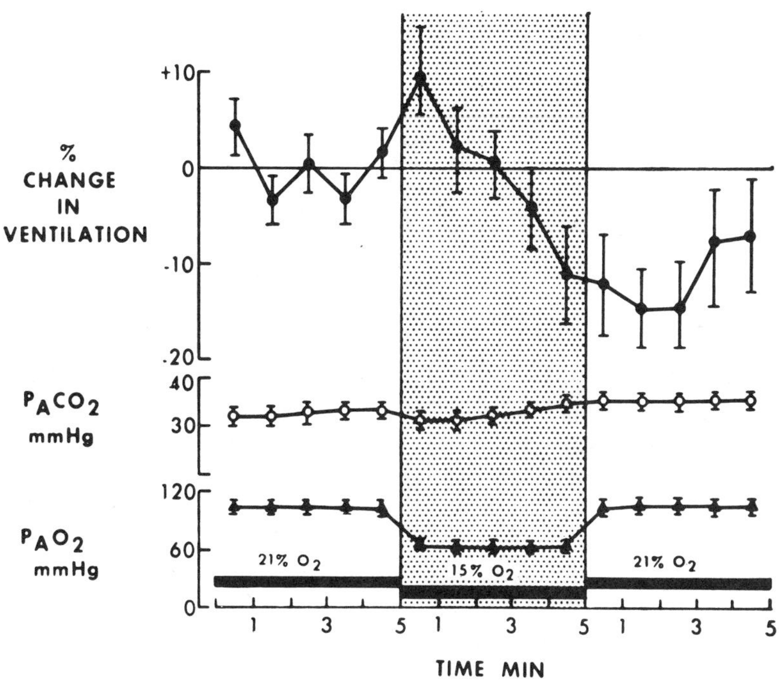

Figure 2.3. Ventilatory response to inhalation of 15% oxygen in 9 preterm infants. (Mean gestational age of 35 ± 1 week). Note the increase in ventilation followed by hypoventilation. Alveolar CO_2 did not significantly change. (Modified from Rigatto H, Brady JP. Periodic breathing and apnea in preterm infants. II. Hypoxia as a primary event. Pediatrics 1972;50:219–228. Reproduced with permission.)

Table 2.1. Apnea of Prematurity: Clinical Associations

Sleep state
Feeding
Thermal stresses
Neck and body position
Anemia of prematurity

the apneic events will terminate without intervention, but others may require oxygen and mask-bag ventilation.

Clinical Associations

Everyday events such as sleep, feedings, thermal stresses, and body position may be associated with apnea (Table 2.1). Apneic infants may also have anemia of prematurity. Some of these associations may be causal, while others may be only coincidental. It is important to remember that apnea is a normal event that occurs in the immature infant and that there is yet no clear demonstration that apnea alone leads to poor outcome. Therefore, it is imperative that the benefit and efficacy of an intervention be weighed critically against the risk.

FEEDINGS

Oral Feedings

Oral feedings may cause apnea by two mechanisms. First, stimulation of laryngeal mucosal receptors with liquid causes reflex cessation of diaphragmatic activity (laryngeal chemoreflex). This reflex has been induced in preterm infants by instillation of saline or distilled water into the oropharynx; however, individual responses varied from arousal at one extreme to swallowing, central apnea, airway obstruction, and prolonged apnea at the other. Aspirations of oral secretions may increase apnea frequency via the laryngeal chemoreflex.

Secondly, ventilatory depression is influenced by the sucking pattern and is more prominent in immature infants. A continuous, as opposed to an intermittent, sucking pattern is observed more frequently in infants at 34 to 35 weeks post conception than in infants between 36 to 38 weeks post conception. Consequently, the younger infants have more episodes of oxygen desaturation, which may lead to hypoxic ventilatory depression and apnea. Thus, apnea can sometimes be reduced by intermittently withdrawing the nipple from the premature infant's mouth to convert a continuous feeding pattern into an intermittent one.

Gavage Feedings

If gavage feedings result in reflux to the level of the larynx, even without obvious aspiration, they can promote central apnea by activation of the laryngeal chemoreflex. Postprandial bradycardia unrelated to apnea is a common finding in premature infants who are gavage fed. Large volumes of gavage feedings may distend the stomach, enhance vagal tone, and promote bradycardia. These apneic and bradycardic episodes are usually brief and self-limiting, but they may be prolonged and require intervention.

Gastroesophageal Reflux

Pathological gastroesophageal reflux (GER) may occur during nipple or gavage feedings in term and premature infants. An association between GER and apnea (central, mixed, and obstructive) was reviewed by Orenstein and Orenstein in 1988. Briefly, GER may promote apnea through activation of the laryngeal chemoreflex. This produces central apnea and/or laryngospasm and results in obstructive apnea. GER may also promote hypoxemia via reflex bronchospasm. Generally, simple alterations in the feeding regimen may decrease the frequency of significant apnea and bradycardia associated with feedings. Small, frequent feeds, thickened feeds, and position (prone upright or upright) may help.

THERMAL STRESSES

Exogenous or endogenous hypothermia or hyperthermia are all associated with an increased frequency of apneic episodes. Increasing the incubator temperature to the upper end of the infant's neutral thermal environment may increase apnea frequency. Similarly, the infant who is dressed too warmly in an open crib may have more apnea. Endogenous temperature instability and apnea may of course also be secondary to incipient sepsis.

POSITION

Neck and body position may alter apnea frequency. Neck flexion and hyperextension, as well as supine positioning, are associated with an increased frequency of mixed and obstructive apnea. Simply repositioning an infant who is curled up into a little ball and is having frequent apnea may decrease the number of apneic events.

ANEMIA OF PREMATURITY

Anemia is frequently observed in growing, stable, premature infants. There are no data to support the concept or the practice of keeping the hematocrit at a set level for any population or disease. No level of hematocrit has been associated with a greater or lesser frequency of apnea in premature infants. In fact, it is not uncommon to see premature infants with hematocrits of 25% who do not have apnea, whereas otherwise similar infants with hematocrits over 35% may have significant and prolonged apnea. The normal developmental process in premature infants with regard to apnea and anemia is that anemia develops and apnea frequency decreases with increasing postnatal age. It is thus *not* recommended that the hematocrit be kept at any given level to hypothetically optimize the reduction of apnea. On the other hand, if the frequency of apnea increases as the hematocrit decreases, especially at values less than 30%, it is not unreasonable to transfuse that infant.

Pathological Conditions Associated with Apnea of Prematurity

It must be emphasized that, although apnea of prematurity is a developmental phenomenon, it clearly can be one of the first signs of pathology as seen in Table 2.2. A pathological cause of apnea should be considered when there is (*a*) an abrupt increase in the frequency and severity of apnea; (*b*) onset of apnea after the first week of life in a premature infant who did not have respiratory distress syndrome; and (*c*) apnea in a term infant at any time.

Table 2.2. Pathological Conditions Associated with Apnea of Prematurity

Disorders of the upper airway
Pierre Robin
Treacher Collins'
Vocal cord paralysis (unilateral)
Subglottic stenosis
Vascular rings
CNS disorders
Arnold-Chiari malformations
Central hypoventilation syndrome
Intraventricular hemorrhage
Periventricular leukomalacia
Hypoxic-ischemic encephalopathy
Posthemorrhagic hydrocephalus
Metabolic Disorders
Hypoglycemia
Hypocalcemia
Hyponatremia
Inborn errors of metabolism
Infections
Bacterial
Fungal (Candida)
Viral (particularly RSV, CMV)
Other
Thermal instability
Drug withdrawal
Benzyl alcohol
Hypoxemia
Left-to-right shunts (PDA)
Anemia
Chronic aspiration

UPPER AIRWAY DISORDERS

By the time the premature infant is labeled a "feeder and grower," the majority of the anatomical causes of apnea have been diagnosed. However, infants who have been tracheally intubated may develop subglottic stenosis or vocal cord paralysis and present with stridor and obstructive apnea. Similarly, vascular rings and unilateral choanal stenosis, congenital or acquired, could easily have been missed in the immediate newborn period.

CENTRAL NERVOUS SYSTEM DISORDERS

Infants who have sustained hypoxic-ischemic insults or who have had significant periventricular-intraventricular hemorrhage with or without periventricular leukomalacia may have significant and prolonged apnea. Infants with Arnold-Chiari malformations may have all types of apnea. Infants with congenital central hypoventilation syndrome usually have central apnea that occurs during quiet sleep and worsens with maturation. With the increased use of recreational drugs, neonatal apnea from drug withdrawal continues to be a problem. Apnea associated with drug withdrawal is usually observed in the immediate newborn period, but it may present later, especially in infants born to mothers who were treated with methadone.

METABOLIC DISORDERS

Hypoglycemia, hyponatremia, hyperammonemia, and hypocalcemia must also be considered in the pathogenesis of apnea. Hypocalcemia in particular may present as significant and prolonged apnea in the recovering premature infant. Diaphragm function is dependent on extracellular calcium. Thus, a low ionized calcium can be associated with profound diaphragmatic fatigue. Hypocalcemia may occur in the rapidly growing premature infant who is born with inadequate calcium stores and who is not receiving adequate calcium for catch-up growth. Soy formulas should be avoided in recovering premature infants because of minimal calcium absorption. The infant who is recovering from necrotizing enterocolitis and whose nutrition has consisted primarily of intravenous hyperalimentation and elemental formulas is at particular risk for significant and severe hypocalcemia.

SEPSIS PRESENTING AS APNEA

It is crucial to rule out sepsis in any premature infant who presents with increased frequency or severity of apnea. The infection may be bacterial, fungal, or viral, and appropriate cultures should be obtained. Very small and immature infants frequently have indwelling central venous catheters. These catheters can become colonized with organisms that are resistant to pencillins and aminoglycosides. Premature infants who are infected with respiratory syncytial virus (RSV) may present with severe apnea prior to any evidence of respiratory distress. Similarly, premature infants who have perinatally acquired cytomegalovirus (CMV) infection may present with profound apnea at 4 to 12 weeks of age. Any upper respiratory tract infection that causes an increase in nasal pharyngeal secretions can increase apnea frequency. Apnea and bradycardia either from sepsis or abdominal distension may be the first sign of necrotizing entercolitis. Conversely, frequent and severe apnea and bradycardia may compromise intestinal blood flow and oxygenation, thus increasing the risk of developing NEC. For both these reasons, feedings should be held until the evaluation is complete.

CARDIOVASCULAR SHUNTS

Many premature infants have a patent ductus arteriosus (PDA). The majority of these are not hemodynamically significant; however, as pulmonary vascular resistance falls in the growing premature infant, a small PDA may become clinically significant. Apnea and bradycardia may begin or, if already present, may increase in frequency. Echocardiography should confirm the diagnosis. Treatment with fluid restriction and/or indomethacin may be sufficient. Some infants will require surgical ligation.

In summary, the diagnosis of apnea of prematurity should be a diagnosis of exclusion. The evaluation of a premature infant with significant and prolonged apnea is similar to that outlined in Table 2.3.

TREATMENT OF APNEA OF PREMATURITY

Therapy should be directed toward the cause of the apnea: antibiotics or antifungals for infections; closure of the symptomatic PDA; calcium for hypocalcemia; glucose for hypoglycemia; oxygen for hypoxia; etc. However, there will be a large subgroup of premature infants who have no discernible cause of apnea. The severity and frequency of apnea and bradycardia will determine which of these infants should be treated. Those with only a few episodes per day, most of which require no intervention, are usually not treated. On the

Table 2.3. Evaluation of the Premature Infant with Apnea[a]

Physical examination
Electrolytes, calcium, and glucose
Hematocrit
Oxygen saturation, capillary blood gas
White blood cell count
Viral and bacterial cultures
Chest and abdominal x-ray

[a]Modification of these recommendations is appropriate as clinically indicated

Table 2.4. Proposed Mechanisms of Treatment Modalities used in Apnea

Methylxanthines
Improves central respiratory drive
Improves ventilatory responses to CO_2
Improves oxygenation
Increases minute ventilation
Stabilizes the oscillations in breathing
May improve diaphragmatic contractility
Decreases central, mixed, and obstructive apnea
CPAP
Pneumatically splints the upper airway; effective in mixed and obstructive apnea
Doxapram
Improves respiratory drive by enhancing peripheral chemoreceptor output

other hand, those with several episodes per day that require at least tactile stimulation are treated. If apnea and bradycardia occur only with feedings, treatment is not recommended.

Apnea of prematurity usually ceases by the time the infant reaches 34 to 37 weeks postconceptional age. Generally, if the infant has reached 34 weeks gestation and has been free of apnea and bradycardia for longer than 1 week, pharmacological therapy (see below) is stopped, and the infant is monitored for an additional 5 to 7 days. It rarely becomes necessary to discharge an infant home while still being treated with methylxanthines.

Although over the last decade we have developed a better understanding of the mechanisms that contribute to unstable breathing patterns in premature infants, treatment has not significantly changed. Therapy is directed toward optimizing ventilation. This is achieved by several different mechanisms, which are outlined in Table 2.4.

Treatment with Methylxanthines

Methylxanthines, either caffeine or theophylline, have become the mainstay for the treatment of apnea of prematurity. Both are effective stimulants of the central nervous system and are associated with improvement in several ventilation parameters (see Table 2.4). Caffeine may have several advantages over theophylline in that it (*a*) has a much wider therapeutic index; (*b*) is a more potent stimulant of the medullary respiratory center; (*c*) has less fluctuation in plasma concentrations; (*d*) is rapidly absorbed from the gastrointestinal tract; and (*e*) may be dosed once daily. On the other hand, the major disadvantage is the fact that caffeine is not commercially available, although it can be prepared in the hospital pharmacy as caffeine citrate. Caffeine sodium benzoate should be avoided in premature infants because of the concern regarding competitive inhibition of bilirubin albumin binding. Another disadvantage is that caffeine plasma levels may be more difficult to obtain.

Theophylline is similar to caffeine with regard to its respirogenic effects. About 30% of theophylline is metabolized to caffeine. Metabolism to caffeine and decreased protein binding in the relatively hypoproteinemic premature infant may account for observed efficacy of theophylline for apnea of prematurity at plasma levels as low as 3 to 4 mcg/ml. Aminophylline can be given intravenously, but it is a theophylline salt and is only 80% theophylline. Dosage recommendations and target plasma levels for caffeine and theophylline are outlined in Table 2.5.

Therapeutic levels of methylxanthines for apnea of prematurity are also associated with (*a*) increased renal blood flow and diuresis; (*b*) relaxation of smooth muscles and stimulation of skeletal muscles; (*c*) increased O_2 consumption; (*d*) hyperglycemia; (*e*) dilation of pulmonary and systemic blood vessels and constriction of cerebral vessels; (*f*) exacerbation of gastroesophageal reflux; (*g*) tachycardia; and (*h*) an increase in cardiac output.

Toxic side effects of methylxanthines are more frequently observed with theophylline than with caffeine, provided caffeine levels are less than 50 mcg/ml. Associated toxicities with theophylline are listed in Table 2.6.

Continuous Positive Airway Pressure (CPAP)

Theophylline has been shown to reduce central, mixed, and obstructive apneas in premature infants. Continuous positive airway pressure (CPAP) improves mixed and obstructive apnea. Because greater than 50% of prolonged apneas may be associated with airway obstruction, nasal CPAP may be an effective treatment for apnea of prematurity. CPAP probably improves airway obstruction by pneumatically splinting the airway. In addition, it may alter the Hering-Breuer inflation reflex by increasing lung volume or inhibit the intercostal-phrenic reflex by stabilizing the chest wall. Nasal CPAP is generally safe. However, mechanical obstruction of the nares from the nasal prongs, irritation, and even necrosis of the nasal septum have been reported. It may also be difficult to keep the prongs

Table 2.5. Dosage Recommendations for Caffeine and Theophylline in Neonates[a]

	Caffeine Base[b]	Theophylline Base[c]
Recommended Dosage:		
Loading	10 mg/kg IV or PO	5 mg/kg IV
Maintenance	2.5 mg/kg IV or PO q24 hr (first dose given 24 hr after loading dose)	2 mg/kg IV q12 hr[d] (first dose given 12 hr after loading dose)
Serum Concentration:		
Therapeutic	5 to 25 μg/ml	2 to 15 μg/ml
Toxic	>40 to 50 μg/ml	>20 μg/ml

[a]Modified from Roberts RJ. Drug therapy in infants. Pharmacologic principles and clinical experience. Philadelphia: Saunders, 1984. Used with permission.
[b]The amount of active caffeine base can range from 40 to 50% of the actual weight, depending upon the chemical material utilized (e.g., caffeine citrate, caffeine sodium benzoate).
[c]A variety of oral preparations available contain from 50 to 100% theophylline base along with a variety of additives. Changing from IV to PO therapy may require an increase in dose.
[d]Maintenance dose requirements for theophylline will vary among neonates, generally ranging between 1 to 4 mg/kg/dose. Serum theophylline concentration monitoring should be accomplished within 48 hours of initiating the loading dose and maintenance therapy to avoid toxicity.

Table 2.6. Toxicity Associated with Theophylline Therapy

Failure to gain weight
Tachycardia
Hyperglycemia
Vomiting
Diuresis/dehydration
Jitteriness
Cardiac arrhythmias
Seizures

in place. Occasionally, an infant refractory to methylxanthine therapy and CPAP may need to be mechanically ventilated. Low ventilator pressures and rates between 10 to 15 breaths/min are usually adequate.

Doxapram

Doxapram is another respirogenic agent. It acts at the peripheral chemoreceptors at low doses, and it may have central effects at higher doses. It has been shown to be useful in the treatment of premature infants with apnea refractory to methylxanthines. It is administered by continuous intravenous infusion at a dose of 2.5 mg/kg/hr but may have therapeutic effects at 1 mg/kg/hr in infants who are concurrently being treated with methylxanthines. Side effects include systemic hypertension, hyperexcitability, vomiting, and seizures. Of considerable concern regarding the continuous infusion of doxapram is the accumulation of benzyl alcohol. Benzyl alcohol is used as a preservative in many medications and fluids used for parenteral therapy. The injectable form of doxapram comes in a concentration of 20 mg/ml and contains 9 mg/ml benzyl alcohol. For continuous intravenous infusion, it is diluted to achieve a concentration of 1 mg/ml of doxapram, which also dilutes the benzyl alcohol to 0.45 mg/ml. The "gasping syndrome" has been reported in premature infants who received 99 mg/kg of benzyl alcohol. There have been no published reports of the "gasping syndrome" in premature infants receiving doxapram for apnea of prematurity. However, the recent report of Jardine et al. suggests an increased incidence of kernicterus and intraventricular hemorrhage in premature infants receiving *any* concentration of benzyl alcohol. Therefore, doxapram should not be used for the treatment of apnea in premature infants until it has been more critically evaluated.

Oxygen Therapy

Hypoxia clearly can induce apnea and periodic breathing. However, there is no reason to administer supplemental oxygen to premature infants who are not hypoxemic. Furthermore, while oxygen supplementation decreases the frequency of apnea, it may also prolong the duration of the apneic episodes. Despite the routine use of pulse oximetry in premature infants, the temptation to use supplemental oxygen to treat apnea should be avoided, even though the apneic episodes themselves may result in a dramatic, although brief, decrease in oxygen saturation. This is more evident in the smaller infants. In the event that mask and bag ventilation is required for apnea termination, the oxygen concentration used should be the same FIO_2 the infant normally receives.

MONITORING

It is generally recommended that any infant less than 1800 grams and/or 34 weeks gestation be monitored for at least the first week of life and until no apneas have occurred for 5 to 7 days. The impedance and heart rate monitors that are used by many nurseries do not directly detect apneic episodes with upper airway obstruction because airflow is not measured. In the event that airway obstruction is prolonged, bradycardia frequently develops in addition to cyanosis and hypotonia. The monitor will alarm for bradycardia. Thus, indirectly, bradycardia and cyanosis with chest wall movement represents a mixed or obstructive apnea. The monitor is usually set to alarm for a respiratory pause ≥15 to 20 seconds and a heart rate of ≤100 beats/min. Some monitors have the capability to alarm for a low respiratory rate in addition to apnea. Although some monitors are set to alarm immediately when the infant becomes bradycardic, many of them will have an internal delay. The duration of this delay for the monitor being used should be known. If any given infant has a low baseline heart rate, it may be reasonable to set the bradycardia alarm at 80 beats/min.

Pneumograms and Polysomnography

A pneumogram is a hard copy of an infant's cardiac and respiratory activity over 12 to 24 hours. It does not measure airflow and thus cannot specify the type of apnea that the infant may be having. Polysomnography measures airflow in addition to heart rate, chest wall movement, electroencephalogram, oxygen saturation, and esophageal pH. Polysomnography is thus the preferred study if further evaluation is needed to characterize the type of apnea and the effect of sleep state on apnea frequency and to rule out apnea associated with gastroesophageal reflux. In a large, population-based prospective study, the extent of respiratory pauses and periodic breathing on pneumograms did not predict those infants who would die unexpectedly. Therefore, pneumograms and polysomnograms should *not* be used as screening tools in premature or term infants to determine the infant's risk for sudden death. Whether infants who have prolonged obstructive apnea are at increased risk for sudden infant death, as was suggested by a case-controlled, retrospective study, is yet to be determined prospectively.

Home Monitoring

The goal of home monitoring is the ability to intervene in the event of life-threatening apnea and thus to prevent mortality and morbidity. Therefore, home monitoring is recommended for those infants who are at increased risk for an apparent life-threatening event (ALTE) or sudden infant death syndrome (SIDS). Recommendations from the Consensus Development Conference on home monitoring are listed in Table 2.7. Key issues regarding premature infants include the following: (*a*) Prematurity, but *not* apnea of prematurity, is an independent risk factor for SIDS and is associated with an increased incidence of 3 to 5 times that of the general population; (*b*) Infants with a history of apnea of prematurity comprise only 2 to 4% of total SIDS cases; and (*c*) There is no evidence that apnea of prematurity per se causes subsequent morbidity. Therefore, home monitoring of the premature infant who has reached term gestation and is no longer having apnea is not recommended.

Table 2.7. Summary of NIH Consensus Statement on Infantile Apnea and Home Monitoring[a]

Cardiorespiratory monitoring is medically indicated for certain groups of infants at high risk for sudden death:
Infants with one or more severe, acute life-threatening events requiring mouth-to-mouth resuscitation or vigorous stimulation;
Symptomatic preterm infants;
Siblings of two or more SIDS victims;
Infants with certain diseases or conditions such as central hypoventilation syndrome.
Cardiorespiratory monitoring is not medically indicated for normal infants with a risk of SIDS of 2/1000 live births.
Routine monitoring of asymptomatic preterm infants, as a group, is not warranted.
For several groups, currently available evidence on the benefits and risks of monitoring and alternative treatment is inconclusive:
Siblings of SIDS infants;
Infants with tracheostomies;
Infants of opiate or cocaine-abusing mothers.
The pneumogram should not be used as a screening tool for deciding whom and when to monitor.

[a]Modified from Consensus statement. National Institutes of Health Consensus Development Conference on Infantile Apnea and Home Monitoring. Sept. 29 to Oct. 1, 1986. Pediatrics 1987;79:292–299.

On the other hand, home monitoring may be a reasonable alternative to prolonged hospitalization in the premature infant who is still having occasional apnea and/or continues to require methylxanthine treatment for control, but who is thriving, maintaining his or her temperature in an open crib, and nipple feeding. This infant usually is between 34 and 37 weeks postconception and may not need to be monitored for an extended period of time. However, in the infant who is still having apnea or who requires methylxanthines at 37 weeks postconceptional age, home monitoring should be continued for a period of 2 to 3 months. Afterwards it can be stopped if there has been no significant apneic episode despite ordinary stresses (e.g., illnesses, immunizations) and the infant has not received methylxanthines for the 1 to 2 weeks preceding monitor discontinuation. Infants with tracheostomies and chronic lung disease may be considered for home monitoring (see Table 2.7).

When deciding whether or not to monitor at home, the infant's family should be carefully assessed regarding their strengths, weaknesses, and support systems. Once the decision to monitor is made, parents and other caretakers should become skilled in cardiopulmonary resuscitation and monitor use. Specifically, preparation of the family should include a thorough explanation of monitor operation and of what to do when the monitor alarms. They must know when to contact their primary care provider and when to contact the monitor company. They should be aware that having an infant on a cardiorespiratory monitor, although reassuring when indicated, is not problem-free, that false alarms may be frequent, and that common activities such as taking a shower or finding a babysitter may be difficult. Appropriate follow-up and support services should therefore be provided throughout the period of home monitoring and should include a primary care provider or specialist comfortable with the infant and the cardiorespiratory monitor. A monitor company with 24-hour availability for equipment malfunctions, changes, and questions is also essential. Pediatric home nursing may be offered to each family. Finally, it is crucial that the parents understand that infants who are monitored may still die unexpectedly.

SUMMARY

The respiratory control system in premature infants is immature, and ventilation is characterized by unstable breathing patterns (central, mixed, and obstructive apnea) and periodic breathing. Although periodic breathing appears to be a benign breathing pattern, significant and prolonged apnea associated with cyanosis and bradycardia may not be optimal for adequate growth and development. Treatment is usually directed toward improving ventilatory drive until the infant reaches 34 to 37 weeks gestation. By this time, the ventilatory patterns become stable, and significant and prolonged apnea ceases. With advances in modern perinatal and neonatal medicine, the premature infant thus triumphs over one of the major challenges of extrauterine life.

SUGGESTED READINGS

Aranda JV, Grondin D, Sasyniuk BI. Pharmacologic considerations in the therapy of neonatal apnea. Pediatr Clin North Am 1981;28:113–133.

Boggs DF, Bartlett D. Chemical specificity of a laryngeal apneic reflex in puppies. J Appl Physiol 1982;53:455–462.

Carlo WA, Martin RHJ, DeFiore JM. Differences in CO_2 threshold of respiratory muscles in preterm infants. J Appl Physiol 1988;65:2434–2439.

Consensus statement. National Institutes of Health consensus development conference on infantile apnea and home monitoring. Sept. 29 to Oct. 1, 1986. Pediatrics 1987;79:292–299.

Davies AM, Koenig JS, Thach BT. Upper airway chemoreflex responses to saline and water in preterm infants. J Appl Physiol 1988;64:1412–1420.

Eyal F, Alpan G, Saig E, et al. Aminophylline versus doxapram in idiopathic apnea of prematurity: a double-blind controlled study. Pediatrics 1985;75:709–713.

Fenner A, Schalk U, Hoenicke H, Wendenburg A, Roehling T. Periodic breathing in premature and neonatal babies: incidence, breathing pattern, respiratory gas tensions, response to changes in the composition of ambient air. Pediatr Res 1973;7:174–183.

Gauda EB, Miller MJ, Carlo WA, DiFiore JM, Johnsen DC, Martin RJ. Genioglossus responses to airway occlusion in apneic versus nonapneic infants. Pediatr Res 1987;22:683–687.

Gerhardt T, Bancalari E. Apnea of prematurity: I. Lung function and regulation of breathing. Pediatrics 1984;74:58–62.

Gershanik J, Boecler B, Ensley H, McCloskey S, George W. The gasping syndrome and benzyl alcohol poisoning. N Engl J Med 1982;307:1384–1388.

Guilleminault C, Coons S. Apnea and bradycardia during feedings in infants weighing 2000 gm. J Pediatr 1984;104:932–935.

Henderson-Smart DJ. The effect of gestational age on the incidence and duration of recurrent apnoea in newborn babies. Aust Pediatr J 1981;17:273–276.

Henderson-Smart DJ, Pettigrew AG, Campbell DJ. Clinical apnea and brainstem neural function in preterm infants. N Engl J Med 1983;308:353–357.

Hoffman HJ. Apnea, birth weight, and SIDS: results of the NICHD cooperative epidemiological study of SIDS risk factors. Statement presented at the consensus panel public hearing, May 19, 1986.

Jardine DS, Rogers K. Relationship of benzyl alcohol to kernicterus, intraventricular hemorrhage, and mortality in preterm infants. Pediatrics 1989;83:153–160.

Kahn A, Blum D, Rebuffat E, et al. Polysomnographic studies of infants who subsequently died of sudden infant death syndrome. Pediatrics 1988;82:721–727.

Keyes WG, Donohue PK, Spivak JL, Jones MD Jr, Oski F. Assessing the need for transfusion of premature infants and role of hematocrit, clinical signs, and erythropoietin level. Pediatrics 1989;84:412–417.

Kirkpatrick SML, Olinsky A, Bryan MH, Bryan AC. Effect of premature delivery on the maturation of the Hering-Breuer inspiratory inhibitory reflex in human infants. J Pediatr 1976;88:1010–1014.

Knill R, Bryan AC. An intercostal-phrenic inhibitory reflex in human newborn infants. J Appl Physiol 1976;40:352–356.

Martin RJ, Miller MJ, Carlo WA. Pathogenesis of apnea in preterm infants. J Pediatr 1986;109:733–741.

Mathew OP, Roberts JL, Thack BT. Pharyngeal airway obstruction in preterm infants during mixed and obstructive apnea. J Pediatr 1982;100:964–968.

Meyers TF, Milsap RL, Krauss AN, et al. Low-dose theophylline therapy in idiopathic apnea of prematurity. J Pediatr 1980;96:99–103.

Miller HC, Behrle FC, Smull NW. Severe apnea and irregular respiratory rhythms among premature infants. Pediatrics 1959;22:676–685.

Miller MJ, Carlo WA, Martin RJ. Continuous positive airway pressure selectively reduces obstructive apnea in preterm infants. J Pediatr 1985;106:91–94.

Orenstein SR, Orenstein DM. Gastroesophageal reflux and respiratory disease in children. J Pediatr 1988;112:847–858.

Pickens DL, Schefft G, Thach BT. Prolonged apnea associated with upper airway protective reflexes in apnea of prematurity. Am Rev Respir Dis 1988;137:113–118.

Rigatto H. Apnea. Pediatr Clin North Am 1982;29:1105–1116.

Rigatto H, Brady JP. Periodic breathing and apnea in preterm infants. II. Hypoxia as a primary event. Pediatrics 1972;50:219–228.

Rigatto H, Brady JP, de La Torre Verduzco R. Chemoreceptor reflexes in preterm infants. I. The effect of gestational and postnatal age on the ventilatory response to inhalation of 100% and 15% oxygen. Pediatrics 1975;55:604–613.

Rigatto H, Brady JP, de La Torre Verduzco R. Chemoreceptor reflexes in preterm infants. II. The effect of gestational and postnatal age on ventilatory response to inhaled carbon dioxide. Pediatrics 1975;55:614–620.

Roberts RJ, ed. Methylxanthine therapy: caffeine and theophylline. In: Roberts RJ, ed. Drug therapy in infants: pharmacologic principles and clinical experience. Philadelphia: Saunders, 1984:119–137.

Thach BT, Start AR. Spontaneous neck flexion and airway obstruction during apneic spells in preterm infants. J Pediatr 1979;94:275–281.

Warburton D, Stark AR, Taeusch HW. Apnea monitor failure in infants with upper airway obstruction. Pediatrics 1977;60:742–744.

Wilson SL, Thach BT, Brouillette RJ, Abu-Osba YK. Upper airway patency in the human infant: influence of airway pressure and posture. J Appl Physiol 1980;48:500–504.

3

Postnatal Anemia

M. Douglas Jones, Jr.

Postnatal anemia is seen so consistently, not only in humans but in virtually all newborn mammals, that it has long been described as "physiologic." Some clinicians have taken this to mean that red cell transfusion is therefore unnecessary or even meddlesome. While that approach causes little disagreement in the case of the full-term infant, there is considerable controversy as to whether anemia is benign in preterm infants. Some authorities have suggested that preterm infants rarely need red cell transfusion, even when the hematocrit falls to 20 to 25%; others insist that the hematocrit should be meticulously maintained over 30 or even 40%. This chapter will not attempt to provide firm criteria for transfusing preterm infants. Its purpose is rather to provide information for informed clinical decisions in individual infants.

CLINICAL COURSE

The hematocrit in the full-term infant reaches its nadir between 4 and 8 weeks after birth. The lowest value is rarely lower than 30%, and by 4 months of age, the hematocrit has returned to the level at which it will remain for the rest of the first year (Fig. 3.1). In preterm infants, especially in those born before 28 weeks of gestation, it is not unusual to encounter hematocrits of 20 to 25%. Anemia is also prolonged. It may take as long as 8 or 9 months before the hematocrit is equivalent to that of infants born at term.

PATHOPHYSIOLOGY

Erythropoietin

Early investigators quite naturally attributed postnatal anemia, particularly the exaggerated form seen in preterm infants, to nutritional deficiencies. On the basis of what is now a large number of studies, it is clear that, even though physiologic anemia can be exaggerated and prolonged by nutritional and vitamin deficiencies, a deficiency of iron or vitamin E or indeed of any exogenous factor is not its primary cause. Attention has therefore turned to the mechanism by which red blood cells are formed. Anemia might theoretically be due to an abnormality anywhere along the complex chain of cellular development that leads to the mature red blood cell. Erythrocyte precursors might be present in insufficient numbers. They might be unresponsive to erythropoietin, the glycoprotein hormone that regulates erythropoiesis. Alternatively, erythropoietin production might be inadequate; the

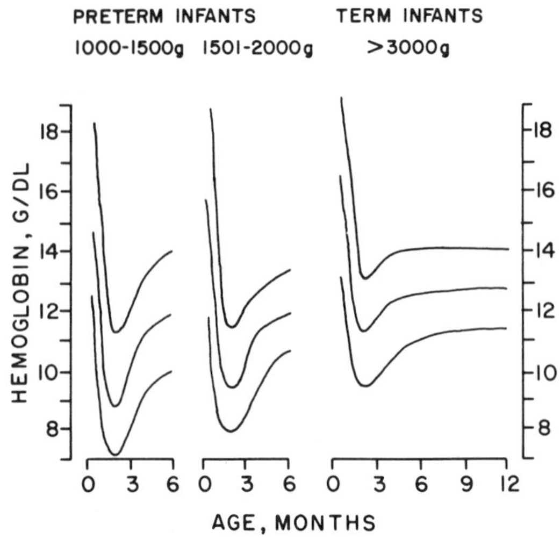

Figure 3.1. Hemoglobin levels in preterm and term infants. Median values and 95% confidence limits are indicated for each of the three birth weight categories. (Modified from Dallman PR. Anemia of prematurity. Ann Rev Med 1981;32:143–160. 1981. Reproduced with permission by Annual Reviews, Inc.)

specific defect could be in the mechanism that senses hypoxia or in processes leading to erythropoietin synthesis and release.

Current evidence indicates that the last of these possibilities, inadequate erythropoietin production, is the most important. In vitro studies have disclosed no defect in the ability of erythrocyte precursors to differentiate in response to erythropoietin stimulation. However, several studies have found that preterm infants have low erythropoietin levels when gauged against comparably anemic older children and adults (Fig. 3.2). The discrepancy between infants and adults is even greater if one allows for differences in fetal and adult oxyhemoglobin affinity. Because the oxygen affinity of fetal hemoglobin is higher than that of adult hemoglobin, anemia in a newborn is associated with correspondingly greater restriction in tissue oxygen availability than in an adult. This remains true over the first several months of life, until fetal hemoglobin is gradually replaced by adult hemoglobin. The deficiency in erythropoietin secretion is most striking in infants who are the least mature. Thus, at comparable levels of "available oxygen," a concept that summarizes the effects of hemoglobin level and oxyhemoglobin affinity, erythropoietin levels are lower in infants born at 27 to 31 weeks postconception than in infants born at 32 to 36 weeks postconception (Fig. 3.3).

DEPRESSED ERYTHROPOIETIN RESPONSE AS A FETAL ADAPTATION

Considered in a broad biological context, inadequate erythropoietin production in the immediate postnatal period is unlikely to represent a simple instance of incomplete or inadequate development. It is more likely that it reflects instead the gradual disappearance of an important intrauterine adaptation, the purpose of which was to limit the erythropoietic response to intrauterine hypoxemia. Initially, this may seem to be an odd concept. The normal newborn infant is polycythemic by adult standards. However, fetal arterial PO_2 is 25 to 40 mm Hg, and in comparison to an adult at the same PO_2, fetal erythropoiesis is

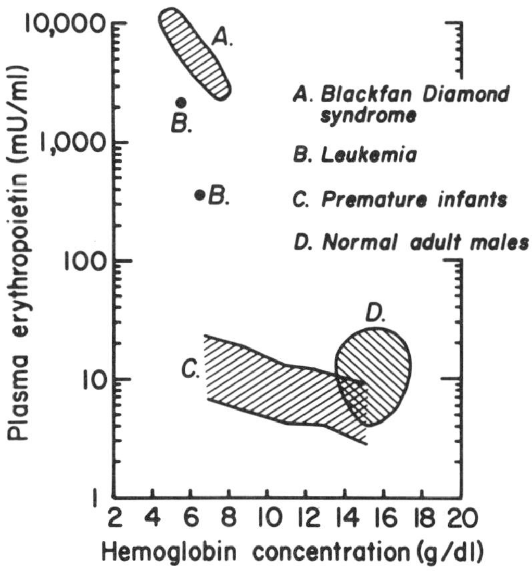

Figure 3.2. Relationship between hemoglobin concentrations and plasma erythropoietin concentration in 21 preterm infants, 7 patients with Blackfan-Diamond syndrome, and two patients with acute lymphocytic leukemia. A encompasses the range of values obtained; C and D represent mean ± 2 SD. (Reprinted with permission from Stockman JA III et al. Anemia of prematurity: determinants of the erythropoietin response. J Pediatr 1984;105:786–792.)

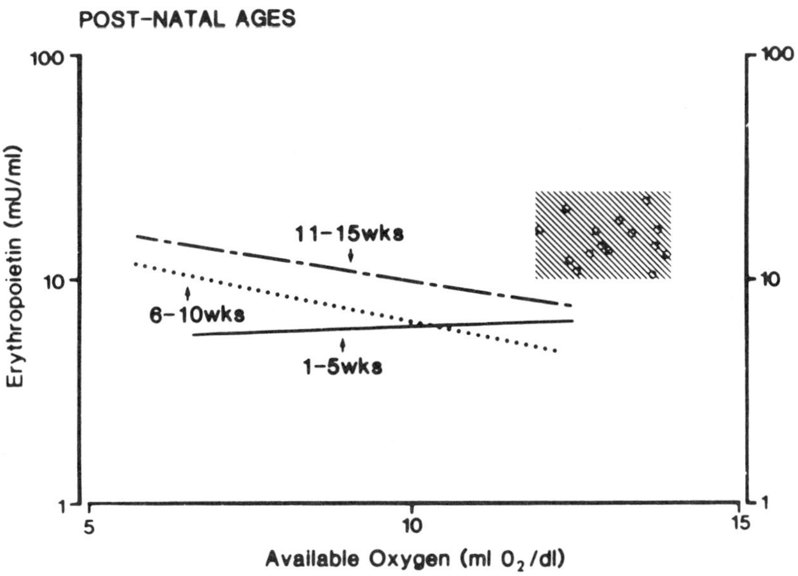

Figure 3.3. Relationship of erythropoietin to "available oxygen" (see text) as a function of maturity. The least mature infants have an erythropoietin response to decreased "available oxygen" that is significantly lower than that in the most mature infants ($P < 0.001$). Boxed values are in adult man, shown for comparison. (Reprinted with permission from Brown MS et al. Decreased response of plasma immunoreactive erythropoietin to "available oxygen" in anemia of prematurity. J Pediatr 1984;105:793–798.)

restrained. Even the comparatively mild hypoxemia of high altitude causes a substantial increase in hematocrit in the adult. More severe hypoxemia, e.g., from cyanotic heart disease or chronic lung disease, causes intense and even life-threatening polycythemia.

The transition from the fetal to the adult pattern of erythropoietin production is gradual rather than immediate. Until the transition is complete, erythropoietin production is suppressed by higher postnatal PO_2s. The result is transient anemia. That does not mean that the fetus is incapable of responding to hypoxemia. Fetal erythropoiesis is brisk enough to allow for the rapid increase in red cell mass that must accompany growth. Furthermore, superimposed hypoxemia, e.g., in a fetus with intrauterine growth retardation or in a fetus born to a mother who resides at high altitude, can cause neonatal polycythemia. In addition, as mentioned, the abnormality of erythropoietin response in postnatal anemia is only quantitative. Severe chronic hypoxemia from cyanotic congenital heart disease or chronic lung disease stimulates erythropoiesis, just as it does in the adult, blunting or even eliminating the postnatal fall in hematocrit. Conversely, erythropoiesis can be suppressed. Exchange transfusion replaces the infant's red blood cells with adult cells that have lower oxyhemoglobin affinity. Thus, tissue oxygen availability will be higher for the same degree of anemia after exchange transfusion. The signal for erythropoiesis is less, and erythropoietin production is suppressed.

In the sense that it reflects the persistence of a response that is essential to fetal well-being, physiological anemia is analogous to physiological jaundice. The fetal liver lacks the ability to conjugate bilirubin with glucuronic acid to create a water-soluble compound. This situation persists transiently after birth, and the result is physiological jaundice. However, the inability to conjugate bilirubin is not a "deficiency" for a fetus. Rather, because water-soluble compounds cross the placenta poorly and because fetal bilirubin must ultimately be metabolized and excreted by the maternal liver, it is to the fetus's advantage *not* to conjugate bilirubin. At birth, the situation changes. The liver of the spontaneously delivered, full-term infant has in some way been prepared for this eventuality, and jaundice is mild and brief. The liver of the preterm infant either misses the signals or fails to respond. The result is more severe and prolonged jaundice. Likewise, postnatal anemia after a full-term gestation is usually mild and brief. And, as with jaundice, in the preterm infant the switch to the postnatal environment is delayed.

SITE OF ERYTHROPOIETIN FORMATION

Animal experiments have shown that liver is the primary site of erythropoietin production throughout fetal and into early postnatal life. This is important to the pathophysiology of postnatal anemia because erythropoietin production by the liver appears to require a greater reduction in oxygen availability than production by the kidneys. The switch to renal production begins prior to birth, but the transition is gradual and is not complete for some time. In animals, the switch is regulated by thyroxine levels, by fetal oxygen availability, and very likely, by other factors. The physiology of the switch in man is unknown, but it is possible that the stresses of infection, poor nutrition, and other disorders common in premature infants can cause variations in timing and thus have their own influence on the duration and severity of physiologic anemia.

Other Factors Affecting Hematocrit

Inadequate production of erythropoietin is not the only determinant of hematocrit in the recovering preterm infant. Early in the hospital course, large amounts of blood are withdrawn for laboratory tests. Even with microanalytical techniques, it is not unusual for repeated blood sampling to amount to 10% (or more) of an infant's blood volume within a few days after birth. Some infants lose additional blood in an intraventricular or abdominal hemorrhage. Although these early losses are usually replaced, replacement is rarely complete. Later, as an infant recovers and begins to grow, growth becomes an important determinant of hematocrit. When a small preterm infant doubles and triples its weight, red cell mass must increase accordingly.

SIGNS AND SYMPTOMS

The principal difficulty in knowing what a low hemoglobin or hematocrit means for an individual infant's well-being is the nonspecificity of most of the long list of signs and symptoms attributed to anemia (Table 3.1). The importance of a nonspecific symptom can be established only when properly designed studies demonstrate that the symptom disappears after red cell transfusion. Several small studies suggest that transfusion of anemic preterm infants decreases heart rate, respiratory rate, and the incidence of apnea and/or bradycardia. However, the evidence is not entirely convincing because investigators have seldom been able to rule out nonspecific effects, e.g., stimulation associated with starting an intravenous line or the effect of an increase in blood volume. Nor is it easy to eliminate investigator bias, especially in the evaluation of apnea and bradycardia.

A further cautionary note, at least with regard to the translation of such studies into nursery policy, is provided by results reported recently by Keyes et al. They found no overall correlation between hematocrit (ranging between 20 and 60%) and heart rate, respiratory rate, or the incidence of apnea and bradycardia. In other words, they did not find that heart rate, respiratory rate, or the incidence of apnea and bradycardia were reliable predictors of hematocrit. They did not deny that a relationship with hematocrit might exist, especially when anemia is severe, but they suggested that any general relationship is obscured by the multiplicity of the determinants of heart rate, respiratory rate, and apnea/bradycardia. Such data do not support the selection, on the basis of the appearance of these symptoms, of any particular hematocrit level as a general indicator for the need for transfusion.

More importantly, Keyes et al. failed to find a reproducible change in heart or respiratory rate or in the incidence of apnea and bradycardia after transfusion. This was true even when they corrected for the highly variable increase in hematocrit that follows a standard packed red blood cell transfusion of 10 ml/kg. Here again, they did not deny the possibility that transfusion might decrease the incidence of apnea and/or bradycardia in some infants (see below). Rather, they suggested that it will not reproducibly decrease the incidence in a population of infants, presumably because other determinants of apnea and bradycardia, in the aggregate, are of greater importance.

Table 3.1. Signs and Symptoms Attributed to Anemia

Pallor
Tachycardia
Tachypnea, dyspnea
Apnea and/or bradycardia
Lethargy, poor feeding
Poor weight gain

MANAGEMENT

Nutritional Deficiencies

Nutritional deficiencies are not the primary cause of postnatal anemia, but care must be taken to ensure that anemia is not exaggerated by nutritional deficiencies. This is especially true in infants born at less than 28 weeks gestation.

IRON

Multiple factors interfere with iron availability in premature infants. The prematurely born infant is deprived of maternal iron that ordinarily both supports the increase in fetal red cell mass and provides for the establishment of iron stores. Most of the premature infant's iron stores are in red cells, and much of that is withdrawn for laboratory analyses. At the same time, the infant's need for iron is enormous. Premature infants double and triple their body weight, and therefore their red cell mass, as they grow at 1.5 to 2.0% of their body weight per day. With this in mind, it is not surprising that infants with birth weights between 1000 and 2000 grams outgrow their iron stores as early as 2 months of age (Fig. 3.4) and that smaller infants are at an even greater disadvantage.

Siimes and co-workers have shown that oral ferrous sulfate in a dose of 2 mg/kg, if started at 2 weeks of age, prevents anemia in infants with birth weights of 1000 to 2000 grams. In infants with birth weights of less than 1000 grams, the same dose started at 2 months and doubled to 4 mg/kg at about 3 months of age (by increasing the dosage or by continuing iron supplementation at the original dose after introduction of an iron-supplemented formula) maintained normal serum iron and iron binding capacity. How-

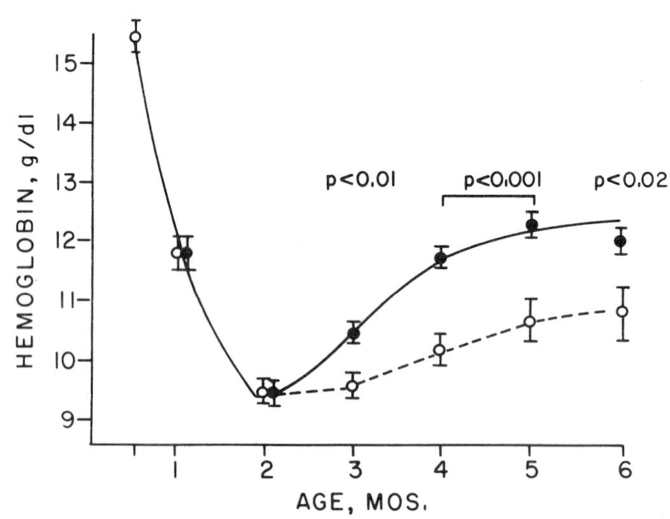

Figure 3.4. Concentration of hemoglobin in low birth weight infants who received no iron supplementation (open circles) and iron supplementation at 2 mg/kg/day starting at 2 weeks of age (closed circles). P values denote significant differences between supplemented and unsupplemented infants. (Reprinted with permission from Lundström U et al. At what age does iron supplementation become necessary in low-birth-weight infants? J Pediatr 1977;91:878–883.)

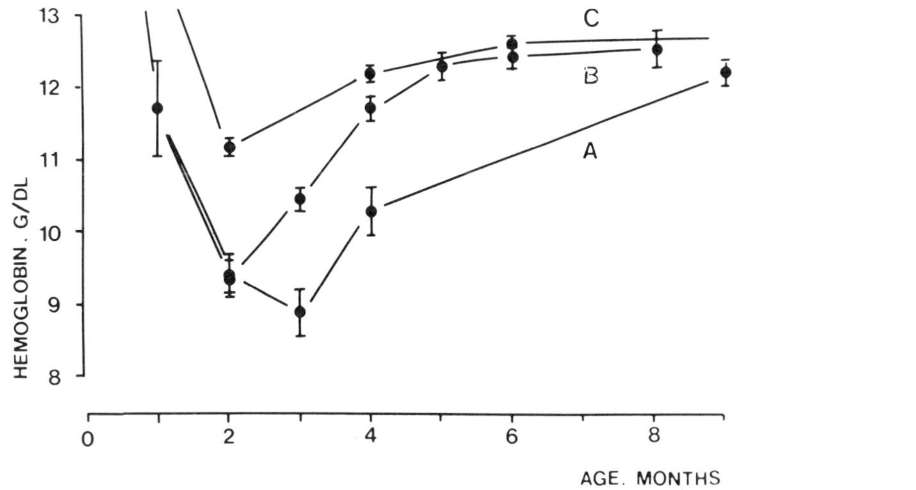

Figure 3.5. Hemoglobin concentrations in healthy infants (Means ± SE). A, Infants with birth weights of < 1000 grams who were supplemented with 4 mg/kg/day of iron; B, Infants with birth weights 1000 to 2000 grams given 2 mg/kg/day of iron; C, Full-term infants supplemented with 1 mg/kg/day of iron. Despite adequate levels of serum iron (data not shown), the anemia was prolonged and more severe in the smallest infants. (Reprinted with permission from Siimes MA, Järvenpää A-L. Prevention of anemia and iron deficiency in very low-birth-weight infants. J Pediatr 1982;101:277–280.)

ever, it still took as long as 9 months for hemoglobin levels to reach those of their full-term peers (Fig. 3.5).

In its most recent (1985) statement, the Committee on Nutrition of the American Academy of Pediatrics recommended that both breast- and formula-fed premature infants receive 2 to 3 mg/kg/day of elemental iron supplementation beginning at 1 to 2 months of age. For formula-fed infants, this dose is roughly equivalent to the dose taken by an infant on iron-supplemented formula. Proprietary formulas contain approximately 1.2 mg of iron/100 ml. An infant taking 150 to 200 ml/kg/day will thus receive approximately 2 mg/kg/day. It is probably unnecessary to keep in mind a specific postnatal age at which iron should be started. Once phlebotomies are at a minimum, the biggest influence on iron requirement is the need to expand red blood cell mass. As a rule of thumb, iron supplementation should be started when an infant begins to grow consistently (1 to 2% of body weight per day).

It is easy to exceed the recommended dose of iron. For example, as usually supplied, ferrous sulfate drops contain 25 mg of elemental iron/ml. The commonly administered dose of 0.6 ml (15 mg) would thus exceed 2 to 3 mg/kg/day in an infant weighing less than 3 kg. The overdose would be even greater in an infant less than 2 kg. Doses approaching 10 mg/kg/day may be deleterious. Iron can promote oxidation of the lipids in red blood cell membranes and cause hemolysis. The risk is particularly high if a high dose of iron is combined with a low dose of vitamin E, a naturally occurring antioxidant. Furthermore, there is some indirect evidence based on the in vitro growth requirements of certain pathogenic bacteria that iron might increase the likelihood of infection. These are not reasons to withhold iron, but they serve as reminders that exceeding the recommended dosage may cause difficulty.

VITAMIN E

Vitamin E is a natural antioxidant. It's biological effects are protean, but for the present discussion, it is important that vitamin E protects lipids in the red blood cell membrane from peroxidation. A number of factors influence the dietary requirement for vitamin E. One is straightforward. All fat-soluble vitamins, including vitamin E, are relatively poorly absorbed by premature infants because fat is poorly absorbed. This is especially true in infants fed proprietary formulas. Correction for this defect is a simple matter of increasing the amount of the supplement. Other issues are more complicated. Polyunsaturated fatty acids are especially susceptible to oxidative damage, and the susceptibility of red blood cell membranes to peroxidation is determined largely by the dietary intake of polyunsaturated fat. Thus, the Committee on Nutrition has recommended that infant formula contain vitamin E, in International Units, in at least a 1:1 ratio to polyunsaturated linoleic acid, in grams. Vitamin E requirement is also a function of the magnitude of the oxidant stress to which the red blood cell membrane is exposed. As mentioned above, iron is one such oxidant, and iron supplementation increases the need for vitamin E.

These factors make the requirement for vitamin E difficult to express in absolute terms and account for much of the confusion in the literature and in the minds of clinicians. The result is that, while the disadvantages of wide departures from a reasonable dietary balance of polyunsaturated fatty acids, supplemental iron, and vitamin E are clear, there is no generally accepted, "optimum" dose of vitamin E. It is common practice on many clinical services, even though premature infant formulas generally contain considerably more than the recommended 1 IU of vitamin E per gram of polyunsaturated fat, to administer supplemental dosages of 25 to 50 IU of Vitamin E. The interpretation of experimental evidence depends on what one selects as the goal of supplementation. Zipursky et al. recently completed a double-blind, randomized, prospective trial in infants with birth weights less than 1500 grams fed both human milk and formula. Formula was supplemented with iron (1.2 to 1.5 mg/liter). The investigators found that a daily dose of 25 IU of *dl*-α-tocopherol produced no difference in hemoglobin or reticulocyte counts at 6 weeks of age. However, they found that some unsupplemented infants had plasma vitamin E levels less than 1 mg/dl. Gross and Gabriel studied a smaller number of similar infants. All infants were given the low dose of vitamin E provided in a standard multivitamin preparation. Beginning at 2 weeks of age, half of the infants were given supplemental iron (2 mg/kg/day). Once again, there was no effect on hematological variables; however, there was chemical evidence of vitamin E deficiency in iron-supplemented infants fed formula (though not in those fed human milk).

If hematological normalcy is the endpoint, there is little evidence that additional vitamin E is of benefit. But if adult vitamin E blood levels are the endpoint, supplementation is justified, especially if an infant is also receiving an iron supplement. Until more is understood about the physiology of vitamin E in premature infants and, in particular, until more is understood about the implications of low blood levels in the absence of other abnormalities, the decision as to whether or not an infant should receive supplemental vitamin E seems best left to the individual clinician.

FOLATE

Folate deficiency has been reported in premature infants, although it is rare. Manifestations are ordinarily limited to hypersegmented polymorphonuclear leukocytes. Chemical evidence of folate deficiency can be prevented by administration of 50 μg/day of folic acid. Premature infant formulas (20 calories/oz) contain approximately 25 μg of folate/100 ml. Folate deficiency has not been reported in infants fed these preparations.

Transfusion Therapy

GENERAL INDICATIONS

Most clinicians would agree that, as hematocrit falls below 25 to 30%, an occasional infant will begin to exhibit poor somatic growth or symptoms that fall into the general category of exercise intolerance (e.g., poor feeding or inability to maintain an airway, i.e., obstructive apnea). However, such manifestations are rare unless the hematocrit falls below 25%, and even then they do not appear consistently. The evidence that such symptoms will be less frequent in a large group of premature infants if the hematocrit is maintained above a certain arbitrary value (e.g., above 30 to 40%) is anecdotal.

There are a number of reasons why the hematocrit might be a poor predictor of symptoms in a chronically anemic, premature infant. First, to the extent that symptoms appear when tissue oxygen sufficiency is compromised, it is important to note that the hematocrit alone is a poor criterion of tissue oxygen sufficiency. The hematocrit provides no information about either tissue oxygen requirements or the cardiovascular determinants of oxygen sufficiency: cardiac output and capillary density. It says nothing about the ease with which hemoglobin will offload oxygen, determined by oxyhemoglobin affinity, and nothing about arterial PO_2 (Table 3.2). Second, symptoms ordinarily attributed to anemia are in part due to complicating conditions that are not usually found with postnatal anemia. For example, the pallor, tachycardia, and tachypnea of acute anemia are more a function of hypovolemia than of anemia.

UNSTABLE INFANTS REQUIRING FREQUENT LABORATORY TESTS

Such infants do not properly fall into the category of a "recovering" NICU infant, and their management is included only for comparison. It is common practice to give blood to unstable infants who are having frequent laboratory tests because without transfusion the hematocrit would decline to unacceptably low levels.

STABLE PRETERM INFANTS (see Table 3.3)

Transfusion should be reserved for infants in whom there is a clear correlation between the development of symptoms and the development of anemia. The symptoms should be of sufficient severity to compromise the infant's well-being, e.g., poor growth, poor feeding, or an increase in the incidence of apnea and/or bradycardia. Tachycardia or tachypnea or the presence of chronic lung disease in themselves seem insufficient indications for transfusion. The infant's response to transfusion should be carefully documented, both imme-

Table 3.2. Determinants of Adequate Tissue Oxygenation

Determinants
Tissue O_2 requirement
Hemoglobin concentration
Cardiac output
Capillary density
Oxyhemoglobin affinity
Arterial PO_2

Table 3.3. Transfusion for Postnatal Anemia

Transfusion Criteria:
- Clear correlation between development of anemia and onset of symptoms
- Insufficient (<2%) reticulocyte response

Be aware of risk of cytomegalovirus transmission with birth weights less than 1200 grams.
Check hematocrit of packed red blood cells.
Document sustained improvement of signs and symptoms.

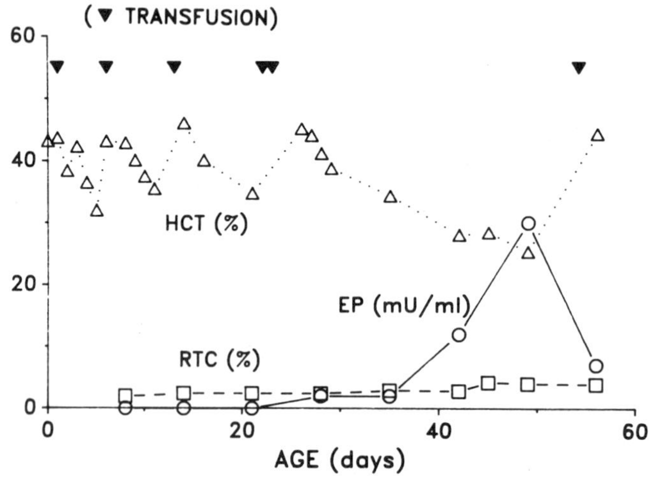

Figure 3.6. A 29 week, 1215 gram boy transfused frequently early in his course to maintain a hematocrit (HCT) over 30%, and also transfused at the nadir of his anemia. Reticulocyte count (RTC) and erythropoietin concentrations (EP) were measured weekly. Hematocrit was determined weekly and when clinically indicated. Note close relationship between EP level and HCT. △, hematocrit; □, reticulocyte count; ○, erythropoietin concentration; ▼, individual transfusions. (Taken from Keyes WG et al. The role of hematocrit, clinical signs and erythropoietin level in assessing the need for transfusion in premature infants. Pediatrics 1989;84:412–417. Reproduced with permission of Pediatrics.)

diately, when a number of factors (handling, stress, blood volume expansion) might produce apparent benefit, and on the following day. Early improvement may not be sustained.

RETICULOCYTE RESPONSE

An important qualification to the need for transfusion is the quality of an infant's reticulocyte response. If the reticulocyte count indicates >2% reticulocytes in an infant with equivocal signs and symptoms, it is reasonable to withhold transfusion. At the same time, transfusion should not be withheld from a symptomatic infant because of fear that the reticulocyte response will be suppressed. Increasing the hematocrit will indeed suppress both erythropoietin production and the reticulocyte response (Fig. 3.6), but this is a manifestation of a normal homeostatic mechanism. There is no reason for erythropoietin to be elevated if the hematocrit has increased to a normal value. The erythropoietin level will increase promptly if the hematocrit falls again (Fig. 3.6).

INFANTS WITH A SYMPTOMATIC LEFT-TO-RIGHT CARDIAC SHUNT

The management of such infants is covered in Chapter 4; however, it should be mentioned here that Lister et al. have shown that transfusion of anemic infants to hematocrit levels of approximately 40% results in clinical improvement in infants with large ventricular septal defects. The benefit would presumably apply in any infant with a cardiac defect resulting in a large left-to-right shunt.

COMPLICATIONS

The increase in hematocrit after a 10 ml/kg packed red blood cell transfusion is surprisingly unpredictable. Keyes et al. found a wide variation in hematocrit after transfusion, even when they controlled for variations in the hematocrit of the packed cells. This demonstrates the poor correlation between hematocrit and red blood cell mass.

The routine risks of transfusions are well known. However, in addition to those routine risks (mismatched blood group, volume overload, transfusion reactions, hepatitis, and HIV infection), premature infants are susceptible to the complications of immunocompromised hosts. One of these is symptomatic cytomegalovirus (CMV) infections. Two factors appear to be important in determining susceptibility: birth weight and the serological status of the mother (and therefore of the infant). Although transfusion-acquired CMV can occur in any susceptible infant, it is rarely a clinical problem in full-term infants. However, in preterm infants, especially those with birth weights less than 1200 grams, transfusion-acquired CMV can lead to serious and sometimes (10% of cases) fatal infection. Up to 24% of seronegative, low birth weight infants may become infected if exposed to seropositive donors. The Standards of the American Association of Blood Banks thus recommend that, if CMV seropositivity is common in the blood supply, seronegative infants weighing less that 1200 grams at birth should receive blood that has been selected or processed to reduce the risk of viral transmission. Because most donor pools contain a substantial percentage of donors who are CMV seropositive, many nursery services have adopted the policy of administering CMV seronegative blood to such infants. A second, and fortunately extremely unusual, disorder is graft versus host disease. The most conservative response to the possibility of graft versus host disease would be irradiation of all blood products given to newborn infants. Information currently does not seem sufficient to justify a general recommendation to that effect. However, that may change as experience accumulates.

Other Therapies

Critical evaluation of the benefits of maintaining hematocrit values within a "normal range" awaits the arrival of a benign means of achieving that end. Administration of human erythropoietin made with recombinant DNA techniques is an interesting possibility if it can be proven to be efficacious and safe.

SUGGESTED READINGS

GENERAL

Dallman PR. Anemia of prematurity. Ann Rev Med 1981;32:143–160.

Stockman JA III. Anemia of prematurity. Ped Clin North Am 1986;33:111–128.

OTHER READINGS

Brown MS, Garcia JF, Phibbs RH, Dallman PR. Decreased response of plasma immunoreactive erythropoietin to "available oxygen" in anemia of prematurity. J Pediatr 1984;105:793–798.

Brown MS, Phibbs RH, Garcia JF, Dallman PR. Postnatal changes in erythropoietin levels in untransfused premature infants. J Pediatr 1983;103:612–617.

Committee on Nutrition of the American Academy of Pediatrics. Nutritional needs of low-birth-weight infants. Pediatrics 1985;75:976–986.

Dallman PR. Iron, vitamin E, and folate in the preterm infant. J Pediatr 1974;85:742–752.

Gross SJ, Gabriel E. Vitamin E status in preterm infants fed human milk or infant formula. J Pediatr 1985;106:635–639.

Joshi A, Gerhardt T, Shandloff P, Bancalari E. Blood transfusion effect on the respiratory pattern of preterm infants. Pediatrics 1987;80:79–84.

Keyes WG, Donohue PK, Spivak JL, Jones MD Jr, Oski FA. The role of hematocrit, clinical signs and erythropoietin level in assessing the need for transfusion in premature infants. Pediatrics 1989;84:412–417.

Lister G, Hellenbrand WE, Kleinman CS, Talner NS. Physiologic effects of increasing hemoglobin concentration in left-to-right shunting in infants with ventricular septal defects. N Engl J Med 1982;306:502–506.

Lundström U, Siimes MA, Dallman PR. At what age does iron supplementation become necessary in low-birth-weight infants? J Pediatr 1977;91:878–883.

Roberton NRC. Top up transfusion in neonates. Arch Dis Child 1987;62:984–986.

Siimes MA, Järvenpää A-L. Prevention of anemia and iron deficiency in very low-birth-weight infants. J Pediatr 1982;101:277–280.

Sanders MR, Graeber JE. Post-transfusion graft-versus-host disease in infancy. J Pediatr 1990;117:159–163.

Shannon KM, Naylor GS, Torkildson JC, et al. Circulating erythroid progenitors in the anemia of prematurity. N Engl J Med 1987;317:728–733.

Stockman JA III, Clark DA. Weight gain: a response to transfusion in selected preterm infants. Am J Dis Child 1984;138:828–830.

Stockman JA III, Graeber JE, Clark DA, McClellan K, Garcia JF, Kavey REW. Anemia of prematurity: determinants of the erythropoietin response. J Pediatr 1984;105:786–792.

Wardrop CAJ, Holland BM, Veale KEA, Jones JG, Gray OP. Nonphysiological anaemia of prematurity. Arch Dis Child 1978;53:855–860.

Zanjani E. Liver to kidney switch of erythropoietin formation. Exp Hematol 1980;8 (suppl 8):29–40.

Zipursky A, Brown EJ, Watts J, et al. Oral vitamin E supplementation for the prevention of anemia in premature infants: a controlled trial. Pediatrics 1987;79:61–68.

4

The Cardiovascular System

Kenneth G. Zahka

The early recognition, evaluation, and management of newborns with cardiovascular disease is now routine. Congenital heart defects are present in approximately 0.8% of live births, and over 50% of these children are diagnosed in the first month of life. The specific cardiovascular questions raised about the premature or term infant in the intermediate care nursery are not necessarily limited to structural heart defects but also include functional murmurs, arrhythmias, cor pulmonale, and hypertension. For those infants with structural heart defects, the vast majority will have been fully characterized and, if appropriate, treated prior to transfer of the infant to the intermediate care unit.

However, there are a number of defects whose presence or severity may only become obvious several weeks after birth. This delay is due to late closure of the ductus arteriosus, gradual fall in the pulmonary vascular resistance, or simply the subtlety of the clinical signs or symptoms. A careful physical examination of the "growing premie" may uncover previously unrecognized heart disease; for example, coarctation of the aorta. An infant initially assumed to have a small ventricular septal defect may develop congestive heart failure as the pulmonary vascular resistance falls and the feedings are advanced over the first weeks of life.

Extensive descriptions of the cardiovascular evaluation of the newborn are found in general pediatric cardiology textbooks. The following section highlights important features of the history and physical examination along with the uses of electrocardiography, two-dimensional and Doppler echocardiography, chest radiography, and pulse oximetry.

CARDIOVASCULAR EVALUATION

History

FAMILY HISTORY

Most epidemiological studies suggest a multifactored etiology for congenital heart disease without a specific pattern of inheritance. The risk of congenital heart disease in the neonate with one affected parent or sibling varies from <1 to 5% depending on the specific defect. However, genetic factors may play a greater role in individual families. This has been noted most often in left-sided lesions (coarctation of the aorta, aortic stenosis, and hypoplastic left heart syndrome). Recognized syndromes with prominent cardiovascular features include pulmonary stenosis in Noonan's syndrome, atrial septal defect in Holt-Oram syndrome, and mitral valve prolapse and regurgitation in Marfan's syndrome.

MATERNAL HISTORY

Maternal diabetes is an important risk factor for structural heart defects. In addition, the increased insulin level in the fetus acts as a myocardial growth factor, producing septal and generalized myocardial hypertrophy. When severe, this interferes with both diastolic filling and systolic emptying of the ventricles. High maternal titer of the Rh antibody associated with subclinical or clinically active systemic lupus erythematosus is strongly associated with congenital complete heart block. Transplacental infection with myotropic enteroviruses may result in myocarditis or arrhythmias. Structural heart defects occasionally follow fetal exposure to lithium or alcohol.

FETAL AND NEONATAL HISTORY

Fetal sonography can now identify structural heart defects, quantify myocardial function, and elucidate arrhythmias. While a number of problems identified in utero require attention in the intensive care nursery, many can be evaluated in the transitional or newborn nursery. Neonatal infection, metabolic disease, and heart disease may all present with nonspecific symptoms, and cardiovascular disorders should be considered as part of the differential diagnosis of any newborn with feeding difficulties, respiratory symptoms, or poor color or activity.

Physical Examination

VITAL SIGNS

There is a broad range of the normal resting heart rate (80 to 175 beats/min) in a healthy premature or term infant. For infants with rates near the limits of normal, it is useful to observe the changes in rate with activity, for example, during sleep in the infant with tachycardia and during crying or feeding in the infant with bradycardia.

The normal respiratory rate may be as high as 60 per minute in the first month of life. Tachypnea associated with congestive heart failure due to increased pulmonary flow or pulmonary venous congestion is often accompanied by retractions and flaring, indicating increased respiratory effort. Tachypnea without retractions, especially in cyanotic infants, suggests increased hypoxic respiratory drive without associated intrinsic lung dysfunction. Primary lung disease due to pneumonia, aspiration, or hyaline membrane disease complicates the assessment of the cardiovascular defect.

Normal blood pressure varies with gestational age and chronological age. Systolic blood pressures between 35 and 65 mm Hg are normal for premature infants, while term infants range between 55 and 90 mm Hg.

COLOR

Central cyanosis is the clinical sign of arterial hypoxia and corresponds to a desaturated hemoglobin concentration of approximately 3 g/dl. In a polycythemic newborn with a hemoglobin of 20 g/dl, this would represent an arterial saturation of 85% ($[(20 - 3) \div 20] \times 100$). In an anemic newborn with a hemoglobin of 10 g/dl, cyanosis would not appear until the arterial saturation fell to 70%.

PULSES

The axillary or brachial and femoral pulses are readily palpable in normal newborns, although dorsalis pedis pulses are easier to feel than the femoral pulses in newborns who are crying with the legs flexed and abducted. The strength of the peripheral pulses is related to the pulse pressure. Wide pulse pressures occur in patent ductus arteriosus and truncus arteriosus. Severe aortic stenosis or myocardial dysfunction results in a diminished stroke volume and a narrow pulse pressure, and all the peripheral pulses are difficult to palpate. Coarctation of the aorta produces a discrepancy in the strength and timing of the pulses in the upper and lower extremities.

PRECORDIAL ACTIVITY

The precordial activity is an excellent reflection of the underlying cardiovascular load. With the normal full-term or premature infant as a reference, an accentuated left ventricular impulse suggests left ventricular volume overload (e.g., patent ductus arteriosus, ventricular septal defect). A persistent right ventricular heave after the first few days of life indicates persistent right ventricular hypertension (e.g., persistent transitional circulation, transposition of the great arteries, large ventricular septal defect).

HEART SOUNDS

The second heart sound is split into aortic and pulmonary components in normal newborns by the second or third day of life when the pulmonary vascular resistance has decreased. A single second heart sound indicates persistent pulmonary hypertension, underdevelopment of either the aortic valve or the pulmonary valve, or abnormal position of the great arteries. A third heart sound indicates increased ventricular early diastolic filling and correlates with increased left-to-right shunting in the infant with a patent ductus arteriosus or ventricular septal defect. Early systolic clicks suggest aortic or pulmonic valve stenosis. Midsystolic clicks suggest mitral valve prolapse.

MURMURS

The *systolic ejection murmur* is a crescendo-decrescendo murmur that begins after the first heart sound, peaks in intensity in midsystole, and ends with the second heart sound. It is produced by blood flow through the aortic or pulmonary outflow tracts. The *holosystolic or pansystolic murmur* begins with the first heart sound, is of approximately equal intensity throughout systole, ends with the second heart sound, and occurs with mitral or tricuspid regurgitation or a ventricular septal defect. An *early systolic murmur* is similar to the holosystolic murmur in that it begins with the first heart sound, but it then tapers in intensity through the first portion of systole. This murmur is characteristic of muscular ventricular septal defects that can be obliterated during the muscular contraction of the septum. A *continuous murmur* begins with the first heart sound, peaks in intensity at the second heart sound, and continues into diastole. A patent ductus arteriosus is the most common etiology of a continuous murmur, although it may be associated with any arteriovenous malformation. *Early diastolic murmurs* due to aortic or pulmonary valve regurgitation are rare in newborns.

The *loudness, quality, location, and radiation* are the additional features required to fully characterize a murmur. The loudness of systolic murmurs has traditionally been graded on a subjective 1 to 6 scale with grade 1 being barely audible, grade 4 being associated with a precordial thrill, and grade 6 being audible with the stethoscope 1 cm from the chest wall. Vibratory murmurs are associated with nonturbulent blood flow. In contrast, harsh quality systolic murmurs are produced by turbulent blood flow from disordered cardiac structure or function.

The location and radiation of murmurs indicate the direction of the blood flow producing them. With normal cardiac and great artery position, murmurs arising from the aortic outflow tract are loudest at the upper right sternal border and radiate to the neck, and murmurs from the pulmonary outflow tract are loudest at the upper left sternal border and radiate to the lungs. Mitral regurgitation is best heard at the lower left sternal border and radiates to the left axilla, whereas tricuspid regurgitation is loudest at the lower right sternal border. The intensity of the murmur influences its radiation. A small ventricular septal defect will produce a well-localized murmur at the lower left sternal border, while the murmur from a larger defect will be heard more widely.

Electrocardiogram

The electrocardiogram is invaluable for the analysis of abnormalities of cardiac rhythm. However, because right axis deviation and dominant right ventricular forces are electrocardiographical features of the normal newborn heart and of many congenital heart defects, the electrocardiogram is an insensitive tool to detect heart disease in the newborn. This is more problematic in the premature infant in whom there is large variation with gestational age in the degree of right ventricular forces on the electrocardiogram.

The electrocardiogram may be diagnostic in specific instances. A positive T wave in V_1 after 5 days of age is a reliable indicator of right ventricular hypertrophy. The absence of the normal neonatal right ventricular hypertrophy, with dominant posterior and leftward forces on the electrocardiogram, suggests hypoplasia of the right ventricle. This is usually associated with left axis deviation and is diagnostic of tricuspid atresia. Left axis deviation, when associated with right ventricular hypertrophy, suggests an endocardial cushion defect.

Two-Dimensional and Doppler Echocardiogram

The echocardiogram permits rapid, accurate diagnosis of nearly all cardiovascular defects in the neonate. The two-dimensional image documents cardiovascular structure and function. Doppler studies demonstrate the direction and the velocity of blood flow.

Three types of Doppler data are available. Pulsed Doppler identifies the direction and the velocity of flow at a specific site. Although it provides well-localized data, the maximum velocity that can be recorded is limited to those in the normal physiological range. The higher velocities found at areas of obstruction or regurgitation must be documented by continuous wave Doppler. Continuous wave Doppler samples along a single ultrasound beam through the heart and documents the velocity of blood flow along that beam. It is, however, relatively insensitive to the beam's location within the heart. Color Doppler codes the direction and the velocity of flow by color. These data are overlayed over a two-dimensional image and provide simultaneous real-time information on cardiac anatomy and blood flow.

Doppler echocardiography has the potential for estimating arterial flow and pressure gradients using a modification of the Bernoulli equation. The pressure gradient (P_1-P_2) between heart chambers or arteries is related to the maximum velocity ($4 \cdot V_{max}^2$) distal to the obstruction. This equation applies to pressure gradients across the aortic or pulmonary arteries or valves (stenosis, banding, coarctation), between the ventricles (septal defect), or between the ventricles and atria (mitral or tricuspid regurgitation).

Chest Radiograph

Due to the refinements in cardiac ultrasound, the chest radiograph has assumed a screening rather than a diagnostic role for pediatric cardiovascular disease. It provides an estimate of overall heart size and pulmonary vascularity and an indication of the position of the heart and the aortic arch.

Pulse Oximetry and Arterial Blood Gases

Noninvasive measurement of arterial oxygen saturation using pulse oximetry is an excellent screening tool for cyanotic heart disease. Desaturation that does not improve with supplemental oxygen suggests an intracardiac right-to-left shunt. Normal saturation, above 95%, while breathing 100% oxygen does not necessarily exclude structural heart defects. Neonates with complete mixing lesions and unrestricted pulmonary blood flow (e.g., single ventricle without pulmonary stenosis) will have a pO_2 >150 mm Hg and 100% saturation on oxygen. Critical aortic stenosis may be associated with left ventricular dysfunction and pulmonary edema, which will cause hypoxemia in room air. Assessment of the acid-base status in arterial blood is important in following the impact of diminished systemic blood flow with left heart obstruction.

SPECIFIC PROBLEMS

Congenital Heart Disease and Chromosomal Syndromes

TRISOMY 21 (DOWN'S SYNDROME)

Approximately 40% of children with Down's syndrome have structural heart defects. Over 60% of these defects are complete or partial atrioventricular canals (Table 4.1). Persistent high pulmonary vascular resistance may initially limit the left-to-right shunt with atrioventricular canal or ventricular septal defect. As a result, a typical murmur may not be present. Clinical signs of right ventricular and pulmonary artery hypertension (palpable right ventricular impulse and a loud, single second heart sound) may be the only clue to the presence of heart disease. Mild hypoxemia, due to right-to-left atrial shunting, occurs in newborns with atrioventricular canal and persistently elevated pulmonary vascular resistance.

Table 4.1. Heart Defects in Down's Syndrome[a]

Defect	%
Complete or partial atrioventricular canal	64%
Ventricular septal defect	16%
Atrial septal defect	10%
Tetralogy of Fallot	6%
Patent ductus arteriosus	4%

[a]Reprinted with permission from Schneider D et al. Patterns of cardiac care in infants with Down's syndrome. Am J Dis Child 1989;143:363–365.

OTHER TRISOMIES

Ventricular septal defect and other cardiovascular defects are present in over 90% of children with trisomy 13 and trisomy 18. However, more complicated defects, including those that are ductal dependent, can also be associated with trisomy 13 or trisomy 18.

TURNER'S SYNDROME

Left heart obstruction defects, most frequently aortic stenosis and coarctation of the aorta, occur in one-third of children with Turner's syndrome. Hypoplastic left heart is present in at least 15% of newborns with Turner's syndrome. The phenotypic severity does not correlate with the occurrence or severity of the cardiovascular defects. Severe aortic stenosis and hypoplastic left heart syndrome also occur in children who are mosaic 45XO/46XX.

Functional Murmurs

PHYSIOLOGICAL PERIPHERAL PULMONARY ARTERY STENOSIS

Physiological peripheral pulmonary artery stenosis is a common source of functional murmurs in premature and full-term infants. The systolic ejection murmur has a vibratory quality and is equally loud across the precordium, in the axillae, and across the back. It is loudest during quiet breathing and is difficult to hear during a valsalva maneuver. The precordial activity, second heart sound, and pulses are normal.

The etiology of this murmur has been assumed to be nonturbulent blood flow through the branch pulmonary arteries. The observation that the murmur is only heard in the first year of life suggests it is due to relative hypoplasia of branch pulmonary arteries, the geometry of the pulmonary arteries, or small chest size. Echocardiography and Doppler studies may suggest branch pulmonary artery hypoplasia with increased blood flow velocity in branch pulmonary arteries.

The differential diagnosis of this murmur is valvular pulmonary stenosis, discrete coarctation of the branch pulmonary arteries, and atrial septal defect. The turbulent main pulmonary artery flow in a newborn with valvular pulmonary stenosis produces a harsh murmur that is loudest at the upper left sternal border with radiation to the lungs. An early systolic ejection click supports the diagnosis of valvular pulmonic stenosis. Discrete coarctation of the branch pulmonary arteries is an unusual defect, and the murmur is often harsh rather than vibratory. The classic clinical signs (right ventricular heave and wide splitting of the second heart sound) of an atrial septal defect are rarely present in the first month of life, but the murmur is similar to physiological peripheral pulmonary artery stenosis. In some instances, the pansystolic murmur of a ventricular septal defect or the abbreviated, continuous murmur of a patent ductus arteriosus may be interpreted as the systolic ejection murmur of physiological peripheral pulmonary stenosis.

Echocardiography is rarely necessary to establish the diagnosis of physiological peripheral pulmonary stenosis. If the murmur is atypical, the precordial activity is increased, or heart sounds are abnormal, an echocardiogram is helpful to exclude other defects. In a well child, persistence of the murmur into the second year of life with strong radiation to the lungs would also warrant further evaluation.

PULMONARY FLOW MURMUR

The pulmonary flow murmur differs from the peripheral pulmonary stenosis murmur only by its more limited radiation. It is usually loudest at the upper left sternal border with radiation to the lower sternal border.

Patent Ductus Arteriosus

PATHOPHYSIOLOGY

Delayed closure of the ductus arteriosus is common in premature infants. After the pulmonary vascular resistance falls, blood flows through the ductus from the aorta to the pulmonary artery in both systole and diastole. The volume overload and enlargement of the left atrium and left ventricle is determined by the size of the ductus arteriosus and the relative systemic and pulmonary vascular resistances. The physical findings are related to the same factors. The aortic pulse pressure, the volume of the peripheral pulses, the precordial activity, the presence of a third heart sound, and the loudness of the murmur reflect the degree of volume loading. Increased pulmonary blood flow can also produce tachypnea, dyspnea, and pulmonary edema.

DIAGNOSIS

Physical Examination

In the newborn with a large shunt as well as low pulmonary artery resistance and diastolic pressure, aortic diastolic pressure is comparable to pulmonary artery diastolic pressure. This produces a wide pulse pressure and bounding peripheral pulses. A third heart sound is associated with increased diastolic left ventricular filling. Increased left ventricular stroke volume results in a prominent left ventricular impulse. In many premature infants, the typical continuous murmur is not present. Rather, they have a murmur that is uneven in intensity throughout systole and is loudest at the upper left sternal border.

A large patent ductus arteriosus with elevated pulmonary vascular resistance is associated with the findings of pulmonary hypertension (right ventricular heave and accentuated pulmonary component of the second heart sound). Because the flow through the ductus arteriosus is limited by the high pulmonary vascular resistance, a murmur is not usually audible. When the pulmonary vascular resistance falls and the left-to-right shunting increases, a continuous murmur develops at the upper left sternal border.

In the premature infant with a small patent ductus arteriosus, the only abnormality on physical examination is the murmur. Normal precordial activity and pulses indicate nearly normal hemodynamics. Tachypnea or dyspnea would not be expected with a small patent ductus arteriosus. The murmur will vary in loudness from exam to exam or with the infant's activity, especially in the infant with a small patent ductus arteriosus.

Echocardiography, Electrocardiography, and Chest Radiography

Confirmation of the presence and severity of a patent ductus arteriosus by two-dimensional echocardiography and documentation of continuous blood flow in the pulmonary artery by Doppler echocardiography is useful. The hemodynamic impact of the shunt may also be judged by the extent of left atrial and ventricular enlargement and by a careful evaluation made for other defects. Similar physical findings are present in infants with arteriovenous malformations, aortic-pulmonary collaterals, aortic-pulmonary windows, and ruptured sinus of valsalva aneurysms.

In the newborn period, the electrocardiogram is insensitive for the evaluation of an infant with a patent ductus arteriosus. Enlargement of the cardiothymic shadow and increased vascularity may be noted on serial chest x-rays.

MANAGEMENT

In the asymptomatic premature infant with a small patent ductus arteriosus, conservative management is warranted with the expectation that spontaneous closure will occur. After 12 months of age, spontaneous closure is unusual, and surgical ligation is currently recommended to prevent the long-term development of pulmonary vascular disease and to decrease the risk of bacterial endocarditis. The recent development of a catheter-delivered ductal closure device may be an alternative to surgical closure in selected children.

Even though eventual spontaneous closure of a patent ductus arteriosus is likely, symptoms of congestive heart failure or respiratory distress are indications for medical or surgical therapy. A trial of modest fluid restriction (100 ml/kg/day) and diuretics (chlorothiazide 20 to 40 mg/kg/day or furosemide 1 mg/kg/day) is indicated if an infant has only mild respiratory distress with or without feeding difficulties. Infants who are anemic with a hematocrit less than 30% may show improvement after transfusion raises the hematocrit above 40%. If the response to these conservative measures is not prompt, with improvement over 3 to 4 days, or continued fluid and, therefore caloric, restriction is necessary to maintain improvement, one should consider pharmacological closure of the patent ductus with indomethacin, a prostaglandin synthetase inhibitor. Unfortunately, indomethacin is often not effective in the recovering premature infant. The drug is most likely to be effective in the first several weeks of life; thereafter, success becomes progressively less likely. If indomethacin therapy fails to close the ductus arteriosus, especially if the infant has more severe congestive heart failure characterized by reappearance or worsening of pulmonary dysfunction and/or apnea and bradycardia, surgical ligation of the ductus arteriosus may be required. Surgical ligation is effective, rapid, and safe in infants of any age or size.

For the infant whose symptoms are being controlled by diuretics or fluid restriction, a trial off medications with normal fluid intake and ad lib feedings prior to hospital discharge is strongly recommended. If the infant remains stable over 4 to 5 days, he or she can be safely discharged home with close follow-up. If, however, signs of respiratory distress or congestive heart failure return, surgical ligation is recommended prior to discharge.

Ventricular Septal Defect

PATHOPHYSIOLOGY

Ventricular septal defect, occurring in 3 to 4/1000 live births, is the most common congenital cardiac malformation. Associated defects that modify the presentation, physical findings, or clinical course include patent ductus arteriosus, atrial septal defect, and coarctation of the aorta.

The relative systemic and pulmonary vascular resistance and the size of the defect determine the clinical presentation and hemodynamic load imposed by a ventricular septal defect. The location of the defect within the septum is not an important factor. Left-to-right shunting across a ventricular septal defect regardless of its size, is minimal immediately after birth because the pulmonary vascular resistance is high. The holosystolic murmur of a ventricular septal defect is produced by turbulent blood flow across the defect; therefore, it is not typical for newborns to have a murmur in the first hours of life. As the pulmonary vascular resistance falls and left-to-right shunting increases, the pulmonary artery, left atrium, and left ventricle are subjected to an increased volume load. If the defect is large, even with low pulmonary vascular resistance, the pressure in the right ventricle and the pulmonary artery may be increased. In those infants, the stimulus for the normal regression of the neonatal right ventricular hypertrophy is lost, and the hypertrophy persists.

DIAGNOSIS

Physical Examination

In the first month of life, a murmur is the typical presentation of a ventricular septal defect. The murmur is harsh, holosystolic, and loudest at the lower left sternal border. The intensity of the murmur is related to the size and the volume of blood across the defect. Large defects provide little restriction to flow and do not tend to produce turbulent flow and loud murmurs. While the blood flow across small, highly restrictive defects is turbulent, the amount of blood crossing the defect is small, and the murmur is also not loud. The loudest murmurs are associated with moderate sized defects with large shunts.

The precordial activity and second heart sound are equally important in the assessment of the size and hemodynamic impact of a ventricular septal defect. The infant with a small defect will have a normally active precordium, a physiologically split second heart sound, and a normal intensity pulmonary component of the second heart sound. A larger defect with pulmonary hypertension causes a hyperactive left and right ventricular impulse and increased loudness and decreased splitting of the second heart sound. Increased diastolic left ventricular filling is suggested by the presence of a third heart sound and a middiastolic mitral flow murmur.

The infant with typical findings usually does not pose a diagnostic dilemma. However, in small infants with rapid heart rates, the systolic ejection murmur of mild pulmonary stenosis may be mistaken for the holosystolic murmur of a small ventricular septal defect. If the systolic murmur is best heard at the upper left sternal border and radiates well to the lungs, it raises the possibility that it originates from the pulmonary valve or pulmonary arteries rather than from a ventricular septal defect. Associated defects should be considered in every infant with a ventricular septal defect. The usual clinical signs of an atrial septal defect or patent ductus arteriosus may be masked by or overlap those of a ventricular septal defect.

Echocardiography

The noninvasive diagnosis of the size and location of ventricular septal defects has been facilitated with the refinement of echocardiography. Investigation is warranted in the first months of life if clinical signs suggest a moderate or large defect or if the diagnosis is in doubt. Echocardiography documents the size and the location of the defect as well as its physiological impact as determined by the degree of left ventricular enlargement, left atrial enlargement, and right ventricular hypertrophy. According to the Bernoulli equation, the right ventricular pressure can be calculated from the velocity of flow across the ventricular septal defect.

Cardiac Catheterization

Cardiac catheterization in a child with a ventricular septal defect is now primarily limited to preoperative evaluation for confirmation of anatomy and measurement of pulmonary and systemic blood flow and resistance.

MANAGEMENT

As many as 40% of ventricular septal defects, including some large defects, undergo partial or complete spontaneous closure. The mechanisms include adherence of the septal leaflet of the tricuspid valve and build-up of the fibrous tissue on the edge of the defect. Muscular defects may close by continued growth of the muscle. Children with large ventricular septal defects that do not close are at risk for the development of Eisenmenger's syndrome with irreversible pulmonary vascular disease and right-to-left shunting.

Diuretics and high calorie formulas have been the mainstay of medical management of congestive heart failure due to a ventricular septal defect. Digoxin may be added for those infants with evidence of poor cardiac output or left ventricular dysfunction.

Persistent pulmonary hypertension at 6 months of age or congestive heart failure in infancy, as manifested by failure to thrive despite adequate caloric and diuretic therapy, are the primary indications for early repair of the ventricular septal defect. Ventricular septal defects, with the exception of apical multiple muscular defects, are usually patched. Mortality is low regardless of age or weight. Pulmonary artery banding in infancy with subsequent total repair in late childhood is now reserved for those children with apical muscular defects. Moderate-sized defects without pulmonary hypertension but with greater than twice normal pulmonary blood flow are usually repaired electively at several years of age. For children with small defects, normal pulmonary artery pressure, and less than twice normal pulmonary blood flow, the only long-term risk is that of bacterial endocarditis. With the exception of appropriate antibiotic prophylaxis, these children need no medications or restrictions.

Left Heart Disease

Left heart disease comprises a group of defects ranging in severity from a bicuspid aortic valve without obstruction to hypoplastic left heart syndrome with aortic and mitral atresia. Mild aortic valve stenosis and coarctation of the aorta are the likely defects encountered in an asymptomatic, recovering premature infant. Severe obstruction of the mitral or aortic valves or critical coarctation or interruption of the aorta will usually present with poor peripheral and organ perfusion in the first days of life coincident with closure of the ductus arteriosus. However, ductal closure may be delayed and may occur after transfer from the intensive care nursery or even after hospital discharge.

PATHOPHYSIOLOGY

Early in utero, left heart obstruction directs flow away from the left heart, and the left ventricle and aorta are underdeveloped. This ranges from complete hypoplastic left heart syndrome in the extreme to mild left heart hypoplasia in some infants with aortic stenosis or coarctation of the aorta.

Left ventricular hypertrophy occurs rapidly in order to maintain cardiac output across the obstruction. However, the ability of the left ventricle to further increase cardiac output with feeding, crying, or other exercise may be compromised with severe obstruction, and cardiac output at rest is impaired with critical obstruction. In infants with critical obstruction and decreased contractility, left ventricular diastolic pressure is increased. This may elevate left atrial and pulmonary venous pressures and cause pulmonary edema.

The status of the ductus arteriosus determines the timing and severity of the presentation of severe forms of left heart disease obstruction (aortic atresia, critical aortic stenosis, or severe coarctation of the aorta) because right-to-left shunting through the ductus arteriosus is the only source of the systemic circulation. Spontaneous closure of the ductus arteriosus results inevitably in renal, hepatic, and gastrointestinal ischemia.

DIAGNOSIS

Physical Examination

An infant with mild aortic stenosis has normal pulses, normal precordial activity, an early systolic ejection click, a normal second heart sound, and a harsh systolic ejection murmur at the upper right sternal border that radiates to the neck. With increasing obstruction, the strength of the pulses diminishes, and the left ventricular impulse and the loudness of the murmur increase. The click and the aortic component of the second heart sound are difficult to hear with more severe obstruction. The classic physical examination is often not present in the newborn, particularly those with severe obstruction and diminished cardiac output, but the combination of poor pulses and a soft murmur suggests severe obstruction with diminished cardiac output.

Poor femoral and distal leg pulses are virtually diagnostic of isolated coarctation of the aorta or interruption of the aortic arch. The discrepancy in pulses should be confirmed by blood pressure measurement, ideally using a standard cuff and manometer with a Doppler flow sensor on a distal pulse. Plethysmographical methods are unreliable when pulsatile flow is poor.

Echocardiography

Confirmation by echocardiography is indicated in all infants with clinically apparent left heart disease. Anatomical definition and velocity measurement of the mitral valve, left ventricle, subaortic area, aortic valve, and aortic arch is necessary to delineate severity.

MANAGEMENT

In the absence of clinical signs of poor cardiac output or echocardiographical evidence of ventricular dysfunction, infants with aortic stenosis or coarctation of the aorta may not require immediate therapy. Poor perfusion, acidosis, or echocardiographical evidence of critical obstruction warrants institution of prostaglandin E_1 to maintain or restore patency of the ductus arteriosus. The timing of spontaneous ductal closure is unpredictable, and its consequences are potentially life-threatening. This is especially important in infants who require transport for tertiary care.

Clinical signs of ventricular dysfunction and pulmonary edema are treated with inotropic drugs and diuretics. The choice of inotropic agents is determined by the infant's condition. Digoxin is suitable for mildly symptomatic infants. Intravenous dopamine or dobutamine are appropriate for those infants with more dramatic congestive heart failure. Furosemide and supplemental oxygen alleviate the effects of pulmonary edema. If the infant has suffered a period of renal, hepatic, and mesenteric ischemia, particular attention must be directed toward the management of electrolyte and fluid abnormalities.

Table 4.2. "Silent" Cyanotic Congenital Heart Disease

Tetralogy of Fallot with pulmonary atresia
Truncus arteriosus
Total anomalous pulmonary venous return
Single ventricle without pulmonary stenosis

Early surgical repair is indicated when severe obstruction results in congestive heart failure. Milder obstruction without clinical or noninvasive evidence of hypertension or left ventricular failure in the neonatal period usually progresses and requires correction in the first few years of life. Because of a high incidence of recurrent obstruction, resection of the coarctation and end-to-end anastomosis of the proximal and distal aorta has been largely replaced by techniques in which the coarctation shelf is excised and the aorta is enlarged either by a patch of synthetic material or by a subclavian artery flap.

The role of balloon angioplasty in the treatment of neonatal coarctation of the aorta is still undefined. In selected infants, the short-term results are comparable to surgery. However, the associated disruption of the aortic wall creates a weakened area prone to aneurysm formation, and the large arterial catheters required for balloon angioplasty increase the risk of intimal damage and thrombosis at the site of entry.

The short-term results of surgical or balloon aortic valvotomy are affected by the extent of aortic annulus hypoplasia, left ventricular hypoplasia and dysfunction, and associated mitral valve abnormalities. Surgical valvotomy is performed either under direct vision on cardiopulmonary bypass or by dilation from the left ventricular apex. While balloon dilation avoids surgery, the risk of damage to the distal arteries is a disadvantage. Aortic regurgitation following relief of the obstruction by either technique is usually mild but may progress with time.

"Silent" Cyanotic Congenital Heart Disease

Cyanotic congenital heart disease in the preterm infant rarely escapes detection in the intensive care nursery. The challenge in the step-down nursery is to identify newborns who are mildly cyanosed and who lack obviously pathological murmurs. Relatively common defects of this type include tetralogy of Fallot with pulmonary atresia and systemic-pulmonary collaterals, truncus arteriosus, total anomalous pulmonary venous return, and single ventricle without pulmonary stenosis (Table 4.2). The unifying pathophysiological feature of this group is extensive mixing of the systemic and pulmonary venous return without diminished pulmonary blood flow. Cyanosis is thus mild. Lacking a restrictive ventricular septal defect or pulmonary stenosis to generate highly turbulent flow, harsh murmurs are typically not present. More subtle abnormalities of the precordial activity, pulses, and auscultation suggest the presence of structural heart disease in these infants.

TETRALOGY OF FALLOT WITH PULMONARY ATRESIA

When tetralogy of Fallot is associated with pulmonary atresia, all blood returning to the right ventricle streams through the large ventricular septal defect into the overriding aorta. Pulmonary blood flow is supplied either through a patent ductus arteriosus or via collateral arteries from the transverse and descending aorta. If the source of pulmonary blood flow is a patent ductus arteriosus, spontaneous postnatal ductal closure dramatically reduces pulmonary blood flow, and profound hypoxemia ensues. Collateral arteries mimic the pathophysiology of a ductus arteriosus, but they do not spontaneously close. Pulmonary blood flow, especially over the first months of life, is adequate to prevent severe hypoxemia. In some infants with multiple large collaterals, the pulmonary blood flow can become excessive and produce congestive heart failure.

The clinical features of tetralogy of Fallot with pulmonary atresia and systemic-pulmonary collaterals include increased precordial activity and a single second heart sound. The collateral flow produces a continuous murmur that is initially difficult to distinguish from the murmur of an uncomplicated patent ductus arteriosus. Because many collateral arteries originate from the descending aorta, the continuous murmur is heard well in the back and across the precordium. As with a patent ductus arteriosus, the diastolic flow through the collaterals decreases diastolic aortic pressure and produces bounding peripheral pulses.

TRUNCUS ARTERIOSUS

In truncus arteriosus, there is a common origin to the aorta and pulmonary artery from a single semilunar valve. The truncal artery overrides a large ventricular septal defect. As the pulmonary vascular resistance falls, pulmonary blood flow increases, causing congestive heart failure. Despite complete mixing of the systemic and pulmonary venous return in the truncal artery, hypoxemia is mild due to the increased pulmonary blood flow.

Precordial hyperactivity, systolic ejection click, single second heart sound, and bounding pulses are the primary signs of truncus arteriosus. A vibratory systolic ejection murmur from increased truncal valve flow and a middiastolic murmur from increased mitral valve flow may also be present. The presence of a harsh systolic ejection murmur and blowing early diastolic murmur suggests associated truncal valve stenosis and regurgitation.

TOTAL ANOMALOUS PULMONARY VENOUS RETURN

Total anomalous pulmonary venous return comprises a group of defects in which the pulmonary veins enter the right side of the heart instead of passing directly into the left atrium. The common sites of insertion are the innominate vein leading to the superior vena cava, the right atrium and coronary sinus, and the portal venous system to the inferior vena cava. Pulmonary venous return mixes completely with systemic venous return in the right atrium. Blood flow to the left heart is accomplished entirely by shunting from the right atrium to the left atrium through the foramen ovale. In the absence of pulmonary venous obstruction, pulmonary blood flow is increased and hypoxemia is mild.

The clinical presentation is variable. Cyanosis and respiratory distress occur with obstructed pulmonary venous return. Infants without obstruction gradually develop tachypnea and a right ventricular heave due to increased pulmonary blood flow. Pulmonary artery pressure is not necessarily elevated, and the second heart sound may be split. A systolic ejection murmur at the upper left sternal border with radiation to the lungs is usually present due to increased flow, but it need not be harsh or obviously pathological.

SINGLE VENTRICLE WITHOUT PULMONARY STENOSIS

There are a number of anatomical varieties of single ventricle without pulmonary stenosis. The unifying pathophysiology is the mixing of the systemic and pulmonary venous returns at the ventricular level. Both great arteries may arise from a single ventricle, or the aorta may arise from a hypoplastic outflow chamber. The timing of symptoms in these infants is similar to that of newborns with isolated large ventricular septal defects or those with truncus arteriosus. Hypoxemia is mild, and congestive heart failure gradually develops as pulmonary vascular resistance falls and pulmonary blood flow increases.

In the absence of atrioventricular valve regurgitation of aortic outflow obstruction, systolic murmurs arise from increased pulmonary flow and are not particularly loud or harsh. Precordial activity is increased, and the second heart sound is single. Arterial oxygen saturation and the chest radiograph suggest the presence of a defect, but Doppler and two-dimensional echocardiography are necessary to establish the diagnosis.

Arrhythmias

The normal heart beat begins in the sinus node at the junction of the superior vena cava and right atrium. The electrical impulse is carried through the atria to the atrioventricular node, the His bundle, and finally along the right and left bundles to the ventricular myocardium. These specialized conducting tissues permit the sequential activation of the atria and ventricles and are responsive to the neural and hormonal stimuli that match the heart rate to the infant's activity.

Conduction abnormalities include delay or blockage of the impulse along the normal pathway of conduction or conduction along accessory pathways as in the Wolff-Parkinson-White syndrome. Arrhythmias result from a deviation from the normal origin of the heart beat at the sinus node and include premature atrial and ventricular beats, supraventricular tachycardia, ventricular tachycardia, and complete heart block.

SINUS RHYTHM

Sinus arrhythmia, the normal deceleration in the heart rate coincident with inspiration, is less dramatic in the first few months of life than in later childhood. More problematic is the wide variation in resting heart rate in apparently normal newborns. Because heart rate and respiratory monitoring are so often utilized for the detection of apneic episodes in step-down nurseries, recognition of tachycardia or bradycardia in otherwise asymptomatic infants is virtually unavoidable.

Bradycardia during sleep, even to 80 to 90 beats/min (bpm), is not necessarily a cause for evaluation. More severe bradycardia should be documented by 24-hour monitoring. These episodes are often related to hypoventilation or to gastroesophageal reflux. Persistent bradycardia also occurs in newborns with hypothyroidism or hypothermia.

Tachycardia, a normal cardiovascular response to feeding or crying, should abate during sleep. The common etiologies of tachycardia are associated with increased cardiac output and include anemia, infection, aminophylline administration, hypoxemia, fluid overload, and a patent ductus arteriosus. If the tachycardia persists, documentation of the actual rhythm by electrocardiography is important to exclude the rare newborn with an ectopic atrial tachycardia or atrial flutter. Decreased variability of the heart rate or abrupt changes in the rate are the clinical clues that there is a primary arrhythmia.

PREMATURE BEATS

Premature Atrial Beats

Isolated premature atrial beats are common both in utero and over the first several weeks of life. They occur when a focus in the atrium depolarizes before the sinus node. The impulse is then conducted down the normal pathway to depolarize the ventricles.

Because the atrial depolarization originates at a site other than the sinus node, the P wave is both early and has a different morphology from the P wave preceding a sinus beat. The impulse travels through normal pathways to the ventricles, and the QRS complex is early but identical in morphology to the normal beats. At the neonatal heart rate, the premature P wave is frequently partially fused with the preceding T wave. In this circumstance, inspection of simultaneous electrocardiographical leads, usually II, V_1, and V_5, facilitates identification of the abnormal P wave.

Aberrant ventricular conduction of premature atrial beats results in a wide QRS complex beat following the premature P wave. The aberrant conduction, usually right or left bundle-branch block, occurs because that part of the conducting system is still refractory from the previous normal beat. The identification of the premature P wave is the best means of differentiating these beats from premature ventricular beats. If the atrioventricular node is refractory, then the premature atrial beat will be blocked. In this case, the abnormal P wave is not followed by a QRS complex. These beats should be differentiated from sinus pauses or, if they occur in a bigeminal pattern, from sinus bradycardia.

Premature Ventricular Beats

Isolated premature ventricular beats also occur in healthy newborns. These are early beats without a preceding P wave and with a wide QRS complex. If the premature ventricular beat is only slightly early, it will combine with the normal sinus beat to produce a fusion beat. Fusion beats are not preceded by a premature P wave, and the QRS morphology is a mixture of the normal sinus beat and a premature ventricular beat.

A 12-lead electrocardiogram and 3-lead rhythm strip is usually diagnostic. If there are clinical signs of heart failure suggesting an underlying myocarditis, an echocardiogram is needed to document the severity of the myocardial dysfunction. Twenty-four-hour Holter monitoring or intensive care monitoring is worthwhile only for those infants with symptoms or signs of sustained tachycardia.

Prognosis

The prognosis of premature atrial or ventricular beats in healthy newborns is excellent if there is no underlying structural heart disease. If they are associated with fetal myocarditis, perinatal asphyxia, central nervous system disease, or metabolic abnormalities, the prognosis is related to the underlying disease. Pharmacological suppression of the arrhythmia, even when the premature beats are frequent, is not necessary in a healthy newborn. Management of an arrythmia in the newborn with myocarditis must be tailored to the clinical state.

SUPRAVENTRICULAR TACHYCARDIA

Supraventricular tachycardia is the most common atrial tachycardia in the fetus and newborn. The mechanism is usually a reentry of the electrical impulse back into the conducting system through an accessory pathway (Wolff-Parkinson-White syndrome) or within the atrioventricular node itself. It occurs in children with structurally normal hearts, congenital heart disease, or myocarditis. The newborn with supraventricular tachycardia has a heart rate of approximately 300 bpm. The tachycardia starts and stops abruptly. It may be tolerated for hours in infants with otherwise normal hearts. In infants with congenital heart defects or myocarditis, symptoms and signs of congestive heart failure develop more rapidly.

The electrocardiogram shows that heart rate varies little with respiration. The QRS complex is usually normal, and P waves, if present, are superimposed on the T wave. When the infant is not tachycardiac, the electrocardiogram is either normal or shows the short PR interval and slurred upstroke of the QRS complex typical of Wolff-Parkinson-White syndrome.

If the tachycardiac infant is hemodynamically stable, maneuvers to increase vagal tone may be tried. Brief facial stimulation with a cold, wet cloth or ice pack stimulates the "diving reflex" and produces a marked vagal stimulus that is particularly effective in terminating the tachycardia in newborns. Other maneuvers include gagging, valsalva, or carotid massage. Any critically ill infant with supraventricular tachycardia should be electrically converted using synchronized DC countershock (0.25 to 1.0 W/sec/kg). Atrial overdrive pacing using an esophageal or transvenous lead is another technique for terminating the tachycardia.

Many drugs are effective for the short- and long-term management of supraventricular tachycardia. There is extensive clinical experience with digoxin in children. Its major drawback is a relative slow onset of action, even when given intravenously. It remains useful for the acute treatment of newborns and is excellent for their chronic treatment. Alternatively, intravenous propranolol, a β-blocker, has a rapid action and minimal effect on blood pressure. The calcium-channel blocker verapamil has become the intravenous drug of choice for the treatment of acute, symptomatic episodes of supraventricular tachycardia in older children. However, it is *not* recommended for children under one year of age due to a high incidence of severe hypotension.

The prognosis of supraventricular tachycardia in infancy is good. Many infants, including some with accessory pathways, have only a single episode, and treatment is discontinued by 1 year of age.

COMPLETE HEART BLOCK

Congenital heart block is now frequently detected in utero and diagnosed by fetal echocardiography. It is often associated with maternal connective tissue disorders and the presence of maternal Rh antibody. There is presumed immunological damage to the fetal conducting system by transplacental transmission of the antibody. In the absence of congenital heart disease, the ventricular rate is usually adequate for normal growth and activity through early childhood and adolescence. Congestive heart failure, due to a combination of the slower than normal ventricular rate and the abnormal hemodynamic load, may occur in newborns with associated structural heart disease. Temporary or permanent ventricular pacing to maintain a physiological heart rate or repair of the underlying defect may be necessary in selected newborns.

Cor Pulmonale

The cardiovascular sequelae of chronic lung disease, cor pulmonale, are mediated through elevation of the pulmonary vascular resistance with pulmonary artery and right ventricular hypertension. Increased pulmonary vascular resistance may be related to hypoxic vasoconstriction or to loss of arterioles due to parenchymal lung damage. Right ventricular hypertrophy is the primary compensatory response to pulmonary hypertension. When chronic and severe, pulmonary hypertension is associated with right ventricular dilation and congestive heart failure.

PHYSICAL EXAMINATION

Early clinical signs of cor pulmonale include a palpable right ventricular impulse, an accentuated pulmonary component of the second heart sound, and hepatomegaly. With progressive right ventricular hypertension and dilation, a harsh holosystolic murmur or a high-pitched diastolic murmur signals the development of tricuspid or pulmonary regurgitation. Peripheral edema, unless it is caused by hypoproteinemia or sodium overload, is usually a sign of severe, right-sided congestive heart failure. The examination may vary with activity, especially if there is fluctuation in the arterial oxygen saturation.

ECHOCARDIOGRAPHY AND ELECTROCARDIOGRAPHY

Serial electrocardiograms and echocardiograms are an excellent adjunct to the clinical evaluation of cor pulmonale. In some infants, right ventricular hypertrophy diagnosed either by electrocardiogram or echocardiogram may provide the initial clue of cor pulmonale. This may be particularly important in infants with severe arterial desaturation during feeding or sleep but with relatively normal saturations at other times. The right ventricular systolic time interval (RSTI) correlates with pulmonary hypertension in some infants. The RSTI, measured from the pulmonary valve mode on the m-mode echocardiogram, is the right ventricular preejection period (RPEP) divided by the right ventricular ejection time (RVET). The RPEP is the time from the onset of the QRS to pulmonary valve opening, and the RVET is the time from pulmonary valve opening to closing. The normal ratio is 0.19 to 0.29, and elevated pulmonary artery pressure is suggested by an increased ratio. For those infants who develop tricuspid regurgitation, the maximum velocity of the regurgitant jet accurately predicts the systolic pressure gradient between the right ventricle and the right atrium. Similarly, the velocity of pulmonary regurgitation predicts the diastolic pressure gradient between the pulmonary artery and the right ventricle. Moderate or severe elevation of the right ventricular systolic pressure or the pulmonary artery diastolic pressure is indicated by regurgitant velocities of 3 and 4 m/sec, respectively.

TREATMENT

Treatment of right heart failure in cor pulmonale is directed toward optimizing the pulmonary status using supplemental oxygen and high-dose diuretics. Nifedipine, a calcium-channel blocker, decreases pulmonary vascular resistance, decreases mean pulmonary artery pressure, and increases cardiac output when administered acutely to children with cor pulmonale. The role of long-term administration of pulmonary vasodilators remains to be elucidated. Inotropic drugs, including digoxin, are indicated for infants with echocardiographical evidence of decreased ventricular function.

SUGGESTED READINGS

General Readings

Adams FH, Emmanouilides GC, Riemenschnieder TA, eds. Heart disease in infants, children, and adolescents. Baltimore: Williams & Wilkins, 1989.

Long WA, ed. Fetal & neonatal cardiology. Philadelphia: Saunders, 1990.

Moller JH, Neal WA, eds. Fetal, neonatal, and infant cardiac disease. Norwalk: Appleton & Lange, 1990.

Specific Readings

Allan LD, Anderson RH, Sullivan ID, et al. Evaluation of fetal arrhythmias by echocardiography. Br Heart J 1983;50:240.

Ascher DP, Rosen P, Null DM, de Lemos RA, Wheller JJ. Systemic to pulmonary collaterals mimicking patent ductus arteriosus in neonates with prolonged ventilatory courses. J Pediatr 1985;107:282.

Brownlee J, Beekman R, Rosenthal A. Acute hemodynamic effects of nifedipine in infants with bronchopulmonary dysplasia and pulmonary hypertension. Pediatric Res 1988;24:186.

Deal B, Keane JF, Gillette PC, Garson A Jr. Wolff-Parkinson-White syndrome and supraventricular tachycardia during infancy: management and follow-up. J Am Coll Cardiol 1985;5:130.

Dunkle L, Rowe R. Transient murmur simulating pulmonary artery stenosis in premature infants. Am J Dis Child 1972;124:666.

Freed MD, Hegmann MA, Lewis AB, Roehl SL, Kensey RC. Prostaglandin E_1 in infants with ductus arteriosus-dependent congenital heart disease. Circulation 1981;64:899.

Garson A Jr, Bink-Boelkens M, Hesslein PS, et al. Atrial flutter in the young: a collaborative study of 380 cases. J Am Coll Cardiol 1985;6:871.

Garson A Jr. Medicolegal problems in the management of cardiac arrhythmias in children. Pediatrics 1987;79:84.

Ghisla RP, Hannon DW, Meyer RA, Kaplan S. Spontaneous closure of isolated secundum atrial septal defects in infants: an echocardiographic study. Am Heart J 1985;109:1327.

Goodman G, Perkin RM, Anas NG, Sperling DR, Hicks DA, Rowen M. Pulmonary hypertension in infants with bronchopulmonary dysplasia. J Pediatr 1988;112:67.

Hagler DJ, Tajik AJ, Seward JB, Ritter DG. Noninvasive assessment of pulmonary valve stenosis, aortic valve stenosis and coarctation of the aorta in critically ill neonates. Am J Cardiol 1986;57:369.

Kramer HH, Majewski F, Trampisch HJ, Rammos S, Bourgeois M. Malformation patterns in children with congenital heart disease. Am J Dis Child 1987;141:789.

Ludomirsky A, Huhta JC, Vick GW, Murphy DJ Jr, Danford DA, Morrow WR. Color Doppler detection of multiple ventricular septal defects. Circulation 1986;74:1317.

Mahoney LT, Truesdell SC, Krzmarzick TR, Lauer RM. Atrial septal defects that present in infancy. Am J Dis Child 1986;140:1115.

Moe D, Guntheroth W. Spontaneous closure of uncomplicated ventricular septal defect. Am J Cardiol 1987;60:674.

Murphy D Jr, Ludomirsky A, Huhta J. Continuous-wave Doppler in children with ventricular septal defect: noninvasive estimation of interventricular pressure gradient. Am J Cardiol 1986;57:428.

Pelech AN, Dyck JD, Trusler GA. Critical aortic stenosis. Survival and management. J Thorac Cardiovasc Surg 1987;94:510.

Rashkind WJ, Mullins CE, Hellenbrand WE, Tait MA. Nonsurgical closure of patent ductus arteriosus: clinical application of the Rashkind PDA Occluder System. Circulation 1987;75:583.

Reller MD, Ziegler ML, Rice MJ, Solin RC, McDonald RW. Duration of ductal shunting in healthy preterm infants: an echocardiographic color flow Doppler study. J Pediatr 1988;112:441.

Schneider DS, Zahka KG, Clark EB, Neill CA, and the Baltimore-Washington Infant Study Group. Patterns of cardiac care in infants with Down's syndrome. Am J Dis Child 1989;143:363–365.

Scott JS, Maddison PJ, Taylor PV, Esscher E, Scott O, Skinner RP. Connective-tissue disease, antibodies to ribonucleoprotein and congenital heart block. N Engl J Med 1983;309:209.

Thoele D, Muster A, Paul M. Recognition of coarctation of the aorta. Am J Dis Child 1987;141:1201.

5

Temperature Regulation

Christine A. Gleason

BASIC PRINCIPLES

Neutral Thermal Environment

The goal of proper temperature regulation in growing preterm infants is to maintain core body temperature constant at approximately 36.5 to 37.5°C while maintaining optimal growth and development. The term "neutral thermal environment" (NTE) is often used to describe the ambient temperature at which these goals may be achieved; that is, "the range of ambient temperature within which metabolic rate is at a minimum, and within which temperature regulation is achieved by nonevaporative physical processes alone" (Bligh and Johnson, 1973). The metabolic rate or basal oxygen consumption varies with gestational and postnatal age, body size, shape, and body weight. Such dynamic variability makes it difficult to predict an appropriate ambient temperature in which to nurse a growing preterm infant. Several tables have been published and revised to give the appropriate NTE for preterm infants at various weights and gestational and chronological ages. Such tables appear to simplify the problems of temperature regulation in the newborn. But the problems may actually be more complex and do not lend themselves to easy tabulation and biomedical instrumentation. For example, an infant may be maintaining a stable core body temperature within the published NTE guidelines for a double-walled incubator, but may have a higher resting heart rate and a slower rate of growth because he or she is producing an unacceptably high amount of heat from basal life-sustaining metabolic processes.

The Clinical Physics of Heat

Thermoregulation involves balancing heat losses with heat gains. Heat is lost from evaporation, convection, conduction, and radiation (see Table 5.1). The three latter losses are all greater in the preterm infant than in the term infant because of the relatively greater body surface area to body mass ratio in the preterm infant and because of their immature thermoregulatory mechanisms, including insufficient stores of brown fat. The extremely low birth weight infant has very poor skin integrity, and initially may have very large evaporative water losses. With increasing chronological age, skin integrity improves. However, sweating ability also improves; therefore, evaporative losses still account for a significant percentage of total heat loss in the growing preterm infant.

Table 5.1 Modalities of Heat Loss

Modality	Heat Lost From:	Heat Goes To:
Convection	Body surface	Cooler surrounding air
Radiation	Body heat	Cooler solid object *not* in contact with infant
Conduction	Body surface	Cooler solid objects in contact with infant
Evaporation	Transepidermal water generation	Air (water vapor)

Homeostatic Mechanisms

When heat losses are greater than heat gain from the environment, infants must generate their own heat to maintain body temperature. This is accomplished by shivering and by nonshivering thermogenesis. Shivering is controlled by the posterior hypothalamus, which responds to cold stress by activating supraspinal motor pathways. Such pathways are not well developed in preterm infants. Nonshivering thermogenesis is controlled by the sympathetic nervous system; brown fat is the primary organ for this type of chemical thermogenesis, and its metabolism is modulated by thyroid hormones. Brown fat stores are decreased in preterm infants, and thyroid hormone levels are often transiently low.

TEMPERATURE INSTABILITY

Instability of an infant's temperature can take several forms:

1. Fever: core temperature $>$ 37.5 to 38.5°C;
2. Stable core temperature, but requiring decreasing incubator temperature;
3. Hypothermia: core temperature $<$ 36 to 36.5°C; or
4. Stable core temperature, but requiring increasing incubator temperature.

Each of these forms of temperature instability may be a sign of serious illness such as infection (altered endogenous heat production) or a sign of equipment malfunction or changes in the environment (exogenous over- or underheating). To differentiate between these conditions, one needs the following information:

1. Incubator temperatures over the past 24 hours;
2. Physical examination of the incubator ("trouble-shooting");
3. Information about any recent environmental changes; and
4. Physical examination of the infant.

Trouble-shooting the incubator should include checking to make sure it is on, that the control dial is set properly, that the portholes are closed, that the power light is on, that any necessary probes are attached, unbroken, and uncovered, and that any humidity required is being delivered properly. A number of changes in the environment can stress the infant's thermoregulatory capabilities. Common stresses include sunlight shining directly onto the incubator, incubator portholes left open for an extended time (as for a procedure), cooling or heating of the nursery, excessive bundling of the infant (in preparation for weaning), recent feeding of cool food, or holding the infant outside the incubator.

The physical examination of the infant should include both rectal and skin temperatures, assessment of dilation or constriction of peripheral blood vessels, assessment of cardiovascular stability, and assessment of the activity and neurological responses of the infant. A fever may be caused either by exogenous overheating of the infant or by increased endogenous heat production, as with infection. Important differentiating signs on physical examination are shown in Table 5.2.

If an infant is judged to have unstable temperature because of changes in endogenous heat production, then sepsis must be the primary consideration, and the appropriate diagnostic studies should be done. If an infant is judged to have unstable temperature because of exogenous factors, the appropriate equipment and/or environmental changes should be made to normalize the infant's temperature. Although there is some debate over whether cold infants should be rewarmed slowly or more rapidly, there is little debate over the treatment of the overheated infant. Clothing should be removed, if indicated, and the incubator temperature should be adjusted if that is a problem. If an overheated infant demonstrates cardiovascular instability such as tachycardia, apnea, tachypnea, etc., then tepid water baths or sponging may also be indicated.

WEANING FROM THE INCUBATOR

There are no strict guidelines regarding how or when (at what age, weight, gestation, etc.) to wean a preterm infant from the incubator. An infant may be ready when the conditions listed in Table 5.3 are met. General guidelines for weaning are given in Table 5.4.

HOME RECOMMENDATIONS

From the parents' perspective, temperature regulation is a major focus of the last few days or weeks of their infant's hospital stay, so it is not surprising that they often have

Table 5.2 "Fever", T > 37.5 to 38.5°C[a]

Exogenous Overheating	Endogenous Heat Production
Flushed	Pale
Peripheral vasodilation	Peripheral vasoconstriction
Hot hands and feet	Cold hands and feet
Skin temp > Core temp	Core temp > Skin temp
Irritable; hyperactive	Quiet; lethargic
Sweating (more mature infant)	Clammy, mottled

[a]Modified from Perlstein PH. The thermal environment. In: Fanaroff AA, Martin RJ, eds. Neonatal-perinatal medicine. 4th ed. St Louis: Mosby, 1987:398–416.

Table 5.3 Weaning from the Incubator: When?

Incubator temperature < 32°C easily maintains infant's core temperature.
Infant is growing well.
Infant has outgrown significant apnea and bradycardia so that close observation and easy access are no longer necessary.
Infant tolerates being held outside incubator without hypothermia.
Infant is 33 to 35 weeks postconceptional age. (Growth retarded or malnourished infants may wean at the later end of the range because of decreased body fat.)

Table 5.4 Weaning from the Incubator: How?

Bundle infant with blankets, hat, booties, and T-shirt.
Turn incubator temperature down to 25° to 26°C (75° to 80°F).
Infant should maintain normal temperature for 24 hours before being moved to an open bassinet.
Follow daily weight gain, oxygen requirements, apnea and bradycardia episodes to see if the infant can adapt.

Table 5.5 Discharge Advice

The infant should be dressed in the same number of layers of clothing/blankets as the parent needs to maintain comfort. Caution against overbundling.
If the weather is cool, the head should be covered when the infant is outdoors or when in drafty rooms for the first month after discharge.
In winter months or in cold climates, keep the room temperature at 70°F.
Warm bottles and solid food before feeding for first 2 months.
If the infant feels too hot or too cold to the touch, take a rectal temperature. If it is too high (>38°C) or too low (<36°C), call the pediatrician.

many questions about how they should regulate temperature at home. Suggestions for discharge advice are given in Table 5.5.

SUGGESTED READINGS

Agate FJ, Silverman WA. The control of body temperature in the human premature infant by low energy infra-red radiation. Anat Rec 1963;136:152.

Bell EF, Gray JC, Weinstein MR, et al. The effects of thermal environment on heat balance and insensible water loss in low-birth-weight infants. J Pediatr 1980;96:452.

Bligh J, Johnson KG. Glossary of terms for thermal physiology. J Appl Physiol 1973;35:941.

Darnall RA. The thermophysiology of the newborn infants. Med Instum 1987;21:16.

Eckberg JJ, Bell EF, Rios GR, et al. Effects of formula temperature on postprandial thermogenesis and body temperature of premature infants. J Pediatrics 1987;111:588.

Frigoletto FD, Little GA, eds. Thermal regulations. In: Guidelines for perinatal care. 2nd ed. Elk Grove Village, IN: American Academy of Pediatrics and American College of Obstetricians and Gynecologists, 1988:274–281.

Hammarlund K, Stomberg B, Sedin G. Heat loss from the skin of preterm and fullterm newborn infants during the first weeks after birth. Biol Neonate 1986;50:1.

Heimler R, Sumners JE, Grausz JP. Thermal environment change in growing premature infants: effect on general somatic growth and subcutaneous fat accumulation. Pediatrics 1981;68:82.

Hey E., Scopes JW. Thermoregulation in the newborn. In: Avery GB, ed. Neonatology. 3rd ed. Philadelphia: Lippincott, 1987:201–211.

Hey NE, Katz G. The optimum thermal environment for naked babies. Arch Dis Child 1970;45:328.

Marks KH. Incubator. Med Instrum 1987;21:29.

Perlstein PH. The thermal environment. In: Fanaroff AA, Martin RJ, eds. Neonatal-perinatal medicine. 4th ed. St. Louis: Mosby, 1987:398–416.

Perlstein PH. Games with children. Pediatrics 1978;61:666.

Polk D. Thyroid hormone effects on neonatal thermogenesis. Semin Perinatol 1988;12:151.

Pomerance JJ, Brand RJ, Meredith JL. Differentiating environmental disease-related fevers in the term newborn. Pediatrics 1981;67:485.

Sauer PJJ, Dane HJ, Visser HKA. New standards for neutral thermal environment of healthy very low birthweight infants in week one of life. Arch Dis Child 1984;59:18.

Silverman WA, Fertig JW, Berger AP. The influence of the thermal environment upon the survival of newly born premature infants. Pediatrics 1958;22:876.

Wu PY, Hodgman JE. Insensible water loss in preterm infants: changes with postnatal development and non-ionizing radiant energy. Pediatrics 1984;54:704.

6

Infectious Disease

John F. Modlin

Serious infections that occur among premature infants during the first days and weeks of life (i.e., early onset bacterial sepsis, infections with candida and other fungi, and necrotizing enterocolitis) have been comprehensively reviewed in other textbooks. The focus of this chapter is infectious disease problems in the NICU infant who has successfully weathered the early problems of prematurity. For convenience, these are grouped according to those infections that are nosocomially acquired and those infections that are vertically transmitted from the infant's mother. The final section briefly describes recommended immunization procedures for preterm infants.

NOSOCOMIAL INFECTIONS

Nosocomial infections are infections that are transmitted within the hospital environment. By definition, neonatal infections that are not vertically acquired are nosocomial. Nosocomial infections occur more frequently, and produce greater morbidity and mortality, in the NICU than in any other pediatric inpatient setting. Infants weighing less than 1500 grams are especially vulnerable. Premature infants are innately more susceptible to nosocomial infection because the mucosal surfaces and skin are less effective natural barriers; because of deficiencies in both humoral and cell mediated immunity; and because natural barriers are often breached by invasive instrumentation. The nursery environment contributes to the risk of nosocomial infection by serving as a reservoir for pathogenic organisms and by providing an efficient means of spread, predominantly via the hands of medical personnel. Finally, the generous use of broad spectrum antibiotics contributes to colonization of the skin and mucosal surfaces by fungi and by pathogenic bacteria with variable degrees of antibiotic resistance.

Nosocomially Acquired Bacterial Infections

COLONIZATION OF THE NEWBORN INFANT

Unless infection in utero occurs because of maternal chorioamnionitis, the newborn infant's first exposure to microorganisms occurs at birth. Regardless of the route of delivery, the skin, upper respiratory tract, and gastrointestinal tract are colonized by a week of age with normal bacterial flora, including *Staphylococcus epidermidis*, diphtheroids, *Escherichia coli*, and anaerobic bacteria. Because these organisms are largely acquired from the mother's genital tract, skin, and upper respiratory tract, the flora of normal newborns resembles that of healthy adults. In contrast, neonates admitted to an intensive care setting become colonized with *Klebsiella*, *Enterobacter*, *Citrobacter*, and other potentially pathogenic Gram-negative bacilli. This is in addition to virulent bacteria such as group B streptococci and certain strains of *E. coli* that may be acquired from the maternal genital tract.

While there are virtually no data regarding the bacterial flora of the recovering NICU infant, one must presume that pathogenic bacteria and fungi are very slowly replaced by normal flora. It is possible that feeding breast milk hastens the return of normal gastrointestinal flora. Conversely, continued antibiotic therapy likely encourages colonization with unwanted microorganisms.

SEPSIS

The risk of bacterial sepsis among recovering infants is lower than among NICU infants under intensive care. Nonetheless, they can occur, principally due to "late onset" infections with group B streptococci, *Listeria monocytogenes*, enterococci, or Gram-negative enteric bacilli. "Late onset" sepsis is generally defined as onset of signs of infection after the first week of life.

Group B Streptococci

Group B streptococci are most commonly acquired from heavily colonized mothers during parturition, but nonmaternal sources also exist. Spread from maternally colonized infants to previously noncolonized infants via the hands of hospital personnel has been well documented. Late onset infections are mostly caused by type III group organisms. Low levels of maternally derived anticapsular antibody are though to put infants at risk of type III, group B streptococcal sepsis.

Most late onset group B streptococcal infections occur between 7 and 28 days of age. Meningitis is the most common clinical manifestation; focal infections of joints and bone also occur. Septic arthritis preferentially involves the hip and knee joints; involvement of the proximal humerus is characteristic of group B streptococcal osteomyelitis. In addition, bacteremia without a focus, cellulitis, lymphadenitis, and a variety of other focal sites of infection are reported.

Diagnosis is based on the recovery of the organism from the blood, CSF, or other focal site. Commercially available latex agglutination (LPA) assays for group-specific capsular antigen, which achieve sensitivities of 88% in CSF and 96% in concentrated urine, often provide specific evidence of group B streptococcal infection within hours. The administration of either penicillin G (400,000 U/kg/day) or ampicillin (300 mg/kg/day) and gentamicin (7.5 mg/kg/day) is recommended for suspected group B streptococcal infections. Proven infections should be treated for a minimum of 14 to 21 days. Approximately 5% of clinically important group B streptococcal isolates exhibit in vitro tolerance to ampicillin, but the clinical significance of such isolates is not known. When these isolates are associated with meningitis, continued use of gentamicin would theoretically enhance the killing of organisms.

Gram-Negative Organisms

The recovering premature infant is also at risk of sepsis from Gram-negative enteric bacilli that colonize the upper respiratory and gastrointestinal tracts. Gram-negative organisms occasionally cause outbreaks of disease in newborn nurseries, although attention to hand washing by personnel has reduced this risk, particularly among infants no longer requiring intensive care. The organisms most often responsible for nursery outbreaks include *Klebsiella pneumonia*, *Serratia marcescens*, *Pseudomonas aeruginosa*, and *Citrobacter diversus*. The common presenting features of infection with these organisms are sepsis and meningitis. Occasionally, these organisms will present with pneumonia, tracheitis, or soft tissue infections (e.g., omphalitis). Suspected Gram-negative infection requires empirical therapy with an aminoglycoside antibiotic (e.g., gentamicin, tobramycin, or amikacin) and either a third generation cephalosporin (cefotaxime, ceftriaxone) or an extended spectrum penicillin (ticarcillin, piperacillin). If *Pseudomonas* is isolated, then ceftazidime should be used with an aminoglycoside. Newer antibiotics such as imipenem and aztreonam should be reserved for treatment of infections caused by broadly resistant organisms.

CATHETER-RELATED INFECTIONS

Central venous catheters are widely used in NICUs to augment or replace enteric caloric intake. The therapeutic value of such catheters is limited by relatively frequent bacterial and fungal infections. The risk of infection is a function of the site of insertion, the duration of catheterization, and the care given to the catheter and catheter insertion site.

Two types of catheter-related infections are recognized; colonization of the intravascular portion of the catheter (i.e., "catheter tip" infections), and infection of the skin and subcutaneous tissues at the site of catheter insertion (i.e., "exit site" infections). Catheter tip infections are documented by isolation of the organism in a blood culture obtained at a site distant from the catheter. Both types of catheter-related infections are caused by resident skin flora, which often includes microbial organisms acquired nosocomially. Gram-positive cocci are most commonly isolated, especially coagulase-negative staphylococci, but many other organisms may cause catheter-related sepsis, including corynebacteria, Gram-negative enteric bacilli, and fungi. Catheter tip infections caused by *Candida sp*. may be especially difficult to manage. *Malassezia furfur* is a lipophilic yeast that may colonize central venous catheters used to infuse lipid emulsions.

The management of catheter-related infections includes parenteral antibiotic therapy, usually through the involved line. Removal of the catheter is mandatory whenever bacteremia persists, an exit site infection fails to clear, there is evidence of thrombosis, persistent thrombocytopenia develops, or fungal infection is documented or suspected.

Nosocomially Acquired Viral Infections

RESPIRATORY VIRUSES

Nosocomial respiratory infections occur commonly in the NICU setting with the spread of infection facilitated by either infection of nursery personnel and visitors or indirect virus transmission via the hands of personnel. Respiratory syncytial virus, influenza viruses, parainfluenza viruses, and rhinoviruses are implicated most frequently. For most, if not all, of these agents, passively acquired maternal antibody is thought to provide some protection against serious disease. However, the recovering premature infant may have deficient levels of antibody because of low titers at birth and loss of antibody during the first weeks of life. Clinical involvement ranges from asymptomatic infection to fatal lower respiratory tract disease. The consequences of respiratory virus infection are more likely to be severe among infants with congenital heart disease or chronic lung disease.

Respiratory Syncytial Virus

Outbreaks of *respiratory syncytial virus (RSV)* disease usually involve premature infants who are more than 3 to 4 weeks of age, thus placing recovering infants at particular risk. Attack rates among both infants and hospital staff may be quite high. Fever, tachypnea, coryza, cough, wheezing, cyanosis, and apnea are characteristic clinical signs. Lower respiratory tract involvement is suggested by an increased oxygen requirement and chest x-ray evidence of hyperinflation or pneumonia. RSV-infected infants under a month of age are more likely to have nonspecific clinical manifestations such as cough and coryza, and less likely to have lower respiratory tract disease. Aerosolized ribavirin may reduce virus shedding and hasten recovery from lower respiratory tract RSV infection, but the degree of benefit is controversial. Strict compliance with glove and gown precautions will reduce the rate of nosocomial transmission.

Influenza

Influenza viruses cause widespread illness in the general population during annual outbreaks from November to March. In contrast to RSV, influenza is highly communicable via the airborne route. Several outbreaks of influenza have been reported in NICU settings. It is likely that many more would be recognized; however, the clinical features of influenza in neonates are relatively mild and nonspecific. Although fatal cases in this age group are described, most neonates with proven influenza virus infection experience self-limited fever, irritability, coryza, and cough. Lethargy, apnea, and poor feeding may lead to suspicion of bacterial sepsis. X-ray evidence of interstitial pneumonia can be found in a few infants.

As with RSV infections, it may be that hospitalized infants more than a month of age have a greater risk of lower respiratory tract disease. Hall and Douglas noted a high rate of fever, leukocytosis, lower respiratory tract disease, and secondary bacterial pneumonia during a nosocomial outbreak of influenza among 1 to 6-month-old infants, many of whom had underlying cardiopulmonary disease.

While such infants might be considered candidates for immunization, influenza vaccines have not been widely tested in this age group, and they are not recommended for infants under 6 months of age.

ENTERIC VIRUSES

Rotaviruses

The rotaviruses are the most important and the best characterized of the viruses that cause gastrointestinal disease in human infants. Rotavirus infections have occurred among recovering newborn infants during outbreaks in neonatal intensive care units, and persistent, endemic rotavirus transmission with high infection rates has also been described in some hospital nurseries. Indirect spread via the hands of personnel is strongly implicated as the major mechanism of transmission. Fifty percent or more of rotavirus-infected neonates remain asymptomatic. Ill infants usually have self-limited, watery diarrhea; however, some will also experience abdominal distention, bloody diarrhea, and signs suggestive of bacterial sepsis. Rotaviruses are among the infectious agents most strongly associated with outbreaks of necrotizing enterocolitis. A policy of limited nursery access and attention to hand washing and gowning in the NICU is thought to reduce the risk of rotavirus infection, particularly during periods of high prevalence in the community and on children's wards elsewhere in the hospital.

TRANSFUSION-ACQUIRED INFECTIONS

The need for frequent transfusion of blood and blood products to neonates results in a considerable risk of transfusion-related infections. In recent years, newborn infants have acquired infections with cytomegaloviruses (CMV), hepatitis B virus, non-A non-B hepatitis (hepatitis C) virus, human immunodeficiency virus (HIV), malaria, and other agents. Routine screening by blood banks has reduced the risk from hepatitis B virus and HIV dramatically, and routine screening for hepatitis C is anticipated soon.

Cytomegalovirus

Even though full-term infants rarely experience symptoms with transfusion-related cytomegalovirus infections, preterm infants receiving intensive care continue to experience considerable morbidity. Infants of CMV seronegative women are at highest risk of severe disease, probably because of an absence of passively acquired CMV antibody. Because of the relatively long incubation period of 3 to 12 weeks, clinical symptoms may not appear until the infant has graduated to level II care or has been discharged home. Increased oxygen requirements, pneumonia, hepatitis, hemolytic anemia, thrombocytopenia, and CNS involvement are known manifestations. Some infants have died of these complications. It is estimated that the risk of CMV transmission is 5% per unit of blood given. This risk can be substantially reduced by limiting donations to only CMV antibody-negative persons, or by use of frozen or leukocyte-depleted blood.

VERTICALLY TRANSMITTED (CONGENITAL) INFECTIONS

When the mother is the source of infection for the fetus or neonate, the infectious agent is said to be vertically transmitted. While vertically transmitted bacteria such as group B streptococci or *Listeria* usually cause disease within the first 7 to 10 days of life, there are many agents that may not produce signs of infection until several weeks of life, or even later. Among the most important of these are cytomegalovirus, human immunodeficiency virus, hepatitis B virus, herpes simplex virus, *Chlamydia trachomatis*, and syphilis. The persistent infections established by some of these agents may affect the developing central nervous system and cause serious, lifelong disability. This section reviews the pathophysiology, diagnosis, and management of vertically transmitted infections that are most likely to arise in the recovering NICU infant.

Cytomegalovirus

The human cytomegalovirus (CMV) is a member of the herpesvirus family that infects 40 to 100% of persons by the time they reach adulthood. The initial (primary) infection in the normal host is usually asymptomatic, although young adults will sometimes have a mononucleosis-like syndrome. Afterwards, periodic reactivation of CMV replication may occur throughout life, particularly during periods of immunosuppression and pregnancy. Asymptomatic excretion of CMV can be found in the urine of 2 to 7% and cervical secretions of 3 to 28% of pregnant women at term. Both intrauterine and intrapartum CMV transmission occur, the latter being the most common. Infection acquired by either route may have important consequences for the premature infant.

The overall rate of intrauterine CMV infection is 0.5 to 2.5%, as defined by the presence of CMV viruria at birth. Both primary and reactivation CMV infections during pregnancy result in intrauterine transmission. The risk of intrauterine transmission is approximately 30 to 40% after primary maternal infection, whereas the estimated risk of intrauterine infection after reactivation of CMV infection is less than 10%. However, because reactivation infection is far more common than primary infection, most congenitally infected infants are born to women having recurrent CMV infections. Fetal infection presumably follows maternal CMV viremia. The virus is disseminated throughout fetal tissues, infecting the lung, liver, reticuloendothelial system, ventricular ependyma, and the organ of Corti. Healing is accompanied by complete resolution of the inflammatory changes in nonneural tissues. However, residual fibrosis and calcification persists within the brain and sensory organs.

Only 5 to 10% of infants infected in utero appear abnormal at birth. Infants presenting with infection at birth are virtually always associated with primary maternal infections. The most common clinical manifestations are low birth weight, hepatomegaly, splenomegaly, jaundice, petechiae, and hemolytic anemia. Pneumonitis occurs in 30 to 40% of symptomatic cases, but it is usually not present within the first few days of life. Central nervous system and ocular defects consist of microcephaly, chorioretinitis, microphthalmia, and cataracts. Laboratory studies often demonstrate atypical lymphocytosis, thrombocytopenia, and mildly elevated transaminase levels. Characteristic periventricular intracerebral calcifications are noted on skull x-rays in about one-third of the cases.

Intrapartum acquisition of CMV occurs in 8 to 18% of all newborn infants as a result of exposure to the virus in maternal cervical secretions or in breast milk. While clinical disease following intrapartum infection is unusual among term infants, premature infants are at risk of considerable morbidity and long-term sequelae. Infected premature infants begin excreting CMV between 4 and 12 weeks of age; excretion may coincide with loss of passively acquired maternal antibody, which disappears more rapidly in the premature infant than in the term infant. Hepatomegaly, splenomegaly, lymphocytosis, thrombocytopenia, neutropenia, and hepatitis may accompany onset of viral excretion. More importantly, pneumonitis may increase or prolong oxygen requirements, particularly among infants with preexisting pulmonary disease.

DIAGNOSIS

The diagnosis of CMV infection is best accomplished by isolation of virus from urine, oropharyngeal secretions, or the buffy coat of preservative-free, heparinized blood. Isolation of CMV in the first 3 weeks of life is diagnostic of intrauterine infection. After 3 weeks of age, virus isolation cannot distinguish intrauterine from perinatal infection. The introduction of monoclonal antibodies has markedly enhanced the speed with which CMV can be identified in cell culture. Simple staining of a centrifuged urine sediment with Wright or Giemsa stain for inclusion-bearing renal epithelial cells is a less sensitive, but an extremely specific, rapid, and simple means of detecting the presence of CMV viruria. Serological methods are more complicated and less useful. Passively acquired maternal CMV antibody must be taken into account when serological tests are interpreted. The sensitivity and the specificity of CMV-specific IgM antibody assays available in many laboratories have been disappointing.

SEQUELAE

Few infants with CMV inclusion disease die in the postnatal period. Pneumonitis may produce a life-threatening illness, but this and other non-CNS manifestations usually clear within the first few weeks of life. Unfortunately, residual CNS defects remain in more than

80% of infants with overt, intrauterine-acquired CMV disease, including microcephaly, mental retardation, seizures, hearing loss, and visual deficits. The prognosis for infants wh have no neonatal manifestations is far better. Nevertheless, diminished intelligence and hearing loss occur more often in these infants than in uninfected siblings. Similar neurodevelopmental sequelae have been demonstrated among low birth weight infants with perinatally acquired infection who begin excreting CMV during the first 8 weeks of life.

TREATMENT

The treatment of congenitally infected infants consists of only supportive care. Antiviral agents, including adenine arabinoside, acyclovir, and interferon, have been administered to infected infants without altering the course of disease.

Human Immunodeficiency Virus

The human immunodeficiency virus (HIV) is a retrovirus that causes the acquired immunodeficiency syndrome (AIDS) and a wide range of other clinical manifestations in infected infants and children who do not meet the clinical definition for AIDS. The current worldwide epidemic of HIV infection is widely considered the most significant public health problem of the past decade and the foreseeable future. Circumstantial evidence suggests that the prevalence of HIV infection may be quite high in some nursery settings. In some centers in the United States, HIV seroprevalence among parturient women exceeds 3%. Because many HIV-positive pregnant women are intravenous drug abusers, have other sexually transmitted infections, or have inadequate prenatal care, they have an increased risk of premature labor and delivery and other perinatal complications.

Because HIV infection rarely causes symptomatic disease until 3 months of age or older, it is not certain how knowledge of the infant's infection status would affect care of the infant in the NICU. Infants known to be infected would become candidates for use of inactivated poliovirus vaccine and for prophylaxis against *Pneumocystis carinii* pneumonia when they are 2 months of age or older. In the future, infected infants may be treated with antiviral agents such as zidovudine from an early age in order to delay the onset of HIV-related disease and prolong life. Studies are now underway to determine whether peripartum administration of zidovudine can actually prevent intrapartum HIV transmission to neonates of HIV seropositive mothers. Although universal infection control policies are applicable to all nursery patients, extra caution would likely be used by nursery personnel caring for an infant known to be infected with HIV.

Although women with all stages of HIV infection have given birth to infected infants, in the U.S. most women have been asymptomatic at the time of delivery. Women who abuse drugs are more likely to give birth to low birth weight infants and more likely to suffer perinatal complications. A study from Montifiore Hospital in New York indicates that asymptomatic HIV infection confers no additional risk of adverse pregnancy outcome; i.e., no effect on gestational age, birth weight, Apgar score, or perinatal complication rate.

The rate of transmission of HIV from mostly asymptomatic, seropositive mothers appears to be in the range of 15 to 35%. Women with more advanced HIV infection are more likely to give birth to infected infants. The recovery of HIV from fetuses aborted as early as early as 15 weeks of gestation indicates that intrauterine infection occurs. Intrapartum transmission, as occurs in hepatitis B infection, is also considered a potential route of transmission, although direct evidence for this mechanism is lacking. Breast feeding represents another mode of vertical transmission, although the extent to which breast feeding contributes to the overall vertical transmission rate is unknown.

DIAGNOSIS

The diagnosis of HIV infection during infancy is confounded by the obligatory passive transfer of maternal antibodies to the newborn infant. Maternal antibodies may persist at detectable concentrations into the second year of life in an uninfected child. Thus, confirmation of infection for younger, asymptomatic infants requires HIV isolation or p24 antigen detection, and these tests have thus far proven rather insensitive. It is expected that more sensitive HIV isolation techniques and introduction of the polymerase chain reaction (PCR) for widespread use will markedly enhance the early diagnosis of HIV infection in the newborn infant.

CLINICAL MANIFESTATIONS

Although virtually all HIV-infected infants appear normal at birth, most develop signs of HIV infection within the first 12 months of life. The most common presenting manifestations are nonspecific, including generalized adenopathy, growth failure, hepatomegaly, splenomegaly, persistent oral candidiasis, or recurrent infections of the middle ear, respiratory tract, or gastrointestinal tract. Neurological disease ultimately occurs in 30 to 60% of HIV-infected children. Reported central nervous system abnormalities include acquired microcephaly, loss of developmental milestones, intellectual deterioration, and motor deficits with weakness, pyramidal tract signs, spastic quadriparesis, dysphagia, dysarthria, ataxia, seizures, and myoclonus. Lymphocytic interstitial pneumonitis (LIP) is an AIDS-defining pulmonary complication that is extremely common in children who survive the first year of life, occurring in at least half of such children. Symptoms of LIP develop slowly and insidiously; they include tachypnea, cough, and progressive hypoxia, but little or no fever. The chest x-ray typically has a diffusely nodular infiltrate with hilar adenopathy, a pattern that is considered sufficiently diagnostic for clinical and surveillance purposes.

The occurrence of opportunistic infections reflects the most severe degree of underlying immunodeficiency and represents the most serious life-threatening events for HIV-infected children. *Pneumocystis carinii* pneumonia (PCP) is the most common and one of the most serious opportunistic infections. PCP is seen most frequently in the first year of life, occasionally as the initial clinical manifestation of perinatal HIV infection. Even when successfully managed, the occurrence of PCP indicates a poor prognosis. Other important opportunistic pathogens include CMV, *M. avium-intracellularae*, *candida sp.*, and *Cryptococcus neoformans*. Recurrent bacterial infections are most often due to encapsulated organisms such as *Streptococcus pneumoniae* or *Hemophilus influenzae*, which cause bacteremia, meningitis, pneumonia, and other serious infections. In addition to opportunistic infections, HIV infection is associated with abnormal function of multiple organs, including the brain, gastrointestinal tract, heart, liver, and kidneys. The dominant laboratory findings include anemia, hypergammaglobulinemia, and depression of the absolute helper T4 lymphocyte count. A wide range of other hematological and biochemical abnormalities are also observed.

TREATMENT

The management of children with HIV infection is complex and challenging. Most pediatric AIDS experts consider the future of specific therapy of human HIV infection to lie with a growing number of antiviral and immunomodulating agents. Zidovudine (azidothymidine, AZT) was the first promising drug to reach widespread clinical testing in both adults and children, and this agent is now the only licensed anti-HIV drug available in the United States. It is well absorbed orally and penetrates into the CSF. Controlled trials have demonstrated zidovudine efficacy in homosexual males with AIDS, and there is now considerable evidence of efficacy in children.

Hepatitis B Virus

In the United States and other developed countries, the overall prevalence of antibody to hepatitis B virus (HBV) is 5 to 10%. HBV infection is transmitted largely by blood or blood products or by sexual contact with infected individuals. Adults at high risk include hemophiliacs and others who require transfusion with large quantities of blood (e.g., cardiac surgical patients), intravenous drug abusers, medical personnel sustaining accidental trauma from needles or other instruments contaminated with blood or blood products (especially surgeons, dentists, surgical nurses, or hemodialysis and laboratory personnel), homosexual males, and heterosexual contacts of chronic HBV carriers. The overall risk to healthy adults of becoming chronic carriers after acute HBV infection is about 6%. Persons infected in infancy or during periods of immunosuppression have much higher rates of chronic hepatitis B surface antigen (HB_sAg) carriage. The overall chronic carrier rate in the United States is low, i.e., less than 1%. The carrier rate is higher among the aforementioned increased-risk groups as well as among immigrants from parts of the world where HBV infection is endemic.

Vertical transmission may occur with acute maternal HBV infection during pregnancy or when the mother is a chronic HBV carrier. In the former case, the major risk to the newborn exists when onset of maternal hepatitis occurs during the last trimester or shortly after delivery. Under these conditions of exposure, the risk of neonatal infection is more than 75%. In contrast, the risk of perinatal transmission is close to zero when maternal hepatitis occurs early enough in pregnancy and maternal antibody to HB_sAg develops before parturition.

A greater number of infants are at risk from mothers who are chronic carriers than from mothers who have acute infection in late pregnancy. Among chronic carrier mothers, the risk of vertical transmission depends greatly on whether or not maternal serum hepatitis B e antigen (HB_eAg), an indicator of high infectivity, is present. In the United States, women who are HB_eAg-positive have more than a 90% chance of transmitting HBV to their newborn infants. In contrast, the probability of infection among infants of HB_eAg-negative mothers is less than 5%. About 20% of women of childbearing age who are chronic carriers are HB_eAg-positive. Breast feeding does not increase the risk of perinatal infection.

CLINICAL MANIFESTATIONS

Less than 10% of HBV-infected newborns acquire infection in utero. Because HBV is usually transmitted during parturition, markers for HBV infection do not appear in the infant's blood until 8 to 15 weeks after exposure. At this time, acute, icteric hepatitis may occur in some perinatally infected infants. Some clinically well infants who have been carefully followed have developed mild hepatic enlargement and modest elevation of serum transaminases. The elevation of serum transaminase levels is accompanied by the appearance of serum antibody to the hepatitis B core antigen (HB_cAb). Infants with self-limited clinical disease tend to clear HB_sAg from the serum and later develop antibodies to HB_sAg.

However, 80 to 90% of perinatally infected infants remain asymptomatic. Subclinical hepatitis is the rule among the majority who are destined to have persistent infection and to become chronic carriers of HB_sAg. Chronic carriers do not make antibody to HB_sAg, but they tend to have persistently high levels of HB_cAg. The chronic carrier state may persist for many years, perhaps for life. As yet, there are no firm data on which to predict the consequences of the chronic carrier state that follows infection acquired during infancy. It is likely that perinatally infected neonates are at risk of developing chronic active hepatitis, cirrhosis, and primary hepatocellular carcinoma (hepatoma) later in life.

DIAGNOSIS

The diagnosis of hepatitis B depends on demonstration of one or more serological markers for HBV infection. The presence of HB_sAg in serum indicates current infection. Persistent infection has been defined as the presence of HB_sAg in serum specimens taken at least 6 months apart. HB_sAb is indicative of past infection and permanent immunity. Patients with permanent natural immunity also have low levels of HB_cAg.

MANAGEMENT

Studies in populations in which HBV infection is endemic have shown that perinatal transmission can be substantially reduced by administration of either hepatitis B immune globulin (HBIG) or hepatitis B vaccine to the newborn infant. Because administration of both HBIG and HBV vaccine provides a level of protection superior to that obtained when either is used alone, the Committee on Infectious Diseases of the American Academy of Pediatrics recommends administration of both HBIG and HBV vaccine to infants of mothers who are either acutely infected in the last two trimesters of pregnancy or who are chronic carriers of HB_sAg. HBIG is given in a dose of 0.5 ml IM as soon as possible after birth, and HBV vaccine is administered in 3 IM doses of 0.5 ml each. The first dose is recommended either at the same time as HBIG (but with a separate syringe and at a different site) or within 7 days of birth and prior to hospital discharge. Unlike HBIG, the administration of HBV vaccine can be delayed if necessary. However, if it is delayed for as long as 3 months, a second 0.5 ml dose of HBIG should be given. The second and third doses of HBV vaccine are given at 1 month and 6 months after the first.

Infants receiving perinatal HBV prophylaxis must be followed in order to assess the effect of these preventive measures and to determine the status of the infants with respect to HBV. This is most reliably accomplished by testing serum for HB_sAg at 9 months of age or later.

Herpes Simplex Viruses

The herpes simplex viruses, type 1 and type 2, are closely related human herpesviruses that cause self-limited, recurrent mucocutaneous infections in many persons, and persistent and sometimes severe visceral disease in persons who are immunocompromised, including newborn infants. Newborn infants are most often infected via intrapartum exposure to virus that is shed from the maternal genital tract. HSV type 2 causes 70 to 80% of neonatal HSV infections, reflecting the predominance of this type as a cause of genital herpes infections. Neonatal HSV type 1 infections may be acquired from the maternal genital tract or from oral virus shed by either the mother or another person having close contact with the neonate during the postpartum period.

The risk of transmission depends on the stage of maternal genital tract infection. Primary genital HSV infections during the perinatal period are associated with a 40 to 50% rate of vertical transmission. In contrast, women with recurrent lesions of the genital tract transmit infection to their newborn infants in fewer than 5% of recognized cases. In either case, delivery of the infant via cesarean section reduces the risk of neonatal infection. Unfortunately, a high proportion of infants with neonatal HSV infections are born to women who have no apparent genital lesions or who give no history of prior genital herpes infection. In these cases, the mother is presumed to shed HSV from the genital tract in the absence of signs or symptoms of genital infection.

Regardless of the mode of transmission, premature infants are considered to have increased risk of infection. Scalp electrodes and other breaks in the skin may promote infection beginning at the site of trauma. The presence or absence of passively transferred maternal antibody may also be an important determinant of infection.

CLINICAL MANIFESTATIONS

The first symptoms or signs of perinatally acquired HSV infection are often observed between 6 and 21 days of age, although the onset of disease in younger infants is widely recognized and disease in infants up to 6 weeks of age has been reported. The characteristic skin or mucous membrane lesion is a single vesicle or a cluster of vesicular lesions. Approximately 40% of infected infants present initially with one or more local lesions, and 70% of these infants will progress to systemic infection if not treated with an appropriate antiviral drug.

Approximately 25% of infants present with signs of systemic infection, with or without mucocutaneous lesions. These infants initially have nonspecific manifestations such as fever, lethargy, apnea, and poor feeding, and they rapidly develop signs of hepatitis, pneumonitis, encephalitis, renal failure, acidosis, and diffuse bleeding. The diagnosis of disseminated HSV disease in the absence of mucocutaneous lesions may be delayed without a high index of suspicion. The clinical picture is indistinguishable from bacterial sepsis and systemic enterovirus infection.

Encephalitis in the absence of cutaneous or other systemic disease occurs in about 35% of HSV-infected newborns. Infants with isolated encephalitis tend to be slightly older (i.e., 2 to 4 weeks old) than infants with localized or systemic infection.

Pneumonitis represents a fourth, less recognized, mode of presentation. Infants with HSV pneumonitis tend to present at less than 7 days of age and then rapidly develop signs of systemic disease. Neonatal HSV pneumonitis is associated with a poor prognosis, in part because of delayed recognition.

TREATMENT AND PROGNOSIS

The mortality of untreated neonatal HSV infection is 50 to 80%, depending on the type of disease; permanent neurological sequelae among survivors is common. The efficacy of adenine arabinoside (Ara-A) as an antiviral agent was established for neonatal HSV infection over a decade ago. Acyclovir is more widely used to treat neonates because it is less toxic and because it can be given intravenously in a smaller volume of fluid. With a 10-day course of intravenous acyclovir, infants with HSV disease localized to the skin and mucous membranes virtually all survive. Survival rates are lower for infants with disseminated disease (35 to 45%) or encephalitis (85 to 90%).

The success of antiviral treatment is relative. Infants who recover have a frequency of neurological sequelae that varies from 7 to 15% for infants surviving local disease to 65% for infants that survive HSV encephalitis. Overall, the risk of neurological sequelae is higher following type 2 HSV disease than following type 1 infection. Some infants experience early systemic or CNS recurrences of disease after a 10-day course of apparently successful antiviral therapy, and others have frequent cutaneous recurrences extending through the first several years of life. Because infants with recurrent disease are more likely to manifest neurological sequelae, studies are underway to assess the efficacy of longer courses of initial antiviral therapy and prolonged courses of oral acyclovir following initial intravenous treatment.

Chlamydia Trachomatis

Chlamydia trachomatis is an obligate intracellular bacterium that is transmitted sexually and colonizes both the female and male genital tracts. In males, chlamydia is a dominant cause of nongonococcal urethritis. Infected females may experience cervicitis, urethral syndrome, and salpingitis, although most infections in women are asymptomatic. An average of 4 to 5% of pregnant women are infected at term, but prevalance may exceed 30% in some high-risk populations.

Vertical transmission occurs during parturition via contact with maternal cervical secretions. Cesarean delivery may be protective, but cases of neonatal disease following cesarean delivery occur, perhaps due to ascending intrauterine infection. Approximately 60 to 70% of infants of culture-positive women become infected, but not all develop symptoms. Chlamydia can be recovered from neonatal conjunctivae, upper respiratory tract, lungs, rectum, and vagina at various times after delivery. The rate of asymptomatic infection is unknown.

CONJUNCTIVITIS

Among infants born to colonized women, 17 to 50% will develop inclusion body conjunctivitis, and 11 to 20% will develop pneumonitis. Chlamydial conjunctivitis generally occurs between 5 and 14 days of age, somewhat later than gonococcal conjunctivitis. Chlamydial pneumonitis generally presents between 2 and 8 weeks of age. Passively acquired maternal antibody does not prevent either conjunctivitis or pneumonitis, although the onset of pneumonitis may be delayed by the presence of maternal antibody. Routine silver nitrate ocular prophylaxis does not prevent chlamydial conjunctivitis. Erythromycin or tetracycline prophylaxis may be more effective.

Conjunctivitis begins as erythema and a thin, watery discharge. With progression, the exudate may become purulent, the lids edematous, and a pseudomembrane may form. If untreated, the conjunctival inflammation may persist for several weeks before spontaneously resolving. Involvement of the cornea is rare.

Simple swabbing of the conjunctival exudate provides an inadequate specimen for examination and culture. Indirect immunofluorescence of conjunctival scrapings using a highly specific monoclonal antibody to *C. trachomatis* is the most sensitive and specific diagnostic procedure. Many laboratories can also isolate and identify the organisms in cell culture. Serological techniques are less useful, in part because of the presence of passively acquired maternal antibody. Chlamydial conjunctivitis is usually treated with a 14-day course of oral erythromycin in a dose of 40 to 50 mg/kg/day q.i.d. Topical antibiotic therapy is also effective, but it is not recommended because it does not eradicate colonization of the respiratory mucosa and does not prevent the later development of pneumonitis.

PNEUMONITIS

Chlamydial infection of the lung produces interstitial inflammation and small airway disease. Clinical symptoms begin insidiously between 2 and 8 weeks of age. A consistent pattern of nonproductive cough, congestion, tachypnea, inspiratory rales, and expiratory wheezing is usually observed. The cough may be paroxysmal. The most common chest x-ray abnormalities are hyperexpansion and bilateral, perihilar, interstitial infiltration. Eosinophilia is often present, and serum immunoglobulins are often elevated. The natural course of untreated chlamydial pneumonia is slow resolution over a period of 4 to 6 weeks. During this time, the infant may gain weight poorly. A small number of infants have serious infections that require mechanical ventilation. CMV and other respiratory viruses can be recovered from the tracheal aspirates or lungs of a significant subset of chlamydia-positive infants. It is not clear if this predicts more serious disease.

The diagnosis of chlamydial pneumonitis depends on the demonstration of chlamydial antigen or isolation of the organism in secretions aspirated from the nasopharynx or trachea. An elevated IgM antibody titer is also diagnostic.

Chlamydial pneumonitis responds to oral erythromycin, which is conventionally administered for 14 days. Complete recovery is the rule, although some infants may have long-term obstructive abnormalities on pulmonary function testing.

Syphilis

The recent dramatic increase in primary and secondary syphilis in the United States has produced a steady increase in the number of cases of congenital syphilis. Congenital syphilis occurs most frequently among infants born to women who have had inadequate or no prenatal care.

Many infected infants are asymptomatic at birth. The early clinical manifestations of congenital syphilis are observed between 3 and 8 weeks of age, and virtually all infected infants develop symptoms by 3 months of age. Common early manifestations include anemia, bone lesions, hepatosplenomegaly, mucocutaneous lesions, pseudoparalysis, jaundice, rhinitis, and generalized lymphadenopathy. Hemolysis may contribute to both anemia and jaundice. Osteochondritis is manifested by widened, irregular metaphyses, dactylitis, and periostitis with new bone formation. Pseudoparalysis, observed in about 15% of cases, is thought to be due to severe bone pain. Two types of generalized skin lesions are well known; copper-colored, annular maculopapular lesions and vesicular or bullous lesions (pemphigus neonatorum). Condylomata may be found at mucocutaneous junctions. Uncommon clinical manifestations include thrombocytopenia, nonimmune hydrops, and the nephrotic syndrome.

Infection of the central nervous system, as defined by CSF pleocytosis, occurs in approximately 60% of infected infants, but most CNS infections are initially asymptomatic. The natural history of CNS involvement in congenital syphilis is not well understood because the inflammatory changes in the CSF usually resolve without therapy.

DIAGNOSIS

Diagnosis is based on serological testing or the demonstration of spirochetes in skin lesions or nasal secretions. Specific monoclonal antibodies make immunofluorescent microscopy a sensitive and specific method for identifying spirochetes in clinical specimens. The presence of serum antibody detected either by nonspecific reagin tests (e.g., VDRL) or by specific tests (e.g., FTA-ABS) may indicate either newborn infection or antibody acquired passively from the mother. On the other hand, the presence of any type of antibody in the CSF indicates CNS infection.

MANAGEMENT

The management of infants with laboratory confirmed, symptomatic congenital syphilis consists of examination of the CSF and administration of penicillin G (aqueous crystalline or aqueous procaine) in a dose of 50,000 U/kg once daily for a minimum of 10 days. Treatment is the same for asymptomatic infants with a positive CSF antibody titer or with a CSF pleocytosis.

The management of asymptomatic infants with a positive serological test for syphilis is more complex. If the mother has received adequate treatment for syphilis during pregnancy, the infant may be followed without therapy as long as a repeat VDRL can be obtained at 3 to 6 months of age to confirm the absence of infection. Adequate maternal therapy consists of 2.4 million units of benzathine penicillin IM and documentation of a drop in VDRL antibody titer. Treatment of maternal syphilis with erythromycin may not be curative. In cases where adequate maternal therapy cannot be documented, examination of the CSF and treatment with penicillin is recommended.

Treatment failures are rare, but infants treated for congenital syphilis should be followed to document a fall in VDRL antibody titer at 3 to 6 months of age.

ROUTINE IMMUNIZATION

Diphtheria-tetanus-pertussis (DTP) vaccine and trivalent oral poliovirus vaccine (TOPV) are routinely recommended for all infants, regardless of gestational age at birth, when they reach 8 weeks of age. This section briefly addresses the use of each of these vaccines for infants recovering from complications of premature delivery. In addition to DTP and TOPV, hepatitis B vaccine is administered to infants born to HB_sAg positive women in the first week of life, regardless of the infant's gestational age. The rationale and the use of hepatitis B vaccine is discussed above.

Diphtheria-Tetanus-Pertussis (DTP) Vaccine

Recent studies indicate that DTP vaccine is both safe and immunogenic for infants born as early as 28 weeks gestation when administered in three doses beginning at 8 weeks of age, as recommended by the American Academy of Pediatrics Committee on Infectious Diseases. Infants should be medically stable at the time they receive their first dose of DTP vaccine. The occurrence of an intraventricular hemorrhage is not a contraindication. The rate of local and systemic reactions following DTP is no different for preterm infants when compared with term infants. Furthermore, diphtheria, tetanus, and pertussis antibody titers are comparable to those in term infants after the second dose of vaccine, which is generally administered at 4 months of age.

Trivalent Oral Poliovirus Vaccine (TOPV)

Like DTP, trivalent oral poliovirus vaccine (TOPV) is both safe and effective when administered to preterm infants according to the schedule recommended by the AAP. As with all newborns, TOPV should not be given to premature infants who may be immunocompromised, especially infants with a family history of a hereditary immunodeficiency syndrome. Furthermore, TOPV should not be administered to hospitalized infants because of consequent fecal viral shedding. The vaccine may be given at the time of discharge, as the infant is literally "going out the door." Infants who will return to households with immunocompromised children or adults should be given inactivated poliovirus vaccine (IPV) instead. IPV is given according to the same schedule as TOPV. Infants born to women who are infected with HIV should receive IPV.

SUGGESTED READINGS

General

Remington JS, Klein JO, eds. Infectious diseases of the fetus and newborn infant. Philadelphia: Saunders, 1983.

Nosocomial Infections

Bacterial

Ford-Jones EL, Mindorff CM, Langley JM, et al. Epidemiologic study of 4684 hospital-acquired infections in pediatric patients. Ped Infect Dis J 1989;10:668–675.

Goldmann DA, Leclair J, Macone A. Bacterial colonization of neonates admitted to an intensive care environment. J Pediatr 1978;93:288–293.

Nelson JD. Control of infection acquired in the nursery. In: Remington JS, Klein JO, eds. Infections of the fetus and newborn infant. Philadelphia: Saunders, 1983:1035–1052.

Salzman TC, Clark JJ, Klemm L. Hand contamination of personnel as a mechanism of cross-infection in nosocomial infections with antibiotic-resistant *Escherichia coli* and *Klebsiella-Aerobacter*. Antimicrob Agents Chemother 1967;7:97–100.

Group B Streptococci

Baker CJ, Edwards MS. Group B streptococcal infections. In: Remington JS, Klein JO, eds. Infections of the fetus and newborn infant. Philadelphia: Saunders, 1983:820–881.

Baker CJ, Edwards MS, Kasper DL. Role of antibody to native type III group B streptococcus in infant infection. Pediatrics 1981;68:544–549.

Band JD, Clegg HW, Hayes PS, Gacklam RR, Stringer J, Dixon RE. Transmission of group B streptococci. Am J Dis Child 1981;135:355–358.

Paredes A, Wong P, Mason EO, Taber LH, Barrett FF. Nosocomial transmission of group B streptococci in a newborn nursery. Pediatrics 1976;59:679–682.

Catheter-Related Infections

Aschner JL, Punsalang A, Maniscalco WM, Menegus MA. Percutaneous central venous catheter colonization with *Malassezia furfur*: incidence and clinical significance. Pediatrics 1987;80:535–539.

Viral

Respiratory Viruses

Dagan R, Hall CB. Influenza A virus infection imitating bacterial sepsis in early infancy. Ped Infect Dis 1984;3:218–221.

Goldson EJ, McCarthy JT, Welling MA, Todd JK. A respiratory syncytial virus outbreak in a transitional care nursery. Am J Dis Child 1979;133:1280–1282.

Hall CB, Douglas RG. Nosocomial influenza infection as a cause of intercurrent fevers in infants. Pediatrics 1975;55:673–677.

Hall CB, Kopelman AE, Douglas RG, Geiman JM, Meagher MR. Neonatal respiratory syncytial virus infection. N Eng J Med 1979;300:393–396.

Joshi VV, Escobar MR, Stewart L, Bates RD. Fatal influenza A_2 viral pneumonia in a newborn infant. Am J Dis Child 1973;126:839–840.

Leclair JM, Freeman J, Sullivan BF, Crowley CM, Goldmann DA. Prevention of nosocomial respiratory syncytial virus infections through compliance with glove and gown precautions. N Eng J Med 1987;317:329–334.

Mintz L, Ballard RA, Sniderman SH, Roth RS, Drew WL. Nosocomial respiratory syncytial virus infection in an intensive care nursery: rapid diagnosis by direct immunofluorescence. Pediatrics 1979;64:149–153.

Wald ER, Dashefsky B, Green M. *In re* ribavirin: a case of premature adjudication? J Pediatr 1988;112:154–158.

Enteric Viruses

Dearlove J, Latham P, Dearlove B, Pearl K, Thomson A, Lewis IG. Clinical range of neonatal rotavirus gastroenteritis. Br Med J 1983;286:1473–1475.

Rotbart HA, Levin MJ, Yolken RH, Manchester DK, Jantzen J. An outbreak of rotavirus-associated neonatal necrotizing enterocolitis. J Pediatr 1983;103:454–459.

Transfusion-Acquired Infections

Ballard RA, Drew L, Hufnagle KG, Riedel PA. Acquired cytomegalovirus infection in preterm infants. Am J Dis Child 1979;133:482–485.

Perham TGM, Caul EO, Conway PJ, Mott MG. Cytomegalovirus infection in blood donors: a prospective study. Br J Haematol 1971;20:307–320.

Yeager AS, Grumet FC, Hafleigh EB, Arvin AM, Bradley JS, Prober CG. Prevention of transfusion-acquired cytomegalovirus infections in newborn infants. J Pediatr 1981;98:281–287.

Yeager AS, Palumbo PE, Malachowski N, Ariagno RL, Stevenson DK. Sequelae of maternally derived cytomegalovirus infections in premature infants. J Pediatr 1983;102:918–922.

Congenital Infections

CMV

Collaborative Study Group. Cytomegalovirus infection in the North West of England: a report of a two-year study. Arch Dis Child 1970;45:513–522.

Conboy TJ, Pass RF, Stagno S, et al. Early clinical manifestations and intellectual outcome in children with symptomatic congenital cytomegalovirus infection. J Pediatr 1987;111:343–348.

Hanshaw JB. Cytomegalovirus. In: Remington JS, Klein JO, eds. Infections of the fetus and newborn infant. Philadelphia: Saunders, 1983:104–142.

Kumar ML, Nankervis GA, Cooper AR, Gold E. Postnatally acquired cytomegalovirus infections in infants of CMV-excreting mothers. J Pediatr 1984;104:669–673.

Paryani SG, Yeager AS, Hosford-Dunn H, et al. Sequelae of acquired cytomegalovirus infection in premature and sick term infants. J Pediatr 1985;107:451–456.

Stagno S, Pass RF, Cloud G, et al. Primary cytomegalovirus infection in pregnancy. Incidence, transmission to fetus, and clinical outcome. JAMA 1986;256:1904–1908.

Stagno S, Pass RF, Dworsky ME, et al. Congenital cytomegalovirus infection. The relative importance of primary and recurrent infection. N Eng J Med 1982;306:945–949.

Stagno S, Reynolds DW, Huang E-S, Thames SD, Smith RJ, Alford CA. Congenital cytomegalovirus infection. Occurrence in an immune population. N Eng J Med 1977;296:1254–1258.

Stagno S, Reynolds DW, Pass RF, Alford CA. Breast milk and the risk of cytomegalovirus infection. N Eng J Med 1980;302:1073–1076.

Human Immunodeficiency Virus

Belman AL, Diamond G, Dickson D, et al. Pediatric acquired immunodeficiency syndrome: neurologic syndromes. Am J Dis Child 1988;142:29–35.

The European Collaborative Study. Mother-to-child transmission of HIV infection. Lancet 1988;2:1039–1043.

Italian Multicenter Study. Epidemiology, clinical features, and prognostic factors of paediatric HIV infection. Lancet 1988;2:1043–1046.

Joshi VV, Oleske JM. Pulmonary lesions in children with the acquired immunodeficiency syndrome: a reappraisal based on data in additional cases and follow-up study of previously reported cases. Hum Pathol 1986;17:641–642.

Jovaisas E, Koch MA, Schafer A, Stauber M, Lowenthal D. LAV/HTLV-III in 20-week fetus [Letter]. Lancet 1985;2:1129.

Lapointe N, Michaud J, Pekovic D, Chausseau JP, Dupuy J-M. Transplacental transmission of HTLV-III virus [Letter]. N Eng J Med 1985;312:1325–1326.

Laure F, Courgnaud V, Rouzioux C, et al. Detection of HIV1 DNA in infants and children by means of the polymerase chain reaction. Lancet 1988;2:538–541.

Oxtoby MJ. Human immunodeficiency virus and other viruses in human milk: placing the issues in broader perspective. Ped Infect Dis J 1988;7:825–835.

Pahwa S, Kaplan M, Fikrig S, et al. Spectrum of human T-cell lymphotropic virus type III infection in children: recognition of symptomatic, asymptomatic, and seronegative patients. JAMA 1986;255:2299–2305.

Pizzo PA, Eddy J, Falloon J, et al. Effect of continuous intravenous infusion of zidovudine (AZT) in children with symptomatic HIV infection. N Eng J Med 1988;319:889–896.

Rubinstein A, Morecki R, Silverman B, et al. Pulmonary disease in children with acquired immune deficiency syndrome and AIDS-related complex. J Pediatr 1986;108:498–503.

Selwyn PA, Schoenbaum EE, Davenny K, et al. Prospective study of human immunodeficiency virus infection and pregnancy outcomes in intravenous drug users. JAMA 1989;261:1289–1294.

Hepatitis B

Committee on Infectious Diseases. Prevention of hepatitis B virus infections. Pediatrics 1985;75:362–364.

Ganem D. Persistent infection of humans with hepatitis B virus. Rev Infect Dis 1982;4:1026–1047.

Xu Z-Y, Liu C-B, Francis DP, et al. Prevention of perinatal acquisition of hepatitis B virus carriage using vaccine: preliminary report of a randomized, double-blind placebo-controlled and comparative trial. Pediatrics 1985;76:713–718.

Herpes Simplex Viruses

Amortegui AJ, MacPherson TA, Harger JH. A cluster of neonatal herpes simplex infections without mucocutaneous manifestations. Pediatrics 1984;73:194–198.

Corey L, Whitley RJ, Stone EF, Mohan K. Difference between herpes simplex virus type 1 and type 2 neonatal encephalitis in neurological outcome. Lancet 1988;1:1–4.

Dankner WM, Spector SA. Recurrent herpes simplex in a neonate. Ped Infect Dis 1986;5:582–586.

Hubble C, Dominguez R, Kohl S. Neonatal herpes simplex pneumonitis. Reve Infect Dis 1988;10:431–438.

Overall JC, Whitley RJ, Yeager AS, McCracken GH, Nelson JD. Prophylactic or anticipatory antiviral therapy for newborns exposed to herpes simplex infection. Ped Infect Dis 1984;193–195.

Prober CG, Sullender WM, Yasukawa LL, Au DS, Yeager AS, Arvin AM. Low risk of herpes simplex virus infections in neonates exposed to the virus at the time of vaginal delivery to mothers with recurrent genital herpes simplex virus infections. N Eng J Med 1987;316:240–244.

Whitley RJ, Nahmias AJ, Soong S-J, Galasso GG, Fleming CL, Alford CA. Vidarabine therapy of neonatal herpes simplex virus infection. Pediatrics 1980;66:495–501.

Whitley RJ, Nahmias AJ, Visintine AM, Fleming CL, Alford CA. The natural history of herpes simplex virus infection of mother and newborn. Pediatrics 1980;66:489–494.

Whitley RJ, Yeager A, Kartus P, Bryson Y, Connor JD, Alford CA. Neonatal herpes simplex virus infection: follow-up evaluation of vidarabine therapy. Pediatrics 1983;72:778–785.

Chlamydia

Givner LB, Rennels MB, Woodward CL, Huang S-W. *Chlamydia trachomatis* infection in infant delivered by cesarean section. Pediatrics 1981;68:420–421.

Tipple MA, Beem MO, Saxon EM. Clinical characteristics of the afebrile pneumonia associated with *Chlamydia trachomatis* infection in infants less than 6 months of age. Pediatrics 1979;63:192–197.

Weiss SG, Newcomb RW, Beem MO. Pulmonary assessment of children after chlamydial pneumonia of infancy. J Pediatr 1986;108:659–664.

Syphilis

Beck-Sague C, Alexander ER. Failure of benzathine penicillin G treatment in early congenital syphilis. Ped Infect Dis J 1987;11:1061–1064.

Centers for Disease Control. Congenital syphilis—New York City, 1986–1988. MMWR 1989;38:825–829.

Centers for Disease Control. Guidelines for the prevention and control of congenital syphilis. MMWR 1988;37(suppl S-1):1–13.

Centers for Disease Control. Increases in primary and secondary syphilis—United States. MMWR 1987;36:393–396.

Norgard MV, Selland CK, Kettman JR, Miller JN. Sensitivity and specificity of monoclonal antibodies directed against antigenic determinants of *Treponema pallidum* Nichols in the diagnosis of syphilis. J Clin Microbiol 1984;20:711–717.

Platou RV. Treatment of congenital syphilis. Adv Pediatr 1949;4:39–81.

Immunization

American Academy of Pediatrics. Report of the Committee on Infectious Diseases. Evanston, IL: American Academy of Pediatrics, 1988.

Bernbaum JC, Daft A, Anolik R, et al. Response of preterm infants to diphtheria-tetanus-pertussis immunizations. J Pediatr 1985;107:184–188.

Koblin BA, Townsend TR, Munoz A, Onorato I, Wilson M, Polk BF. Response of preterm infants to diphtheria-tetanus-pertussis vaccine. Pediatr Infect Dis J 1988;7:704–711.

7

Chronic Lung Disease

Susan U. Lipstein and Bonnie B. Hudak

Chronic lung disease (CLD) continues to be a common complication of prematurity despite recent therapeutic advances such as surfactant administration. Management goals for the recovering infant are: (*a*) to maintain optimal oxygenation and energy balance to promote growth and development; (*b*) to avoid complications of therapy; and (*c*) to prepare both the infant and family for discharge (Table 7.1). Assessment of these infants, management in the Neonatal Intensive Care Unit (NICU), preparation for discharge, and follow-up after discharge will continue to be a challenge.

DEFINITIONS

Bronchopulmonary dysplasia (BPD) was originally described by Northway in 1967. He described an orderly progression of changes from the radiographical picture of severe hyaline membrane disease to one characterized by cystic changes and areas of atelectasis. Since that time, the term BPD has gradually been applied to a progressively more diverse group of infants with a wide variety of clinical and radiographical findings. The group of infants reported by Northway were more mature (30 to 39 weeks) and larger (1475 to 3200 grams) than the population of infants that are commonly seen today. In addition, the techniques of resuscitation and ventilation of neonates with hyaline membrane disease (HMD) have changed dramatically since 1967. Not surprisingly, the clinical course and pattern of radiographical changes described by Northway are rarely seen today.

Several alternate definitions of BPD, which is perhaps better termed chronic lung disease (CLD), have been suggested. The first of these was put forth in 1979 and takes into account the infant's condition at 28 days of age. It has been commonly used in studies for defining BPD. Applying this definition, an infant is considered to have chronic lung disease if he or she was ventilated in the first week of life for HMD and has a supplemental oxygen requirement, physical findings of lung disease (retractions, tachypnea), and blood gas and radiographical abnormalities that persist beyond 28 days of age. Although this definition is more general than that of Northway, it still has practical limitations. With the survival

Table 7.1. Goals in Managing Patients with Chronic Lung Disease

Maintain adequate oxygenation
Promote optimal growth and development
Avoid complications of therapy
Prepare infant and family for hospital discharge

of very immature infants, such as those born at 23 weeks gestation, the status at 28 days of age may have little predictive value for condition at discharge and long-term outcome.

More recently, it has been suggested that the requirement for oxygen therapy at 36 weeks postconceptional age is more predictive of an abnormal pulmonary outcome. Although this definition may include infants with a broad spectrum of pulmonary disorders, it is probably the most relevant to condition at discharge and ultimate outcome. However, it is obviously not helpful in infants who have not yet reached 36 weeks postconceptional age.

In this chapter, the term chronic lung disease will be applied to those infants with symptomatic lung disease. This includes infants with clinical and radiographical evidence of lung disease who require therapies such as supplemental oxygen, diuretics, bronchodilators, or fluid restriction.

PATHOGENESIS

Although CLD is commonly thought to result from oxygen toxicity and barotrauma alone, the pathogenesis is complex, very likely involving multiple causes of lung injury in a susceptible host (Fig. 7.1). The premature infant is particularly at risk for lung injury and, in addition, is less capable of repairing injured lung. The third trimester is an important time in the development of lung structure and biochemical maturity. At the beginning of the third trimester, the fetus has few air sacs (the forerunners of alveoli) and comparatively little surface area for gas exchange. The antioxidants required to prevent toxicity from even relatively low concentrations of oxygen are not yet being synthesized in significant quantities. Similarly, the synthesis and release of pulmonary surfactant has not yet begun.

In preparation for birth, the fetus rapidly matures during the third trimester. In the infant born prematurely, structural and biosynthetic immaturities combine to predispose to

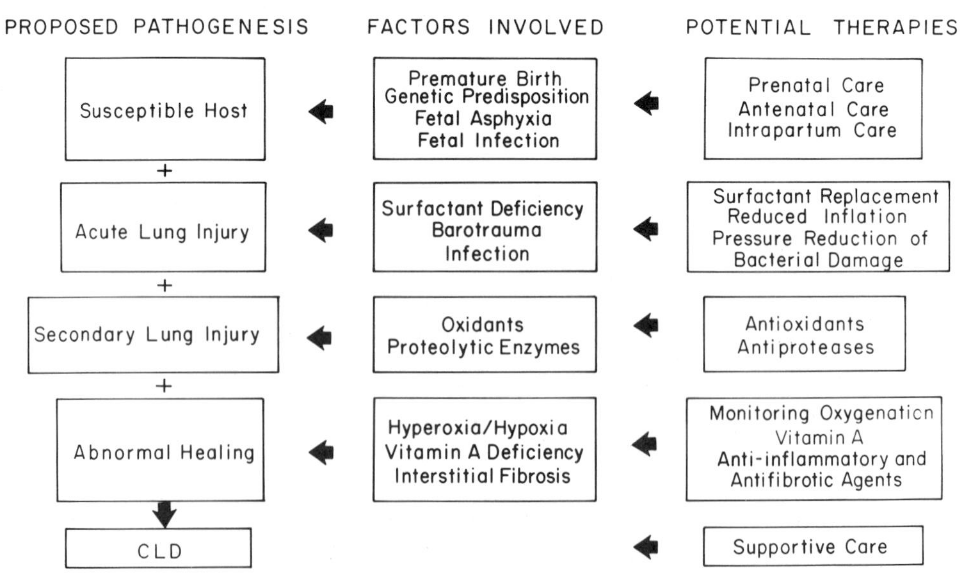

Figure 7.1. Proposed pathogenesis of, factors involved in, and potential therapies for chronic lung disease (CLD). (Reprinted and modified with permission from Goetzman BW. Understanding bronchopulmonary dysplasia. Am J Dis Child 1986;140:332–334. Copyright 1986, American Medical Association.)

lung injury from oxygen, barotrauma, and a variety of other insults. These may include pulmonary edema from a patent ductus arteriosus, trauma from an endotracheal tube, airway damage from incompletely humidified gas, damaging products from polymorphonuclear leukocytes, etc. In addition, the premature infant is relatively poorly nourished and is unable to quickly repair injured lung. Chronic lung disease is, most simply, the result of lung injury and impaired lung growth and repair in a susceptible patient.

ASSESSMENT

Ongoing assessment is critical in the management of CLD. As the infant grows and matures, the problems encountered continue to change. The assessment of clinical status must be combined with chest x-rays, blood gases, pulse oximetry, echocardiography, and other studies to formulate a comprehensive treatment plan.

Clinical Status

The evaluation of the clinical status of the infant includes both a thorough physical examination and the taking of a history relating to recent problems (Table 7.2). This historical information may be the key to the successful management of changes in the infant's condition.

HISTORY

Information gathered from individuals previously involved in the infant's care and from the chart is invaluable. Note should be made of changes in the frequency and/or timing of apnea and bradycardia, feeding tolerance, emesis, or general appearance and behavior. Short- and long-term patterns of weight gain should be assessed.

A sudden increase in the frequency of apnea and bradycardia may result from hypoxemia, neurological immaturity, symptomatic anemia, or other causes such as infection. For example, the infant with an increase in the number of episodes of apnea and bradycardia may have recently had his or her oxygen weaned.

Difficulty with feedings, including apnea and bradycardia, may reflect hypoxemia, immaturity, or gastroesophageal reflux (GER). Infants with CLD may have difficulty feeding for one or more reasons: (*a*) There may be respiratory insufficiency that first becomes apparent during exertion with nipple feeds; (*b*) A full stomach may compromise the infant's ability to breathe effectively; (*c*) The infant may have sustained some neurological damage and have oromotor dysfunction; and (*d*) Premature infants normally begin to coordinate suck, swallow, and breathing between 32 and 36 weeks postmenstrual age. Those with benign NICU courses are more likely to nipple earlier than those with more complicated courses. Clustering of apneic and bradycardic episodes during and after feeds raises the possibility of dysfunctional swallowing or gastroesophageal reflux. If the infant is <36 to 37 weeks, this is most likely the result of immaturity. The likelihood of pathological gastroesophageal reflux increases with postnatal ages >36 to 37 weeks.

Growth is an index of recovery of the infant with CLD. All growth parameters should be followed closely. The long-term pattern of weight gain is the best indicator of true growth. Specifically, normal growth results in a steady gain in weight of 1 to 2% of body weight per day. A large acute weight gain or loss is likely to represent a change in fluid status.

Table 7.2. Important Aspects of History and Physical Examination in CLD

History	Comments
Resting vital signs	
Baseline HR and RR	Assess acute changes
Blood pressure	Hypertension as complication
Apnea and bradycardia	Number, timing, severity
Feeding	Behavior, emesis, tolerance
Growth patterns	Short- vs. long-term changes
General appearance/activity	Assess change from baseline
Examination	
HEENT	
Nasal flaring	Sign of respiratory distress
Cry	Assess quality
Palatal groove	Sign of prolonged intubation
Pulmonary	
Retractions	Change from baseline helpful
Color	Not very sensitive
Auscultation	
Rales, wheezes	Assess acute vs. chronic changes
Air exchange	Note change from baseline
I : E ratio	Prolonged expiration with bronchospasm
Stridor	Indicates vocal cord or airway problem
Cardiovascular	
Precordial activity	Increased with PDA; heave with RVH
Presence of murmur	PPS, PDA, TR possible causes
Second heart sound	Increased P_2 with cor pulmonale
Pulses and perfusion	Correlate with change in examination
Digital clubbing	Indication of chronic hypoxia
Abdomen	
Liver/Spleen	Hyperinflation, right heart failure
Genitourinary	
Inguinal hernia	Occurs in males and females
Neurological	
Tone, posture, reflexes, symmetry	Abnormalities warrant close neurodevelopmental follow-up

EXAMINATION

Vital Signs

Both resting heart and respiratory rates are affected by oxygenation. Tachypnea may be the first and only sign of mild or intermittent hypoxemia. Tachypnea and tachycardia may be symptoms of hypoxemia or pulmonary edema. Infants with chronic lung disease are at risk for hypertension. Resting blood pressures should be followed regularly, and evaluation and treatment should be initiated if the mean blood pressure is consistently greater than 70 mm Hg in infants less than 38 weeks postconceptional age.

General

When noting the general status of the infant, pertinent information includes color, activity, amount of subcutaneous fat, and general sense of comfort. The amount of subcutaneous fat gives an indication of nutritional status and chronicity of the infant's disease. Many infants with complicated NICU courses appear wasted and undernourished.

HEENT

Examination of the head, eyes, ears, nose, and throat discloses additional signs of chronic disease. Nasal flaring may be present with respiratory distress. Palatal grooves and a weak or hoarse cry may be secondary to prolonged intubation. Anxious facies may be seen in infants whose courses have been prolonged.

Pulmonary

The pulmonary examination of the infant with CLD may change from day to day, especially in infants with moderate to severe disease. An appreciation of the infant's baseline examination is important in assessing current clinical status. When examining the chest, the presence and severity of retractions (intercostal, subcostal, suprasternal, or sternal) should be noted. Retractions can be a measure of change in status. Although true pectus excavatum is uncommon, it can be mimicked by sternal retraction in combination with a compliant chest wall.

Attention should be paid to the quality of breath sounds, the amount of air exchange, the inspiratory:expiratory ratio (I:E ratio), and the presence of cough or stridor. Breath sounds are often coarse. Diffuse rales may be heard, representing either pulmonary edema or fibrosis. In moderate to severe disease, there may be poor air exchange, a prolongation of the expiratory phase, and/or wheezing, suggesting bronchospasm. Stridor can result from vocal cord paralysis, subglottic stenosis, edema secondary to prolonged intubation, or laryngomalacia.

Cardiovascular

The cardiovascular examination gives additional information regarding the chronicity and the severity of CLD. The quality and splitting of the second heart sound (S_2), the presence of a murmur, and the quality of pulses and perfusion should be noted. A single, loud, or snappy S_2 or the systolic murmur of tricuspid regurgitation (TR) indicates pulmonary hypertension. A patent ductus arteriosus (PDA) may occasionally become symptomatic in the infant with CLD. The diagnosis is suggested by an increase in peripheral pulses with or without a murmur. Usually, a PDA produces a short systolic murmur, but occasionally, it may produce the classic, continuous "machinery" murmur. An echocardiogram (ECHO) can confirm the diagnosis. Color Doppler may provide an indication of the magnitude of intracardiac shunts. The extremities should be examined for digital clubbing, a sign of chronic hypoxemia.

Abdominal

The liver edge may be depressed secondary to lung hyperinflation or to right-sided congestive heart failure. A thorough cardiopulmonary examination and assessment of liver span may differentiate between these etiologies, but a chest x-ray is occasionally necessary.

Genitals

Inguinal hernias are a common finding in the premature infant of either sex, particularly those with severe CLD (See Chapter 13).

Neurological

Prior to discharge, the infant should be examined for abnormalities of muscle tone, quality of deep tendon and primitive reflexes, asymmetries of tone and/or reflexes, and strength and quality of suck and gag.

Supporting Studies

In assessing the infant with CLD, the infant's history and physical examination are supplemented by supporting information that may include chest x-rays, blood gases, pulse oximetry, echocardiogram (ECHO), electrocardiogram (ECG), pulmonary function testing, and other laboratory studies (Table 7.3).

CHEST X-RAY

The chest x-ray is helpful in assessing and managing CLD, following the progress of the disease, and helping to evaluate acute changes in the infant's status. Findings characteristic of CLD include diffuse opacification, atelectasis, pulmonary interstitial emphysema, and cystic changes. Prominent hyperinflation and increased lung markings suggest a component of reactive airway disease. Increased heart size points to cor pulmonale or to a patent ductus arteriosus.

BLOOD GASES

With the advent of pulse oximetry, frequent blood gases are no longer necessary. There is, however, useful information that can be obtained from a blood gas. PaO_2 is a measure of oxygenation at the moment that the blood is drawn. $PaCO_2$ provides information about ventilation status that cannot be obtained from pulse oximetry.

Table 7.3. Supporting Studies in the Management of Infants with CLD

Pulse oximetry	Useful in assessing oxygenation over the short term or over longer periods and with activity. Good quality of pulse waveform essential for accurate study.
Transcutaneous oxygen and carbon dioxide monitoring	Good for showing trends. Tends to overestimate $PaCO_2$ and underestimate PaO_2. Should be correlated with arterial blood gas.
Blood gases	Both arterial and capillary blood gases provide information about ventilation (pH, PCO_2). ABG is the only way to accurately assess PaO_2, especially at high saturations. The calculated bicarbonate value provides an excellent index of $PaCO_2$. Chronic hypercapnia leads to bicarbonate retention ($>$26 mEq/liter).
Chest x-ray	Intermittent "routine" films can help follow course of disease. Chronic changes frequently present, requiring comparison to previous films.
Electrocardiogram (ECG)	Useful for evaluation of right ventricular hypertrophy (RVH), especially in conjunction with echocardiography.
Echocardiogram (ECHO)	Can assess both dynamic and structural correlates of pulmonary hypertension and RVH.
Electrolytes	Monitoring essential for infants on diuretic therapy. Serum bicarbonate can also provide important information (See Blood gases above).

Measurement of the pH in conjunction with $PaCO_2$ gives an indication of acid-base status and of the chronicity of ventilatory problems. In the case of acute respiratory deterioration, a respiratory acidosis (elevated $PaCO_2$, decreased pH) develops. With gas exchange abnormalities of several days duration, renal retention of bicarbonate becomes apparent. This results in normalization of the blood pH. Elevation of the serum bicarbonate (>26 mEq/liter) indicates hypercapnia even if the $PaCO_2$ has been momentarily depressed by crying. Excessive elevations in bicarbonate sufficient to produce an alkaline blood pH (>7.45) indicates chloride loss from diuretics or loss of gastric juice.

The relative merits of arterial vs. capillary blood gas measurements are often debated. Interpretation of PaO_2 and $PaCO_2$ after a prolonged sampling effort is impossible. On the other hand, there is no alternative method for measurement of arterial PO_2. For example, PaO_2 may be significantly greater than 100 mm Hg when arterial saturation measurements of 98 to 100% are obtained. However, a pulse oximetry reading of arterial saturation (SaO_2), in conjunction with a carefully obtained capillary PCO_2 measurement, generally provides adequate information.

PULSE OXIMETRY

Pulse oximetry has facilitated the assessment and management of the infant with chronic lung disease. It is useful for determining oxygen requirements under various conditions, including sleep, feeding, and wakefulness. Pulse oximetry monitors arterial hemoglobin oxygen saturation (SaO_2) using spectrophotometric principles. It is a continuous, noninvasive technique for monitoring oxygenation and has proven reliable over SaO_2 ranges from 78 to 100%. An SaO_2 of 90 to 95% roughly predicts a PaO_2 of 50 to 100 mm Hg (Fig. 7.2).

ELECTROCARDIOGRAPHY/ECHOCARDIOGRAPHY

Pulmonary vascular abnormalities, either vasoconstriction from hypoxemia or anatomical observations from damage and/or abnormal growth, lead to pulmonary hypertension and cor pulmonale. This makes assessment with electrocardiography (ECG) and echocardiography (ECHO) important in infants with severe CLD. Cor pulmonale can be assessed when the infant is quiet by measuring the size and geometry of the right ventricle, the shape of the left ventricle, the motion of the ventricular septum, and the right ventricular systolic time interval (RSTI). The RSTI is the ratio of the right ventricular preejection period (PEP) to the ventricular ejection time (VET). The normal range is 0.19 to 0.29 with an RSTI of greater than 0.30 suggestive of pulmonary hypertension. However, an RSTI measurement should be interpreted cautiously because it is technically difficult to measure and can change for a variety of reasons, including acute hypoxemia and changes in respiratory pattern. Ventricular hypertrophy on ECG supports the diagnosis of cor pulmonale.

PULMONARY FUNCTION

Recently, techniques have been developed for measurement of pulmonary function in infants. There is also commercially available equipment for making these measurements. While these techniques are based on sound physiological principles, their accuracy and intrasubject reproducibility have yet to be proven, thus limiting their usefulness in clinical decision making.

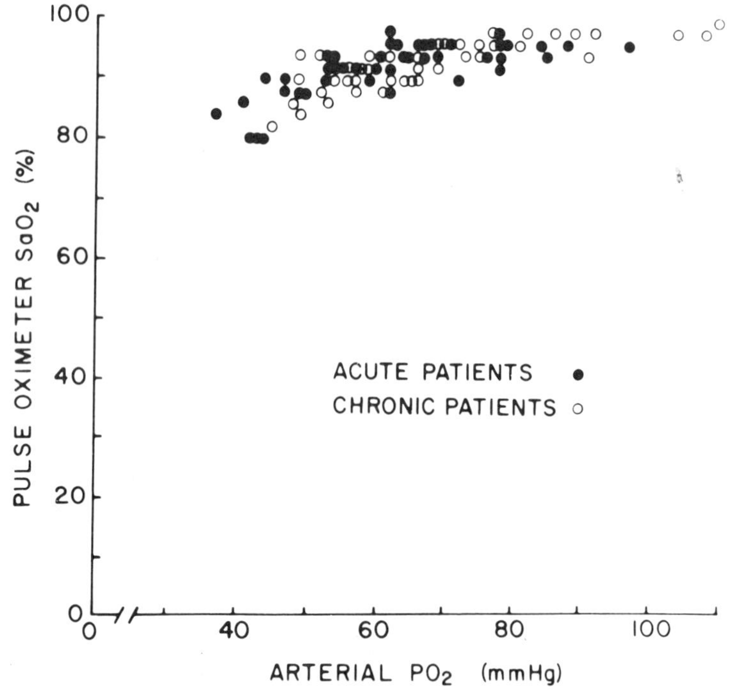

Figure 7.2. Relationship between arterial PO_2 and pulse oximeter arterial oxygen saturation (SaO_2) in patients with acute (●) and chronic (○) lung disease. (Reprinted from Ramanathan R, Durand M, Larrazabal C. Pulse oximetry in very low birth weight infants with acute and chronic lung disease. Pediatrics 1987;79:612–617. Reproduced with permission of Pediatrics.)

DOCUMENTED MONITORING AND POLYSOMNOGRAPHY

Occasionally, infants with severe CLD require more prolonged and detailed study of oxygen saturation, heart rate, respiration rate, and cardiac function. Documented monitoring provides a means of assessing oxygen saturation, respiration rate, and heart rate over a prolonged period of time by recording to a hard disk episodes of desaturation, apnea, and bradycardia. Such monitoring is not able to differentiate central from obstructive apnea because the monitor records chest wall movement in assessing periods of apnea. If more detailed evaluation of these episodes is needed, polysomnography can be utilized. As with documented monitoring, SaO_2 can be evaluated under a variety of activities, including sleep, but in this case, the use of a thermistor to detect air flow from the nares can differentiate central from obstructive apnea. Additionally, a continuous ECG can be monitored. Caution should be used in overreading such studies. Documented monitoring either alone or in conjunction with polysomnography evaluates only the period of time during which the infant is being studied.

LABORATORY STUDIES

Infants with CLD may develop a variety of electrolyte abnormalities. Hypochloremia may occur secondary to diuretic therapy and/or to renal compensation for a primary respiratory acidosis. Hyponatremia and hypokalemia, often the consequence of renal immaturity, may be worsened by diuretic therapy.

Serum calcium and phosphorus levels may be abnormally low in the premature infant with CLD, thus placing the infant at risk for rickets (See Chapter 1). The likelihood of rickets in infants with CLD may be increased because excessive urinary loss of calcium and sometimes phosphorus can occur with the use of diuretics.

The hematocrit and/or reticulocyte count merit periodic measurement. A high hematocrit signifies intermittent hypoxemia.

MANAGEMENT

The management of the infant with CLD is aimed at maintaining optimal pulmonary status and requires frequent adjustment of therapies as the infant's needs change (Table 7.4). This mandates continued reassessment of clinical status and supporting studies. Among the most important therapies in infants with CLD are nutrition, oxygen, diuretics, and bronchodilators.

Nutrition

GROWTH

Improvement in lung function is dependent on both repair of injured lung and growth of new lung tissue. Thus, nutrition should be adequate to support somatic growth. This task is complicated by an increased caloric requirement (as high as 150 kcal/kg/day or

Table 7.4. Complications Seen Prior to Hospital Discharge in Infants with CLD

HEENT
Palatal grooves
Otitis media
Pulmonary
Pulmonary edema
Bronchospasm
Pneumonia
Subglottic stenosis
Vocal cord paralysis
Laryngomalacia
Cardiovascular
Hypertension
Cor pulmonale
Gastrointestinal
GER
Swallowing dysfunction
Gallstones
Genitourinary
Renal calcifications
Inguinal hernias
Neurodevelopment
ROP
Sensory-neural hearing loss
Increased risk for cerebral palsy, cognitive delay
Miscellaneous
Poor growth
Anemia
Rickets

Table 7.5. Evaluation of Poor Growth in the Infant With CLD

Ensure adequate caloric intake
Assess oxygenation during feedings and sleep and over time
Assess caloric expenditures
Consider work-up for swallowing dysfunction or GER if clinically warranted
Consider concurrent medical conditions, especially severe cor pulmonale

more) and/or need for fluid restriction. This need for increased caloric intake may be related to an increased work of breathing and an increased metabolic rate. If high caloric intake or significant fluid restriction are required, concentrated formula may be necessary.

Formula can be concentrated up to 30 kcal/oz if urine output, electrolytes, and renal functions are followed closely. The formula can safely be concentrated to 24 kcal/oz by mixing 5 ounces of concentrated liquid formula with 3 ounces of water. Higher caloric densities are best achieved by adding a combination of polycose (2 kcal/ml) and MCT oil (7.7 kcal/ml), thereby avoiding protein intake in excess of current recommendations. This is best done with the aid of a nutritionist (See Chapter 1).

If an infant will not grow and caloric intake is felt to be adequate, oxygenation should be reassessed with pulse oximetry and, if necessary, adjunctive studies such as polysomnography, an EKG and ECHO, or a hematocrit and reticulocyte count. If indicated, further work-up might include an evaluation of swallowing function, an esophagram, and a pH probe to rule out swallowing dysfunction or GER (Table 7.5).

If the nutritional management of the infant is further complicated by fatigue with feeding (due either to immaturity or exercise intolerance), swallowing dysfunction, or severe gastroesophageal reflux, frequent small, concentrated, feeds may be required. Supplemental tube feedings, either nasogastric (NG) or via gastrostomy (GT) and either intermittent or continuous, can be extremely useful (see Chapter 1). NG tube feedings are particularly helpful in the nursery if instituted for conditions that are anticipated to be of relatively short duration. They must be approached with caution for use in the home because of the risks associated with misplaced NG tubes or tubes that become dislodged during the course of feeding. For severe feeding difficulties that appear to be long-term, gastrostomy tubes can provide a safe and practical route for feeding in the hospital or at home. A thorough evaluation for gastroesophageal reflux should be undertaken prior to GT placement to avoid the need for a Nisson fundal plication at a later date (see Chapter 13).

It seems that infants with severe CLD and cor pulmonale do not grow regardless of how much nutrition they receive. The inability to grow does not appear to reflect poor nutrition. In such infants, continued increases in caloric intake may result in hyperlipemia and azotemia.

RICKETS

The recovering premature infant may be deficient in both calcium and phosphorus. As a result, rickets of prematurity may be present. (See Chapter 1).

GASTROESOPHAGEAL REFLUX

Most premature infants, if evaluated thoroughly, would show signs of GER. Occasionally, an infant will require intervention. Symptoms can include poor feeding; vomiting or coughing, especially at the end of or after completing a feed; bradycardia during or after feeding; and irritability with feeds. Intermittent, mild aspiration events may result in increased oxygen requirement, wheezing, and increased respiratory effort. Evaluation involves careful documentation of quality and timing of emesis, a cine-esophagram, and a pH probe. These studies can also help rule out swallowing dysfunction, a related complication of prematurity. In either case, a chest x-ray may show signs of aspiration. Certain common medical therapies, including the use of theophylline-containing medications and nasogastric tubes, can worsen reflux.

Initial treatment includes maintaining the infant in a prone position with the head of the bed raised after feeds, thickening feeds with rice cereal in the ratio of 1 tablespoon to 4 ounces of formula, and providing small, frequent feeds. The use of medications such as metoclopramide in the premature infant is controversial. If medical management is not effective, a Nisson fundal plication, with or without a gastrostomy tube, may become necessary (see Chapter 13). In all but the most severe cases, GER is a self-limiting condition.

ANEMIA

In an effort to avoid symptomatic anemia and possibly the need for transfusions, premature infants should be started on prophylactic elemental iron at 2 to 3 mg/kg/day once they are tolerating full feeds. If an infant is taking full calorie feeds of regular infant formula with iron, additional iron supplements are usually unnecessary.

Oxygen

The goal of oxygen therapy in the infant with CLD is to promote optimum growth and development while avoiding toxic side effects. The risks of oxygen therapy vary depending on the gestational age of the infant, necessitating a transition in thinking about the infant's management as he or she matures. Until the retina is completely vascularized, which usually occurs near term, the infant remains at risk for the development of retinopathy of prematurity (ROP) (See Chapter 8). But in the infant with CLD, management is further complicated by the risk of developing cor pulmonale, a condition that is exacerbated by hypoxia. The infant's oxygen needs must therefore be balanced with the complications of its use.

During the third trimester and continuing after birth, there is an increase in the number and maturity of alveoli. New lung tissue continues to form until the child is approximately 8 years old, providing a tremendous opportunity for recovery from CLD. In fact, supplemental oxygen therapy may be necessary for only a few weeks to months after hospital discharge.

OXYGEN DELIVERY

Low-flow supplemental oxygen can be delivered to the recovering NICU patient via infant nasal cannula or oxygen hood. There are problems that can occur with each of these delivery systems: (*a*) Although the cannula allows the infant to be handled more easily, it is often difficult to maintain close control of the oxygen flow rate even with the use of special flow meters calibrated to provide low flow; (*b*) The cannula delivers oxygen only through the nares. If there is obstruction of either the nares or the tubing, oxygen delivery will be compromised. Similarly, variable amounts of oxygen will be inspired during crying or mouth breathing; (*c*) The cannula may become dislodged; and (*d*) The cannula is generally not satisfactory for use with infants whose oxygen requirement is greater than 30%.

Difficulties also arise with the oxygen hood: (*a*) Maintaining proper placement of the hood over the infant's head becomes difficult in the active infant; (*b*) The hood restricts movement, visual contact, and access by the NICU staff and family members; and (*c*) As with any oxygen delivery system, the tubing may become dislodged or obstructed. However, for those rare infants whose lung disease is so severe that oxygen requirements are greater than 30% and/or the amount of oxygen delivered must be tightly controlled, the hood can deliver a more consistent amount of oxygen than can the cannula.

Assessment of the infant's oxygen requirements is an ongoing process. It requires periodic reassessment of the history, physical examination, pulse oximetry, chest radiograph, ECHO and ECG, blood gases, and laboratory studies.

PULSE OXIMETRY

The optimal oxygen saturation for a given infant is a function of that infant's condition and postconceptional age. For infants with incompletely vascularized retinas, recommended saturations are in the 88 to 94% range; for infants with vascularized retinas, saturation should be maintained >94%. Once retinas are mature, oxygen saturations of ≥94% (pO_2 >70 mm Hg) are probably optimal to promote growth and prevent cor pulmonale.

When the infant is stable and growing, with oxygen saturations above the appropriate range, an attempt to wean supplemental oxygen should be made. Oxygen saturations for a particular infant will vary depending on the infant's activity. Therefore, saturations should be measured during sleep and feeding and while at rest. Heart and respiration rates should remain stable as oxygen is weaned.

If intermittently measured oxygen saturations do not seem to correlate with the clinical status, a prolonged study may be necessary to rule out intermittent hypoxemia. This study should include either careful observation during pulse oximetry or the use of documented monitoring to record the events surrounding episodes of desaturation, apnea, or bradycardia.

Routine studies for infants on supplemental oxygen are recommended every 7 to 10 days, with initiation of nipple feedings, and prior to discharge. Changes in the amount of oxygen delivered should be gradual. If the retinal vasculature is incomplete and pulse oximetry shows that SaO_2 is >94% on 100% oxygen by nasal cannula at a minimum flow rate (0.1 to 0.125 liter/min), the inspired oxygen concentration can be decreased. This method is not practical for home use because oxygen blenders are rarely available outside the hospital. Therefore, such infants could either be discharged without supplemental oxygen, if ready, or remain hospitalized until retinal vascularization is complete. At that time, if they still require some oxygen, they can be safely discharged at a flow rate of 0.1 liter/min with 100% FiO_2.

Any infant whose supplemental oxygen has been recently reduced or discontinued should be followed closely for signs or symptoms of hypoxemia (Table 7.6). These symptoms include slowed growth rate, change in sleep or feeding patterns, apnea and bradycardia,

Table 7.6. Signs and Symptoms of Hypoxemia

Slowed weight gain
Poor feeding
Awakening from sleep
Irritability
Increase in frequency of apnea and bradycardia
Increase in baseline heart and respiration rates
Change in baseline activity level
Presence of pallor, mottling, or cyanosis
Deterioration of pulmonary or cardiac examination

tachycardia, irritability, lethargy, color changes, or change in the quality of breath sounds or of the second heart sound. The final determination of supplemental oxygen requirement must be based on both clinical status and studies of oxygenation.

Although pulse oximetry is helpful in monitoring oxygenation, there are difficulties with its use. For example, the saturation reported by the oximeter is dependent on the quality of the arterial pulsations received by the probe. The oximeter underestimates SaO_2 when the pulse waveform is poor. In addition, many oximeters will continue to display the previous reading when the probe loses good arterial pulsations. Therefore, the SaO_2 can only be accurately assessed when the probe receives an adequate pulsation. Also, unless a pulse oximeter that has the capability of recording saturations and correlating these with heart rate is used, a prolonged pulse oximetry study is labor intensive, therefore limiting its usefulness.

CHEST RADIOGRAPH

Unless there is an acute change in clinical status, frequent chest films are usually not necessary. Monthly films to follow progress should be adequate in the stable infant with CLD. A final film should be obtained near hospital discharge for comparative purposes in the event that the infant develops respiratory illness after discharge.

ELECTROCARDIOGRAPHY/ECHOCARDIOGRAPHY

Infants with moderate to severe CLD are at risk for cor pulmonale. Indications for obtaining an ECHO and ECG include a snappy second heart sound, tricuspid regurgitation, and/or difficulty weaning supplemental oxygen. In the infant with moderate to severe CLD, a baseline study prior to discharge may be useful. If cor pulmonale does develop, management includes the reassessment of oxygenation with prolonged oximetry and increasing supplemental oxygen accordingly, so that periods of hypoxia are avoided.

BLOOD GASES

Because blood gases are primarily used to monitor progress of the disease, measurements every 1 to 2 weeks should be adequate if the clinical status is stable. More frequent measurements may be indicated by clinical status, following changes in therapy, or if the information obtained will influence clinical decisions.

LABORATORY STUDIES

As part of the general assessment, the evaluation of the infant with CLD includes a hematocrit and a reticulocyte count. The routine timing of these laboratory studies is variable, but once every 1 to 2 weeks is probably adequate in the stable infant. More frequent routine sampling adds to iatrogenic blood loss, thus increasing the chances of the need for blood transfusions.

Fluid Management

Pulmonary edema is a frequent complication of CLD. The goals of fluid management in the infant with CLD are to provide sufficient calories to attain good growth without contributing to pulmonary edema while avoiding problems related to fluid restriction and diuretic use.

Typical findings of pulmonary edema on physical examination vary depending on its chronicity and severity. These range from mild to moderate intercostal retractions with diffuse fine rales to increased tachypnea and tachycardia, pallor or cyanosis, nasal flaring, retractions, poor air exchange, coarse breath sounds, wet rales, wheezing, and/or grunting. These findings can occur either acutely or gradually. Chest radiographs often appear to have fluffy infiltrates; there may also be a decrease in PaO_2 or SaO_2 with an increase in $PaCO_2$.

If pulmonary edema is mild, fluid restriction to 120 to 150 ml/kg/day is often adequate to prevent deterioration. Adequate caloric intake can be maintained by the use of 24 kcal/oz formula. If this magnitude of fluid restriction is insufficient, the addition of diuretic therapy is warranted. More severe pulmonary edema may require further fluid restriction, more concentrated formula, and treatment with chronic diuretics. If treatment with fluid restriction or diuretics becomes necessary, urine output, electrolytes, and renal function should be followed closely.

The development of congestive heart failure secondary to cor pulmonale is a rare but definite indication for chronic diuretic therapy in conjunction with both reassessment of oxygen needs and fluid restriction. A single parenteral dose of diuretic, specifically furosemide, is usually beneficial in the infant with acute worsening of cor pulmonale or pulmonary edema.

Diuretic Therapy

There are three major diuretics used in the treatment of CLD; chlorothiazide (Diuril), spironolactone (Aldactone), and furosemide (Lasix) (Table 7.7). Theophylline is a weak diuretic, but it is rarely used for this purpose.

CHLOROTHIAZIDE

Chlorothiazide acts by increasing the renal excretion of sodium and chloride and an accompanying volume of water. Additionally, chlorothiazide augments the excretion of potassium. It has been shown to decrease airway resistance and increase dynamic compliance. Although less potent than furosemide, it is not associated with side effects such as ototoxicity or nephrocalcinosis and may cause far less electrolyte disturbance than does furosemide. When given in conjunction with spironolactone, electrolyte abnormalities are decreased to the extent that electrolyte supplements may not be necessary.

Chlorothiazide has an onset of action of 2 hours with a peak effect at 3 to 6 hours after dosing. The recommended dose is 5 to 20 mg/kg/day given in divided doses every 12 hours. Occasionally, doses as high as 40 mg/kg/day have been used but usually result in electrolyte imbalances requiring supplements. It is available for oral use as a 50 mg/ml suspension.

SPIRONOLACTONE

The diuretic effect of spironolactone is achieved by competitive antagonism of aldosterone. It causes an increase in the excretion of sodium and water while retaining potassium. As a result, hyponatremia and hyperkalemia may occur. Because it is a weak diuretic, spironolactone's main benefit is its potassium-sparing effect. When used in combination with other diuretics such as chlorothiazide, dosages can be manipulated to reduce the need for electrolyte supplements.

Table 7.7. Respiratory Medications in the Management of Infants With CLD

Diuretics		
Chlorothiazide (Diuril)	5 to 40 mg/kg/day divided q 12 h, PO	Ideal as chronic diuretic, usual dose 10 to 20 mg/kg/day
Spironolactone (Aldactone)	1.0 to 3.3 mg/kg/day divided q 12 h, PO	Weak diuretic, used for potassium-sparing effects
Furosemide (Lasix)	1.0 to 4.0 mg/kg/dose q 6 to 24 hr, PO 1.0 mg/kg/dose, q 12 to 24 hr, IV or IM	Potent diuretic useful for rapid diuresis, more frequent electrolyte disturbances and other side effects
Oral bronchodilators		
Theophylline	0 to 2 months: 3 to 6 mg/kg/day divided q 8 hrs 2 to 6 months: 6 to 15 mg/kg/day divided q 6 hrs	Dose must be individualized, peak serum levels 10 to 20 μg/ml optimal for bronchodilation
Albuterol (Ventolin, Proventil)	0.1 mg/kg/dose q 8 hr	Little experience with this drug in premature infants, side effects may include tachycardia, jitteriness, irritability
Metaproterenol (Alupent)	1.3 to 2.6 mg/kg/day divided q 8 hr	As above
Inhaled bronchodilators		
Albuterol (Ventolin, Proventil)	0.04 to 0.15 mg/kg in 2 ml normal saline (NS), q 2 to 8 hr	Side effects include increase in heart rate and jitteriness, lessened by decreasing dose
Metaproterenol (Alupent, Metaprel)	0.25 to 0.5 mg/kg in 2 ml NS, q 2 to 8 hr	As above
Terbutaline (Breathaire)	0.1 to 0.3 mg/kg in 2 ml NS, q 2 to 8 hr	As above
Isoetharine (Bronkosol)	0.1 to 0.2 mg/kg in 2 ml NS, q 2 to 8 hr	As above

Spironolactone achieves its maximum effect 1 to 2 hours after a single oral dose. The recommended dose is 1.0 to 3.3. mg/kg/day given in divided doses every 12 hours. Dosing to avoid electrolyte supplements is usually in a 1:10 ratio of spironolactone to chlorothiazide. Spironolactone suspension must be made by a pharmacist, and the concentration must be specified.

Furosemide

Furosemide is the most potent of the commonly used diuretics; however, it is also associated with the greatest number of side effects. It acts by inhibiting the reabsorption of sodium and chloride in the proximal and distal tubules as well as in the loop of Henle. It also leads to the urinary excretion of potassium, calcium, and even phosphorus. This drug, therefore, places the infant at high risk for the development of electrolyte abnormalities as well as for nephrocalcinosis and osteopenia. The use of chlorothiazide in conjunction with (or instead of) furosemide causes less calcium excretion than does furosemide alone, and it may contribute to the radiological dissolution of renal stones. Other adverse reactions of furosemide use include hyperglycemia, reversible elevations of BUN, and hearing loss, especially when it is given in conjunction with aminoglycoside antibiotics or in the presence of renal impairment.

Furosemide is especially useful when a potent diuretic is needed acutely. Its primary use in the infant with CLD is in the acute treatment of pulmonary edema, either alone or as a supplement to chronic diuretic therapy.

The onset of action, peak effect, duration of diuretic effect, and dose depend on the route of administration of the drug. Orally, absorption in neonates is erratic, with an onset of action 10 to 60 minutes after the dose and a peak diuretic effect 1 to 2 hours after administration. The diuretic effect lasts 6 to 8 hours. The dose for oral administration is 1 to 4 mg/kg/dose, one to four times per day. Furosemide is available as a 10 mg/ml suspension for oral use.

Intravenously administered furosemide begins to have an effect within minutes. Rapid diuretic effect is also obtained after intramuscular injection. Its peak effect is within 30 minutes, and the duration of its diuretic effect is approximately 2 hours. The dose for both IV and IM administration is 1 mg/kg/dose given every 12 hours. The injectable form contains 10 mg/ml of furosemide.

Fluid restriction remains the first-line treatment for chronic difficulties with pulmonary edema. Chlorothiazide and spironolactone, given together, can be added if fluid restriction alone is unsuccessful. Furosemide can usually be reserved for acute episodes of pulmonary edema. The need for additional doses of diuretics indicates the need for adjustments in the infant's chronic fluid and diuretic regimen. Electrolytes, renal function, and urine output need to be monitored closely until a satisfactory regimen is attained. If electrolyte supplements become necessary, they may often be discontinued prior to discharge because urinary losses will decrease with renal maturation. The infant who is discharged home with electrolyte supplements should be the rare exception.

Bronchodilator Therapy

For many years, it had been thought that infants lacked sufficient musculature in their small airways to develop clinically significant bronchospasm. However, both clinical experience and measurements of pulmonary function in infants have now demonstrated this to be incorrect. CLD, like other forms of severe lung injury, can predispose to bronchospasm.

Bronchodilator therapy is now recognized as having a role in the management of premature infants who develop CLD (Table 7.7). Even the very immature infant, as young as 26 weeks postconceptional age or 10 days chronological age, may have an improvement in lung function following administration of aerosolized bronchodilators. Studies have also demonstrated improvements in pulmonary function measurements (lung resistance and compliance) and gas exchange following treatment with oral or aerosolized bronchodilators.

The indications for beginning therapy with bronchodilators are not as readily apparent in the tiny infant with CLD as in the older child. Bronchospasm in chronic lung disease is often unaccompanied by wheezing. It may be manifested much more subtly, with increased retractions, a prolonged expiratory phase, CO_2 retention, or increasing O_2 requirement. The strategy for therapy must be adapted to the needs of the immature patient with particular attention to side effects.

THEOPHYLLINE

Theophylline has long been a mainstay of treatment in the child with asthma. It has also been used widely for treatment in infants with CLD and suspected bronchospasm.

When used in doses sufficient to maintain a theophylline level of >10 μg/ml, it has been shown to improve lung function in infants with CLD. However, the use of theophylline in doses sufficient to maintain these levels is sometimes associated with unacceptable side effects, including irritability, feeding intolerance, and gastroesophageal reflux.

β-2 AGONISTS

An alternative is the use of either an oral or an inhaled β-2 agonist. These agents have been shown to improve lung resistance, compliance, and gas exchange in infants with CLD. Although experience is limited with oral preparations of β-2 agonists in this population, metaproterenol or albuterol can be administered in weight-appropriate doses and seem to be well tolerated. The dose of an inhaled β-2 agonist such as metaproterenol, albuterol, or isoetharine should also be adjusted for the weight of the infant. There is often a transient increase in heart rate and/or jitteriness following the administration of one of these medications as an aerosol. Dosing must be individualized; some infants will achieve therapeutic benefit with fewer side effects at lower doses.

OTHER THERAPIES

Other therapies commonly used for treatment of asthma in the pediatric patient, such as cromolyn sodium or steroids, have not been well-studied in young infants with chronic lung disease. Based on their mechanisms of action, as they are currently understood, there is reason to expect that they may be of benefit in this group of patients as well.

It is important to carefully assess benefits and side effects in any infant begun on medication for presumed bronchospasm. In the infant without overt wheezing, therapy may result in a decrease in respiratory rate or retractions, an improvement in CO_2 retention, or a lessening of the O_2 requirement. Infant pulmonary function testing has been used to assess the benefits in controlled studies of groups of patients treated with bronchodilators. However, these techniques are still under development, and day-to-day reproducibility within a given subject is not well-established. Results obtained before and after the institution of therapy in an individual should be interpreted with great caution and in view of the overall clinical setting. After a reasonable trial period, perhaps a week, these medications should be discontinued if no clear benefit has been seen.

Steroids

In order to decrease ventilator requirements, dexamethasone is sometimes used in selected preterm infants who continue to require high ventilator and FiO_2 settings after at least 2 weeks of age. The goal of this therapy is to improve pulmonary outcome in those infants at high risk for chronic lung disease secondary to hyaline membrane disease. As recommended by Cummings et al., dexamethasone is given at a starting dose of 0.5 mg/kg/day and is slowly tapered over 42 days. Because the course is prolonged, it is not unusual for the stable infant to continue to receive dexamethasone up to the time of discharge. These infants, therefore, require close observation during and after completion of therapy because of the potential complications of corticosteroid use. Adrenal, immune, and thyroid effects of this therapy in this population are not yet known.

DISCHARGE

Preparation

Discharge planning goals for an infant with CLD are to ensure that the infant will be discharged safely, continue to make progress outside the hospital, and have good, consistent follow-up. These goals raise two important questions: (*a*) How does one decide when an infant is ready for discharge; and (*b*) Is it appropriate for all babies with CLD to be discharged home? Answering these questions requires input from the NICU staff, the family, the primary care provider, support services such as home nursing, and any specialists involved in the infant's care. If the natural history and management of CLD are discussed with the family early in the hospitalization, then discharge planning may be facilitated.

REQUIREMENTS FOR DISCHARGE

There are several basic requirements from the infant and parents whenever the discharge of an infant on supplemental oxygen is contemplated (Table 7.8). The infant must remain on a stable oxygen regimen and generally require an oxygen flow rate of no greater than 0.5 liter/min at rest. This rate gives the infant somewhat of a buffer in the event that an acute illness would require a temporary increase in oxygen. Also, at higher flow rates, infants are at risk for the development of significant hypoxemia should oxygen flow be interrupted. Infants who have CLD severe enough to require more than 0.5 liter/min of oxygen usually require too much physician, respiratory therapy, and nursing intervention to be safely managed at home.

In addition to a stable oxygen requirement, the infant must demonstrate appropriate growth on nipple feeds or, if necessary, nasogastric or gastrostomy tube feeds. Fluid and medication requirements must be well established.

Parents must demonstrate competency in caring for their infant prior to discharge. They should receive training in cardiopulmonary resuscitation (CPR), oxygen and monitor use, medication administration, signs and symptoms of illness, who and when to call for help, and other related information. Involvement of more than one family member and rooming in with the infant and equipment is strongly encouraged. This process often takes a week or more.

The home environment must safely allow for the presence of oxygen. Access to a nearby telephone is essential, although a telephone in the home is not always necessary.

Occasionally, the determination is made that the infant's anticipated medical needs exceed the family's ability to meet them in the home. In addition to medical issues, important social factors may include access to medical care, age and maturity of the parents, support systems, home nursing support, number and ages of other children in the home, and quality of the living space. Temporary placement in a chronic care facility may be an alternative until the infant's condition improves to the point that home care can be further simplified.

Table 7.8. Discharge Criteria for Infants With CLD

Discharge criteria
Oxygen: requirement stable at $\leq$0.5 liter/min
Feedings: schedule and volume well-tolerated
Growth: appropriate on established feeding regimen
Medications: doses well-established, electrolytes stable
Family: informed, competent, ready

Table 7.9. Preparation for Discharge

Discharge Evaluation (as appropriate)
- Laboratory data
  - Hematocrit/reticulocyte count
  - Electrolytes
  - Drug levels
- Assessment of oxygenation
- Chest radiograph
- ECG and echocardiogram

Home Care Planning
- Select equipment company for oxygen and/or monitor
- Select oxygen delivery system
- Adjust medication and feeding regimens for home administration
- Arrange for special formula if necessary
- Arrange home nursing visits as appropriate
- Arrange follow-up:
  - primary care
  - subspecialty
- Inform primary care provider of NICU course and special needs
- Parent training:
  - Oxygen and monitor use
  - Medication administration
  - Signs and symptoms of illness
  - Emergency plans
  - Rooming in

Finalizing Discharge Plans

PREDISCHARGE EVALUATION OF THE INFANT

An overall reassessment of the infant's clinical condition is necessary shortly before discharge (Table 7.9). In addition to a thorough examination and review of growth, laboratory and special studies should be repeated. Laboratory studies should include a recent hematocrit and reticulocyte count. Electrolytes and drug levels should be obtained in those on diuretics and theophylline, respectively. Oxygen needs should be finalized. A chest x-ray should be obtained to monitor progress and to serve as a baseline for future comparisons. For infants with severe chronic lung disease or previously abnormal studies, an ECG and an echocardiogram should be repeated.

OXYGEN

During the week prior to discharge, arrangements should be made for oxygen delivery to the home. The oxygen system should include both a stationary and a portable unit equipped with a low-flow meter. These systems may be either compressed gas or liquid. In the former, the stationary unit is an "H-cylinder"; the portable unit is a small canister that is not refillable but provides up to 60 hours of use at flow rates of ≤0.5 liter/min. With the alternative liquid system, the stationary tank is less cumbersome and can be used to refill the portable unit. However, the portable tank provides only about 8 hours of service at ≤0.5 liter/min before refilling. Disposable equipment, including infant nasal cannulas and oxygen tubing, will also be needed. In addition to providing equipment, the chosen company should have provisions for 24-hour availability of a respiratory therapist.

MONITOR

Although data are limited, most infants who are discharged on supplemental oxygen should be placed on a cardiorespiratory monitor. This recommendation is made because the risk of sudden, unexpected death is greater in infants with bronchopulmonary dysplasia (BPD) than in the general population and hypoxemia may increase this risk.

FLUIDS AND MEDICATIONS

The medical regimen should be simplified for homegoing. If possible, fluids should be liberalized to provide greater satisfaction for the infant and to increase the likelihood of compliance with the prescribed regimen. The medication regimen should also be simplified as much as possible. The total number of medications, doses, and timing of doses must be limited to those that are essential and can be reasonably administered by the family.

FOLLOW-UP

Primary care follow-up for the infant should be arranged. The provider should be contacted prior to discharge to discuss the final medical plan and provisions for after-hours care. Multidisciplinary follow-up is often required for infants with symptomatic chronic lung disease. Follow-up may involve either a pulmonologist or neonatologist. In addition, infants with chronic lung disease are at increased risk for developmental disability and should receive developmental follow-up.

A summary of the infant's hospitalization and discharge chest x-ray should be sent to the primary care provider and appropriate subspecialists. If possible, contact between subspecialists and family should be made prior to hospital discharge.

It is imperative that there be 24-hour access to a medical provider familiar with the infant. In addition, there must be a single provider who is charged with coordinating the various aspects of the infant's outpatient management. This role may be filled by either the primary care provider, a pulmonologist, or neonatologist. Regardless, the family should clearly know whom to contact with questions or problems.

Visiting home nurses can aid in evaluating the home prior to discharge and in providing the family with additional support, advice, and reassurance once the infant is home. They can also relay useful information regarding the infant's condition at home to health care providers.

OUTCOME

Both the pulmonary and neurodevelopmental outcomes of infants with CLD are of great concern. In general, their prognosis is excellent. However, some infants do have ongoing complications related to both their prematurity and their CLD.

Pulmonary Outcome

The rapid advances in neonatal care, particularly surfactant therapy, and the increasing survival of the very tiny premature infant limit long-term follow-up information available regarding pulmonary outcome. Despite the improvements in neonatal care and the increasing use of exogenous surfactant, many very premature infants continue to be discharged with a diagnosis of chronic lung disease and, frequently, to require supplemental oxygen.

Although the spectrum of chronic lung disease at the time of discharge is variable, in general, the short-term outlook for these infants is good. Many are able to be weaned off oxygen within 4 to 6 months after discharge. They often demonstrate catch-up growth as their pulmonary status improves. Respiratory illnesses requiring readmission to the hospital remain common, occurring in approximately 30 to 50% of infants discharged on oxygen.

There is no information available regarding the long-term pulmonary outcome of the extremely premature infants with CLD now being discharged from neonatal intensive care units. There are, however, studies of older, larger infants with classic bronchopulmonary dysplasia (BPD). When evaluated at 10 years of age, children who had developed BPD in the neonatal period demonstrated a predisposition to airway hyperreactivity and pulmonary function abnormalities consistent with obstructive lung disease (such as asthma) but no impairment in exercise tolerance. These reports suggest that there is a great potential for recovery of lung function in NICU survivors.

When counseling the parents of an infant with mild to moderate CLD, including those being discharged on oxygen, it is important to stress that, while all infants are different, the prognosis for a good pulmonary outcome is likely and that the duration of oxygen therapy is usually relatively brief. However, these children are more likely to develop significant symptoms, perhaps requiring hospitalization, with viral illnesses. Preterm infants who were intubated are at increased risk for developing croup. The duration of intubation increases this risk. They are also predisposed to developing asthma in childhood. Careful follow-up and compliance with prescribed therapies are essential.

Neurodevelopmental Outcome

The premature infant with respiratory distress syndrome does not appear to be at increased risk for developmental disability. However, the preterm infant who goes on to develop CLD is at an increased risk of neuromotor dysfunction and of cognitive delay. These risks seem to be affected by the severity of CLD and of intracranial hemorrhage (See Chapter 10).

SUGGESTED READINGS

American Academy of Pediatrics. Nutritional needs of low-birthweight infants. Pediatrics 1985;75:976–986.

Bader D, Ramos AD, Lew CD, Platzker ACG, Stabile MW, Keens TG. Childhood sequelae of infant lung disease: exercise and pulmonary function abnormalities after bronchopulmonary dysplasia. J Pediatr 1987;110:693–699.

Ballard RA. Pediatric care of the ICN graduate. Philadelphia: Saunders, 1988.

Bancalari E, Abdenour GE, Feller R, Gannon J. Bronchopulmonary dysplasia. J Pediatr 1979;95:819–823.

Bancalari E, Gerhardt T. Bronchopulmonary dysplasia. Pediatr Clin North Am 1986;33:1–23.

Blanchard PW, Brown TM, Coates AL. Pharmacotherapy in bronchopulmonary dysplasia. Clin Perinatol 1987;14(4):881–910.

Brown ER. Bronchopulmonary dysplasia. In: Taeusch HW Jr, Yogman MW, eds. Follow-up management of the high-risk infant. 1st ed. Boston: Little, Brown, 1987:213–220.

Cummings JJ, D'Eugenio DB, Gross SJ. A controlled trial of dexamethasone in preterm infants at high risk for bronchopulmonary dysplasia. N Engl J Med 1989;320:1505–1510.

Englehardt B, Elliott S, Hazinski TA. Short- and long-term effects of furosemide on lung function in infants with bronchopulmonary dysplasia. J Pediatr 1986;109:1034–1039.

Escobedo MB, Gonzales A. Bronchopulmonary dysplasia in the tiny infant. Clin Perinatol 1986;13:315–326.

Fiascone JM, Rhodes TT, Grandgeorge SR, Knapp MA. Bronchopulmonary dysplasia: a review for the pediatrician. Curr Probl Pediatr 1989;19:169–227.

Goetzman BW. Understanding bronchopulmonary dysplasia. Am J Dis Child 1986;140:332–334.

Greer FR, Tsang RC. Calcium, phosphorus, magnesium, and vitamin D requirements for the preterm infant. In: Tsang RC, ed. Vitamin and mineral requirements in preterm infants. New York: Marcel Dekker, 1985.

Hudak BB, Allen MC, Hudak ML, Loughlin GM. Home oxygen therapy for chronic lung disease in extremely low birth weight infants. Am J Dis Child 1989;143:357–360.

Kao LC, Durand DJ, Nickerson BJ. Effects of inhaled metaproterenol and atropine on the pulmonary mechanics of infants with bronchopulmonary dysplasia. Pediatr Pulmonol 1989;6:74–80.

Kao LC, Warburton D, Cheng MH, Cedeno C, Platzker ACG, Keens TG. Effect of oral diuretics on pulmonary mechanics in infants with chronic lung disease: results of a double-blind crossover sequential trial. Pediatrics 1984;74:37–44.

Merritt TA, Northway WH Jr, Boynton BR. Contemporary issues in fetal and neonatal medicine. Vol. 4. Bronchopulmonary dysplasia. Boston: Blackwell Scientific Publishers, 1989.

Northway Jr WH, Rosan RC, Porter DY. Pulmonary disease following respirator therapy of hyaline membrane disease—bronchopulmonary dysplasia. N Engl J Med 1967;276:357–368.

O'Brodovich HM, Mellins RB. Bronchopulmonary dysplasia: unresolved neonatal acute lung injury. Am Rev Respir Dis 1985;132:694–709.

Rimsza ME. Complications of corticosteroid therapy. Am J Dis Child 1978;132:806–810.

Ramanathan R, Durand M, Larrazabal C. Pulse oximetry in very low birth weight infants with acute and chronic lung disease. Pediatrics 1987;79:612–617.

Shennan AT, Dunn MS, Ohisson A, Lennox K, Hoskins EM. Abnormal pulmonary outcomes in premature infants: prediction from oxygen requirement in the neonatal period. Pediatrics 1988;82:527–532.

Smyth JA, Tabachnik E, Duncan WJ, Reilly BJ, Levison H. Pulmonary function and bronchial hyperreactivity in long-term survivors of bronchopulmonary dysplasia. Pediatrics 1981;68:336–340.

Werthammer J, Brown ER, Neff RK, Taeusch Jr HW. Sudden infant death syndrome in infants with bronchopulmonary dysplasia. Pediatrics 1982;69:301–304.

Workshop on bronchopulmonary dysplasia. J Pediatr 1979;95(5 pt 2):815–920.

8

Retinopathy of Prematurity

Janet E. Graeber

Retinopathy of prematurity (ROP) is a condition of the underdeveloped eye in which the normal progression of newly forming retinal vessels is interrupted. Vasoconstriction and obliteration of the advancing capillary bed is followed in progressive stages by neovascularization extending out into the vitreous, edema, hemorrhage, fibrosis, traction, and eventual detachment of the retina. In the majority of cases, the process reverses before fibrosis occurs. However, advanced stages may lead to blindness. It is estimated that 450 to 500 children each year may be blinded by ROP. Although some feel this estimate is high, it is widely accepted that a far greater number will suffer significant visual impairment as a result of this potentially devastating and elusive disorder.

When originally described, the condition was seen only in its most advanced form, after extensive fibrosis and scarring had already occurred. In was therefore termed retrolental fibroplasia. There is now an appreciation that a spectrum of changes occurs in the newly developing vasculature before the onset of end-stage fibrosis. The condition is considered a true retinopathy, and because it is found primarily in prematures, it is now called the retinopathy of prematurity, a term first used by Heath in 1950 but advocated in the 1980s. The term cicatricial ROP is similar to the original meaning of the older term, retrolental fibroplasia.

PATHOPHYSIOLOGY

Retrolental fibroplasia, or RLF as it was originally called, was first described by Terry in the 1940s and was positively associated with the use of oxygen in newborn infants by Patz and associates. This association was subsequently confirmed in a large, collaborative trial known as the Kinsey study. The first epidemic, extending from the early 1940s into the 1950s and estimated to be responsible for 30% of the blindness in preschool children by the end of the 1940s, occurred during a period of liberal oxygen administration. Following this recognized association, oxygen use in nurseries was curtailed. Although the incidence of RLF fell, infant mortality rates and morbidity increased. In the 1960s, improved oxygen monitoring techniques paved the way for the cautious reintroduction of oxygen into the nursery.

Despite improved oxygen monitoring, a second epidemic of retrolental fibroplasia, now termed retinopathy of prematurity, became evident in the late 1970s and has continued to the present. The association of ROP with oxygen alone is now not so clear. There have been multiple recorded instances of ROP occurring in infants who have not been exposed to elevated oxygen concentrations. Many other factors such as extreme prematurity, maternal complications, apnea, sepsis, hyper- and hypocarbia, vitamin E deficiency, intraventricular hemorrhage (IVH), anemia, exchange transfusion, hypoxia, lactic acidosis, and light have been implicated. Of particular concern are the increasing numbers of survivors less than 1000 grams who have the highest incidence of ROP and may account for much of the current epidemic.

The precise pathophysiology of ROP is still in question. Based on clinical and morphological findings, Ashton proposed the following sequence of events. In the normally developing retina, there are no retinal vessels until approximately 16 weeks gestation. Until then, oxygen diffuses from the underlying choroidal circulation. At 16 weeks, in response to an unknown stimulus (relative hypoxia as the retina thickens has been suggested), cells derived from mesenchyme traveling in the nerve fiber layer emanate from the optic nerve head. These cells, termed "spindle cells," are the precursors of the vascular system. A fine capillary network advances through the retina to the ora serrata or retinal edge (Fig. 8.1). More mature vessels form behind this advancing network. Vascularization on the nasal side of the ora serrata is complete at about 8 months gestation, while that on the temporal side, having a longer distance to travel, is ordinarily complete at term. Once fully vascularized, the retinal vasculature is no longer susceptible to insults of the type that lead to ROP.

Multiple etiologies have been invoked in the pathogenesis of ROP, but experimental studies have focused primarily on the role of oxygen. There appear to be two phases in the development of ROP as reviewed by Patz: (*a*) early vasoconstriction and obliteration of the capillary network in response to elevated oxygen concentrations (Fig. 8.2), followed by (*b*) vasoproliferation, which follows the period of high oxygen exposure, possibly in response to an angiogenic factor released by the hypoxic retina. Both in vivo and in vitro evidence has been developed in support of this hypothesis. Of particular interest is a study

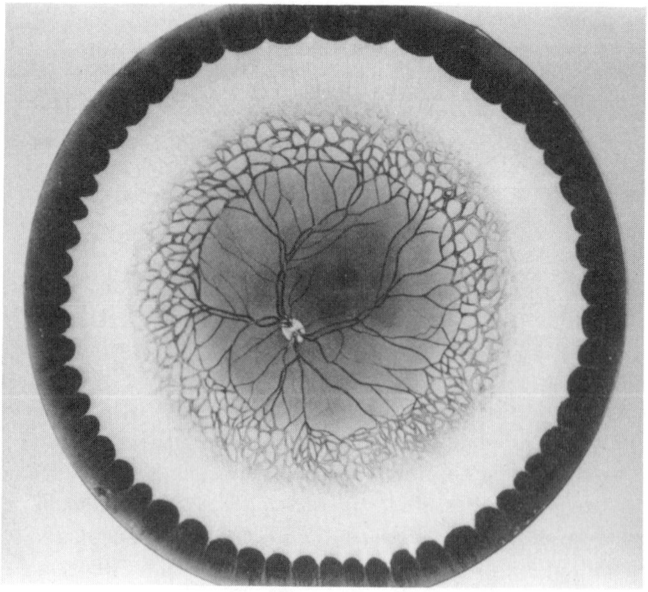

Figure 8.1. Schematic drawing of normal retinal vasculogenesis. Vessels are shown emanating from the optic nerve head with the capillary network advancing toward the periphery of the retina. (Reprinted with permission from Flynn JT, Cassady J, Essner D, et al. Fluorescein angiography in retrolental fibroplasia: experience from 1969–1977. Ophthalmology 1979;86:1700–1723. Published courtesy of Ophthalmology.)

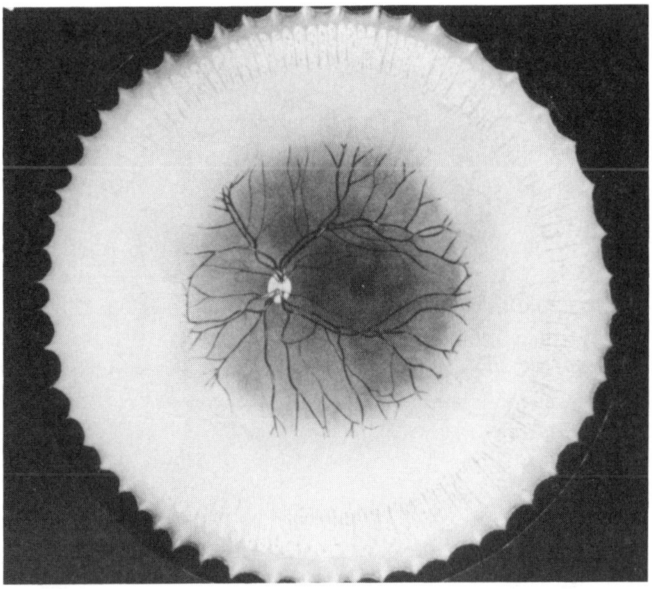

Figure 8.2. Schematic drawing of retinal oxygen exposure in which newly forming vessels in the capillary border are obliterated. (Reprinted with permission from Flynn JT, Cassady J, Essner D, et al. Fluorescein angiography in retrolental fibroplasia: experience from 1969–1977. Ophthalmology 1979;86:1700–1723. Published courtesy of Ophthalmology.)

reported by Phelps and Rosenbaum, in which kittens were made hyperoxic and then allowed to recover in room air or 13% oxygen. Those recovering in the hypoxic environment had worse retinopathy than those recovering in room air, suggesting that hypoxia may indeed play a role in retinal vasoproliferation.

Although oxygen has been used experimentally to induce retinopathy, there is suspicion that endothelial cell injury induced by other causes of altered retinal blood flow and substrate delivery may play a role in the pathogenesis of ROP.

Alternatively, Kretzer et al. have proposed that mesenchymal "spindle cells," precursors of retinal vasculature, form intercellular gap junctions in response to increased oxygen tensions. These increased gap junctions form a barrier to ongoing mesenchymal migration into the retina, and the normal progression of vascularization ceases. In addition, they postulate that these cells produce an angiogenic substance that leads secondarily to abnormal vasoproliferation. They have reported experimental evidence that the administration of vitamin E decreases gap junction formation; however, questions have been raised about this hypothesis.

CLINICAL PRESENTATION

Several methods of classification of ROP have been proposed and used in the past. However, with development of the International Classification of ROP, there has now been general agreement on the staging of active disease. The very first indication of ROP is seen in stage I, in which a thin demarcation line develops between the vascularized region of the retina and the avascular zone. In stage II, this line develops into a ridge protruding into the vitreous. In stage III, vessels behind the ridge may become dilated and tortuous, tufts of neovascularization may be seen behind the ridge, and fibrovascular proliferation

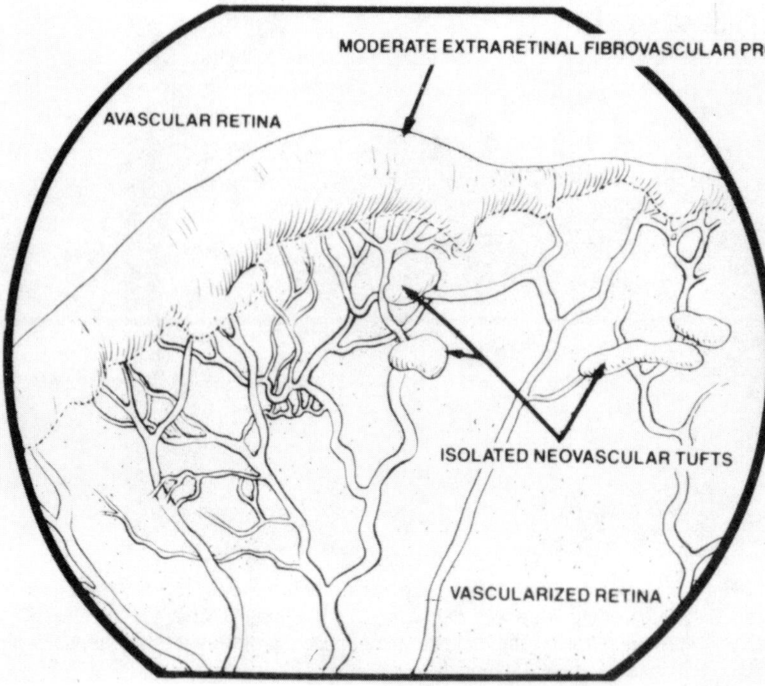

Figure 8.3. Schematic drawing of moderate stage III ROP. Optic nerve head is at the bottom off the drawing and periphery of the retina at the top. (Reprinted with permission from Garner A. An international classification of retinopathy of prematurity. Pediatrics 1984;74:127–133. Reproduced with permission of Pediatrics.)

may extend out into the vitreous (Fig. 8.3). New vessels at this stage are very permeable, resulting in edema and hemorrhage. In "plus" disease, the vessels become increasingly dilated and tortuous, and a vitreous haze may develop. In stage IV disease, fibrosis and scarring occur as the neovascularization extends into the vitreous. Traction occurs on the retina, resulting in detachment. The original International Classification has more recently been expanded to elaborate on retinal detachment. In stage IV, subtotal detachment may be extrafoveal (stage IVA), or it may include the fovea (stage IVB). In stage V, total retinal detachment, which is funnel-shaped as the retina pulls up into the vitreous from around the optic nerve head, occurs. The classification is then subdivided by the shape of the funnel, both anteriorly, just behind the lens, and posteriorly, closer to the optic nerve head. The funnel of fibrotic tissue may be open or narrow, and this shape, sometimes detected by ultrasound, serves to differentiate the types of total detachment.

Each stage of ROP may progress into the next or may regress spontaneously and resolve. About 90% of stages I and II regress spontaneously. Current information suggests that, by stage III+, only about 50% regress spontaneously. The more immature the retina and the more advanced the stage of ROP, the less likely it is to regress. In addition, the more severe the original disease, the more severe the complications following regression. Sequelae of regressed disease, such as strabismus, amblyopia, glaucoma, and late detachment, are possible and require regular follow-up.

Although very little is known about the processes of regression, Flynn speculates that it relates to normal differentiation of the primitive mesenchymal and immature endothelial cells at the site of the shunt. Thus, progressive ROP results from a failure of normal endothelial cell differentiation following the initial injurious event. Recent evidence suggests that vitamin A, a differentiating factor for epithelial cells, may affect the incidence of ROP via this mechanism. Further studies are needed in this area.

It is evident that the incidence of ROP is greater in more immature infants despite careful monitoring of arterial oxygen. Phelps has reported scarring in 2.2% of infants between 1000 and 1500 grams with 0.3 to 1.1% blinded; as many as 22 to 44% of infants <1000 grams have scarring with 5 to 11% blinded. More complete natural history data will be reported when the final results of the natural history arm of the recently concluded national collaborative trial for cryotherapy for ROP become available.

Diagnosis

The American Academy of Pediatrics recommends an ophthalmoscopic examination by a trained ophthalmologist at 5 to 7 weeks of age for all oxygen-exposed premature infants <1800 grams and all infants <1300 grams. Screening criteria suggested by Brown et al. and based on examinations of 2986 neonates attempt to decrease unnecessary examinations by limiting them to those infants <1600 grams or by examining those over 1600 grams only if they have been in oxygen for >50 days. In the recently completed trial of cryopexy for ROP, examinations for infants <1251 grams were begun at 4 to 6 weeks of age and repeated every 2 weeks until maturity or until eyes were prethreshold, just prior to eligibility for treatment. Because rapid progression can occur, prethreshold infants were then examined every week until eligible for treatment at stage III+ or until regression occurred. In view of the known possibility of "rush" disease, an initial examination between 4 to 6 weeks of age in smaller infants seems prudent. In the absence of disease, examinations can then be conducted every 2 to 4 weeks until vascular maturity is reached. Follow-up eye examinations for infants with fully regressed ROP are recommended every 1 to 2 years. For those with cicatricial ROP, follow-up examinations should be scheduled every 6 to 12 months. Report forms have been suggested by the International Committee for Classification of ROP (Fig. 8.4); these include information on the extent of disease as defined by stage, zone, and clock hours. Staging has been defined above. Zone refers to the vascular advancement toward the periphery of the retina. Zone I is least mature with only the medial portion of the retina vascularized. Zone 2 refers to more peripheral vascularization, and zone 3 refers to complete vascularization as occurs in a mature retina. Disease stages II and III would be of much greater concern in an immature retina vascularized only in zone I than in a mature retina vascularized to zone 3 because the potential for advancing disease would be much greater in the less mature retina. Clock hours refer to the extent of circumferential disease around the optic nerve head.

Management

VITAMIN E

The early administration of vitamin E has been advocated in the treatment of ROP. Although vitamin E administration makes theoretical sense because of its action as an antioxidant, data to date are conflicting. Several studies, notably those of Hittner et al. and Finer et al., have shown a beneficial effect. The studies of Pulkin et al. and Phelps showed no effect, and that of Johnson et al. concluded that the risk/benefit ratio did not warrant

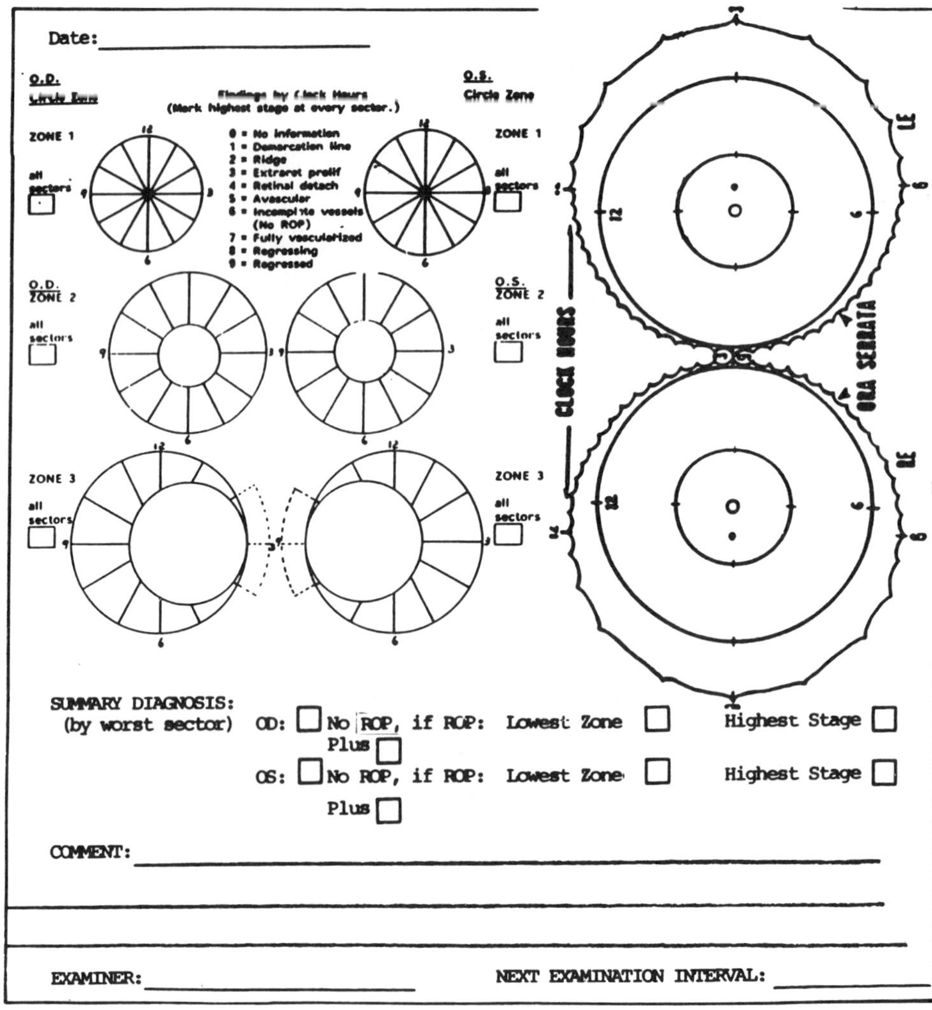

Figure 8.4. ROP ophthalmic examination record suggested by International Committee for Classification of ROP. (Reprinted with permission from Garner A. An international classification of retinopathy of prematurity. Pediatrics 1984;74:127–133. Reproduced with permission of Pediatrics. The form was adapted, with permission, from a data form of the Multicenter Trial of Cryotherapy for Retinopathy of Prematurity.)

its routine use in pharmacological doses. In addition, there have been reports of sepsis, necrotizing enterocolitis, and intraventricular hemorrhage in infants receiving vitamin E who have serum levels generally above the normal range. Because of these reports, vitamin E administration continues to be viewed with skepticism and requires further study. However, maintenance of a normal vitamin E level seems prudent.

LIGHT

Glass et al. have reported a decreased incidence of ROP in infants nursed in an area of reduced light intensity. This report was not conclusive and will require further study, but decreasing light intensity in intensive care nurseries has many proponents.

CRYOTHERAPY

Circumferential cryopexy is now the treatment of choice for progressive (stage III+) disease. During this procedure, which must be performed by an ophthalmologist experienced in the technique, the avascular portion of the retina up to but not including the ridge is frozen. The precise mechanism of action of the technique in limiting the disease is unclear, but it is theorized that cryopexy destroys cells in the avascular region that may be producing angiogenic factors. Results of the recent large, collaborative, NIH-sponsored trial indicate that cryopexy carried out at stage III+ can reduce the incidence of severe visual impairment by approximately 50% if performed within 72 hours of detecting threshold disease. If both eyes are involved, cryopexy is usually offered to one eye only because there are some risks with the procedure (e.g., vitreal hemorrhage). However, if there are enough risk factors for retinal detachment, cryopexy may be offered to both eyes.

It is clear that, to make any significant difference in visual outcome in infants with progressive disease, intervention must occur prior to retinal detachment. Once stage IV is reached, the outcome is bleak. Attempts at retinal reattachment in stage IV disease have met with limited success, although reattachment of late detachments in childhood, a known complication of ROP, has been more successful. Vitrectomy is performed for advanced stage V disease but has not substantially improved outcome.

Once an infant has demonstrated potential visual handicap, it is important to offer services to that infant and the family as quickly as possible. The American Foundation for the Blind, New York, NY is one of many sources for this information.

ROP continues to be an enigmatic disease that we are only beginning to understand. Active research is directed at basic mechanisms that may control this process. Although cryotherapy is the first treatment modality found to be unequivocally beneficial, it still represents rescue therapy. We must develop a better understanding of underlying mechanisms in ROP so that some day we can prevent its development and potentially devastating consequences.

SUGGESTED READINGS

American Academy of Pediatrics. Guidelines for perinatal care. 2nd ed. Elk Grove Village, IL: American Academy of Pediatrics, 1988.

Ashton A. The pathogenesis of retrolental fibroplasia. Ophthalmology 1979;86:1695–1699.

Avery GB, Glass P. Retinopathy of prematurity: what causes it? Clin Perinat 1988;15:917–928.

Brown DR, Biglan AW, Stretavsky MA. Screening criteria for the detection of retinopathy of prematurity in patients in a neonatal intensive care unit. J Pediatr Ophthal Strabismus 1987;24:212–214.

Charles S. Vitreoretinal surgery for retinopathy of prematurity. In: Flynn JT, Phelps DL, eds. Birth defects: original article series. 1988;24:287–293.

Cole CA, Henderson D, Mukherjee T. Vitamin E questioned. Pediatrics 1984;73:734.

Cryotherapy for Retinopathy of Prematurity Cooperative Group. Multicenter trial of cryotherapy for retinopathy of prematurity: preliminary results. Pediatrics 1988;81:697–706.

Finer NN, Schindler RF, Grant G, et al. Effect of intramuscular vitamin E on the frequency and severity of retrolental fibroplasia: a controlled trial. Lancet 1982;1:1087–1091.

Flynn JT, Cassady J, Essner D, et al. Fluorescein angiography in retrolental fibroplasia: experience from 1969–1977. Ophthalmology 1979;86:1700–1723.

Flynn JT. Retinopathy of prematurity. Ped Clin North Am 1987;34:1487–1517.

Garner A. An international classification of retinopathy of prematurity. Pediatrics 1984;74:127–133.

Gibson DL, Sheps SB, Schechter MT, Wiggins S, McCormick AQ. Retinopathy of prematurity: a new epidemic? Pediatrics 1989;83:486–492.

Glaser BM, D'Amore PA, Michels RG, Patz A, Fenselau A. Demonstration of vasoproliferative activity from the mammalian retina. J Cell Biol 1980;84:298–304.

Glass P, Avery GB, Subramanian KNS, Keys MP, Sostek AM, Friendly DS. Effect of bright light in the hospital on retinopathy of prematurity. N Engl J Med 1984;313:401–404.

Hittner HM, Godio LB, Rudolph AJ, et al. Retrolental fibroplasia: efficacy of vitamin E in a double blind clinical study of pre-term infants. N Engl J Med 1981;305:1363–1371.

International Committee for the Classification of the Late Stages of Retinopathy of Prematurity. An international classification of retinopathy of prematurity. II. The classification of retinal detachment. Arch Ophthalmol 1987;105:906–912.

Johnson L, Quinn GE, Abbasi S, et al. Effect of sustained pharmacologic vitamin E levels on incidence and severity of retinopathy of prematurity: a controlled clinical trial. J Pediatr 1989;114:827–838.

Kalina RE, Karr DJ. Retrolental fibroplasia: experience over two decades in one institution. Ophthalmology 1982;81:91–95.

Kinsey VE. Retrolental fibroplasia: cooperative study of retrolental fibroplasia and the use of oxygen. Arch Ophthal 1956;56:481–543.

Lucey JF, Dangman DB. A reexamination of the role of oxygen in retrolental fibroplasia. Pediatrics 1984;73:82–96.

McPherson AR, Hittner HM, Kretzer FL. Retinopathy of prematurity. Current concepts and controversies. Philadelphia: Decker, 1986.

Nissenkorn I, Kremer I, Gilad E, Cohen S, Ben Sira I. 'Rush' type retinopathy of prematurity: report of three cases. Br J Ophthalmol 1987;71:559–562.

Patz A, Hoeck LE, DeLaCruz E. Studies on the effect of high oxygen administration in retrolental fibroplasia. I. Nursery observations. Am J Ophthalmol 1952;24:1248–1253.

Patz A. Current concepts of the effect of oxygen on the developing retina. Curr Eye Res 1984;3:159–163.

Phelps D. Retinopathy of prematurity: an estimate of vision loss in the United States—1979. Pediatrics 1981;67:924–926.

Phelps DL. The role of vitamin E in high-risk neonates. Clin Perinatol 1988;15:955–963.

Phelps DL, Phelp CE. Cryotherapy in infants with retinopathy of prematurity. A decision model for treating one or both eyes. JAMA 1989;261:1751–1756.

Phelps DL, Rosenbaum AL. Effects of marginal hypoxemia on recovery from oxygen-induced retinopathy in the kitten model. Pediatrics 1984;73:1–6.

Phelps DL, Rosenbaum AL, Isenberg SJ, Leak RD, Dorey FJ. Tocopherol efficacy and safety for preventing retinopathy of prematurity: a randomized, controlled, double-masked trial. Pediatrics 1987;79:489–500.

Pulkin JE, Simon RM, Ehrenkranz RA. Influence on retrolental fibroplasia of intramuscular vitamin E administration during respiratory distress syndrome. Ophthalmology 1982;82:96–103.

Purohit DM, Ellison RC, Zierler S, Miettinin OS, Nadas AS. Risk factors for retrolental fibroplasia: experience with 3025 premature infants. Pediatrics 1985;76:339–344.

Second International Retrolental Fibroplasia Conference. Retinopathy of prematurity/idiopathic fibroplasia. Pediatrics 1981;67:751–752.

Shenai JP, Kennedy KA, Chytil F, Stahlman MT. Clinical trial of vitamin A supplementation in infants susceptible to bronchopulmonary dysplasia. J Pediatr 1987;111:269–277.

Silverman WA. Retrolental fibroplasia: a modern parable. New York: Grune and Stratton, 1980.

Tasman W. Late complications of retrolental fibroplasia. Ophthalmology 1979;86:1724–1740.

Taylor CM, Weiss JB, Kissun RD, Garner A. Effect of oxygen tension on the quantities of procollagenase-activating angiogenic factor present in the developing kitten retina. Br J Ophthalmol 1986;70:162–165.

Teplin SW. Development of the blind infant and child with retinopathy of prematurity: the physician's role in intervention. In: Flynn JT, Phelps DL, eds. Birth defects: original article series. 1988;24:287–293.

Terry TL. Extreme prematurity and fibroplastic overgrowth of persistent vascular sheath behind each crystalline lens. I. Preliminary report. Am J Ophthalmol 1942;25:203–204.

9

Neurodevelopmental Outcome and Interventions

Marilee C. Allen

Although quality of life issues are always important, parental and professional concern initially focuses on survival and the acute medical problems of the sick neonate. As the infant's medical condition improves, attention shifts toward preparation for discharge home and toward neurodevelopmental issues: What kind of developmental problems is my child likely to encounter? What are his or her chances of being handicapped? What can I do to help? Who can help us? This is an appropriate shift in focus, and it is the professional's job to help parents make this transition.

This chapter will address many of these issues: the range of neurodevelopmental outcomes, developmental assessment and monitoring, parent counseling, various developmental interventions, and the availability of community services. The next chapter will address the assessment of perinatal risk factors, including abnormalities on examination and on cranial imaging and their use in predicting developmental outcome of high-risk infants.

NEURODEVELOPMENTAL OUTCOMES

High-risk NICU infants demonstrate a wide range of neurodevelopmental outcomes that describe a spectrum of the developmental disabilities (Table 9.1). Developmental disabilities are chronic, nonprogressive disorders of central nervous system function that occur as a result of insult to or a malformation of a developing brain. Types of impairment range from motor to cognitive to sensory impairment, and from severe (cerebral palsy, mental retardation) to the more subtle central nervous system disorders of attention deficits and learning disability.

In neonates, it is difficult or impossible to diagnose the developmental disabilities with certainty. An assessment of perinatal risk factors, the neonatal neurodevelopmental examination, and some laboratory and/or imaging procedures (e.g., EEG, auditory brainstem responses, cranial ultrasound, or CT scan) can be used to select infants at high risk for developmental disability so that their development can be carefully followed during infancy and childhood.

Cerebral Palsy and Mental Retardation

Cerebral palsy is a disorder of movement and posture, and it can be classified according to the type of neurological abnormality, the muscle groups involved, and the severity (Table 9.2). Diagnosis of cerebral palsy is based on delayed motor milestones and

Table 9.1. Range of Neurodevelopmental Outcome: The Spectrum of the Developmental Disabilities

Major handicaps
Cerebral palsy (motor impairment)
Mental retardation (cognitive impairment)
Sensory impairment
Visual impairment
Hearing impairment
Minimal cerebral dysfunction (more subtle central nervous system dysfunction)
Minor neuromotor dysfunction
Language delay
Visual perceptual problems
Learning disability
Attention deficit
Hyperactivity
Behavior problems

Table 9.2. Types of Cerebral Palsy

Physiological (Neurological)
Spastic (hypertonia and hyperreflexia)
Extrapyramidal (variable tone, involuntary movements)
Mixed (combination of spastic and extrapyramidal)
Topographical (Muscle groups)
Quadriplegia (all four extremities involved, lower extremities greater than upper)
Diplegia (primarily lower extremities involved, mild to minimal involvement of upper extremities)
Hemiplegia (ipsilateral upper and lower extremity involved, upper greater than lower extremity)
Severity
Minimal (also known as minor neuromotor dysfunction)
Mild
Moderate
Severe
Profound

abnormal tone and reflexes, in the absence of any progressive disease. Severity of cerebral palsy ranges from mild (delayed motor milestones and mild neuromotor abnormalities in a functional ambulator), to moderate, to severe, and to profound (completely dependent). The infant with mildly delayed or deviant (nonsequential) motor milestones and mild or transient neuromotor abnormalities can be viewed as having minimal cerebral palsy.

Mental retardation is a global impairment of cognitive functioning that affects the child's ability to adapt and function in society. It can be recognized by delays in a child's language and/or problem solving abilities, and it is best diagnosed by formal psychological testing. It also ranges in severity from mild (IQ 55 to 70), to moderate (IQ 40 to 55), severe (IQ 25 to 40), and profound (IQ <25). Borderline intelligence is a mild delay in cognitive abilities (IQ 70 to 85) that may affect school performance and later functioning.

Sensory Impairments

Visual impairments range from loss of visual acuity to legal blindness (acuity of 20/200 or less) to absence of light perception. Causes include congenital malformations, prenatal insults (e.g., from congenital infection), and perinatal damage to the eyes (e.g., retinopathy of prematurity) or the brain (e.g., cortical blindness from perinatal asphyxia).

More subtle visual problems (e.g., myopia, strabismus) may not show up until later in infancy or preschool age.

Hearing loss occurs in approximately 5 to 10% of NICU infants. High-risk infants should have their hearing screened during their first year. For a detailed discussion of the diagnosis and management of hearing loss, refer to Chapter 12.

Minimal Cerebral Dysfunction

The more subtle disorders of central nervous system dysfunction grouped under the umbrella term of minimal cerebral dysfunction (Table 9.1) generally do not become apparent until the preschool and school years. Nevertheless, they may well be due to prenatal and perinatal causes. Early manifestations may include mild delays and deviant (nonsequential) milestone development, mild or transient neuromotor abnormalities, and problematic behavior (e.g., irritability, posturing, feeding problems) in infancy. There are many possible manifestations of minimal cerebral dysfunction (motor, language, perceptual, behavioral), and they are all difficult to measure. Therefore, there are no generally accepted criteria for the various aspects of minimal cerebral dysfunction. Any given child may manifest one, all, or any combination of these various aspects of minimal cerebral dysfunction. Also, the prevalence of minimal cerebral dysfunction or its various manifestations in the general population is not known. For all these reasons, follow-up studies evaluating the incidence of minimal cerebral dysfunction in high-risk NICU populations are time-consuming (requiring follow-up to school-age), expensive (requiring multidisciplinary evaluations and control groups), and difficult to do.

Need for Assessment and Follow-up

Because brain damage tends to be diffuse, not focal, any child who displays evidence of one developmental disability should undergo an interdisciplinary evaluation. This provides an assessment of the child's strengths and weaknesses, and it allows for more accurate parent counseling and the development of a plan for habilitation. Often, the child's presenting problem is not the one that is most handicapping. For example, a one-year-old, 26 week gestation, premature infant had mild motor delay and tight heel cords, requiring bracing. She was diagnosed as having mild spastic diplegia. Nevertheless, she walked at just over 2 years, and she now walks and runs quite well. However, she also has severe myopia requiring glasses and mild mental retardation, which in the long run will be far more handicapping. An evaluation that focused only on her motor disability would have missed her more important disabilities, and early intervention for these other disabilities was more important.

MONITORING THE HIGH-RISK INFANT

As the focus shifts from acute illness, the recovering NICU infant should continue to be carefully monitored in a fashion that reflects long-term concerns.

Growth

Assessments of growth should include not only measurements of weight, length, and head circumference, but also their growth percentile for gestational age and an appreciation of how these change with time. Weight, length, and head circumference should be determined and graphed at least weekly. For preterm infants, specific graphs that represent the normal pattern of growth for healthy, preterm infants should be used. Infants who are not growing appropriately should be reevaluated as to their caloric needs and nutritional balance (see Chapter 1).

Head growth is generally the result of brain growth, and it should be viewed in terms of the other growth parameters and the overall health status of the infant. Inadequate nutrition may result in poor head growth as well as poor weight gain, although head growth is usually the last parameter to be affected. An infant who is gaining weight and length appropriately but is not demonstrating adequate head growth (i.e., moving toward isolated microcephaly) should be evaluated for evidence of brain abnormality and closely followed.

Rapid head growth may be the result of the early growth phase that preterm infants demonstrate. Often their head grows first, before they demonstrate gains in weight and length. However, it may also be a sign of hydrocephalus. The only way to differentiate these two is by a cranial ultrasound and evaluation of ventricular size. If ventricular size is increasing, a neurologist or neurosurgeon should be consulted.

Cranial Imaging Studies

Cranial imaging studies (e.g., ultrasounds, CT scan, MRI) help to determine both prognosis (see Chapter 10) and management. Because periventricular hemorrhages and echodensities can be clinically silent, serial ultrasounds should be performed in all preterm infants (gestational age <32 to 34 weeks). A cranial ultrasound obtained at 4 to 7 days should pick up any periventricular hemorrhage that has occurred, and a cranial ultrasound at 10 to 14 days allows evaluation of ventricular size. If the infant has developed an intraventricular hemorrhage or ventricular dilation, repeat ultrasounds should be obtained on a periodic basis (e.g., q 1 to 2 weeks) to follow ventricular size. Sonograms should be followed more frequently, and a neurologist or neurosurgeon should be consulted if increasing ventricular dilation is noted. Periventricular echodensities or cysts, suggestive of periventricular leukomalacia, generally occur later in the preterm infant's course, and a repeat cranial ultrasound should be obtained at 6 weeks or prior to NICU discharge whether or not the initial studies were normal.

A cranial ultrasound or other imaging study (e.g., CT scan or MRI) should be obtained on any child with any major congenital anomaly or multiple minor anomalies. Asphyxiated infants should have either a CT scan or, if possible, an MRI study to evaluate brain parenchyma. The MRI is particularly good at evaluating posterior fossa lesions and venous infarcts.

Neurodevelopment

A developmental assessment of the recovering NICU infant can be used to help assess the risk of developmental disability, to develop specific interventions, and to counsel parents.

The neurodevelopmental examination is most predictive of later disability when performed at term, but a shortened version of the examination may be helpful to monitor developmental status and to identify specific interventions. It has practical applications, such as helping to determine when an infant is ready to attempt nipple feeds (i.e., when

Table 9.3. Components of the Neonatal Neurodevelopmental Examination

Growth parameters (weight, length, head circumference, and percentiles)
General physical examination
Posture
- In prone (degree of extremity flexion, head control in prone, and hip adduction)
- In supine (degree of extremity flexion and hip adduction, space behind neck)

Tone
- Extremity tone (subjective assessment, recoil, heel-to-ear and popliteal angle maneuvers)
- Axial Tone
  - Neck (head lag or neck extensor hypertonia on pull to sit from supine or rocking in a sitting position)
  - Trunk (ventral suspension)
  - Shoulder (slip through, anterior and posterior scarf signs)
  - Hip tone (subjective assessment)

Deep tendon reflexes (pectoralis, biceps, brachioradialis, knee and ankle jerks)
Pathological reflexes (Babinski, Chaddock, mass reflex, crossed adduction)
Primitive reflexes (asymmetric tonic neck reflex, Moro, Galant, tonic labyrinthine supine and prone, upper and lower extremity grasp reflex, lower extremity placing, positive support, stepping)
Cranial nerve and oromotor function (root, suck, gag, eye movements, facial asymmetry, tongue movements)
Sensory responses (alert to bell, blink to light, habituation, visual fixation, visual attention)
Behavior (range of states of alertness, transition from state to state, irritability, jitteriness, lethargy, consolability, cuddliness)

the infant has up-and-down jaw movement, stripping action of the tongue, a coordinated swallow, and a good gag reflex). This generally occurs at 32 to 34 weeks gestational age.

The neonatal neurodevelopmental examination (Table 9.3) can be used to select neonates who are at high risk for developmental disability so that they can be carefully followed during infancy and childhood. It will also identify opportunities to intervene if an infant demonstrates abnormalities. Although there is controversy as to whether early intervention (e.g., infant stimulation, physical therapy) influences developmental outcome, most developmentalists agree that some interventions appear to be beneficial, inexpensive, and harmless. In some cases, specific interventions may benefit the infant with specific developmental abnormalities (e.g., perioral stimulation and nonnutritive sucking for gavage-fed infants, specific positioning and handling techniques for asymmetric infants).

It is important to determine the interaction between the infant's general health status and his or her neurodevelopment. Chronic conditions may have a profound impact on the neurodevelopmental examination (e.g., hypotonia in the infant with chronic lung disease) and on the child's developmental outcome. For example, preterm infants with chronic lung disease have a higher incidence of developmental disability. The infant's condition at the time of the examination may also have an impact. An infant with exercise intolerance may demonstrate lower muscle tone and increased lethargy, especially toward the end of the examination.

The assessment of tone and reflexes in preterm infants must be viewed in terms of the infant's postmenstrual (synonymous with postconceptional) age. The postmenstrual age is the sum of the child's gestational age from birth and his current chronological age. Because postnatal gestational age assessments (e.g., Dubowitz, Ballard) tend to overestimate gestational age in preterm infants and may be influenced by prenatal neurological insults to the fetus, it is best to use the gestational age calculated from mother's last menstrual

Table 9.4. Common Abnormalities on the Neonatal Neurodevelopmental Examination

Hypotonia
- Extremity (less flexor hypertonia in upper and/or lower extremities for postmenstrual age)
- Axial (low neck, trunk, shoulder, and/or hip tone for postmenstrual age)
- Global (low extremity and axial tone for postmenstrual age)

Extensor hypertonia
- Extremity extensor tone (upper or lower extremities)
- Neck extensor hypertonia
- Arching through back and lower extremities (in supine or prone, or on ventral suspension)

Asymmetry (of posture, tone, deep tendon reflexes, pathological reflexes, or primitive reflexes)
Hyperreflexia (sustained clonus)
Cranial nerve abnormalities (sunsetting of eyes, markedly disconjugate gaze, facial asymmetry)
Oromotor abnormalities (absent gag, weak or absent suck, tongue thrust, tongue fasciculations)
Abnormal sensory responses (poor response to bell or light, poor habituation, abnormal visual attention)
Abnormal behavior (jittery, irritable, lethargic)

period (if accurately recalled) and/or an early sonogram (<20 weeks gestation). What is normal at one point in time may be very abnormal at another time.

For example, the evolution of tone and reflexes prior to term proceeds in caudocephalad (lower to upper extremity) and centripetal (distal to proximal) directions. Thus, greater flexor tone in the lower extremities than in the upper extremities is normal in a preterm infant at 34 to 36 weeks postmenstrual age. However, it would be abnormal at 1 to 2 months postterm. The purpose of the examination is to recognize deviations from the normal patterns of development (Table 9.4).

COMMON PATTERNS OF ABNORMALITIES AND THEIR SIGNIFICANCE

Hypotonia

The presence of hypotonia (Table 9.4) is determined by comparing the infant's tone to what is normal for the infant's gestational or postmenstrual age. Although there are some individual differences in the development of tone, marked delays or abnormal patterns of tone (e.g., normal extremity and trunk tone but nuchal hypotonia) are abnormal. Hypotonia may be related to the infant's nutritional status, medical status (e.g., chronic lung disease), medications (e.g., phenobarbital), or to an abnormal central nervous system. Infants with nuchal and truncal hypotonia require careful handling to protect their neck and airway. Infants with hypotonia at the hips can develop hip abduction contractures (i.e., tensor fasciae latae contractures) and should be positioned for at least part of their day with their legs flexed and adducted.

Neck Extensor Hypertonia and Extremity Extensor Tone

Neck extensor hypertonia is one of the better single predictors of neuromotor outcome, but many infants who demonstrate mild neck extensor hypertonia are normal. Factors such as prolonged intubation and frequent gastroesophageal reflux may contribute to this finding.

Because most neonates also have a strong tonic labyrinthine reflex (in which the shoulders are retracted and the legs are extended if the neck is extended), infants with neck extensor hypertonia also often develop increased shoulder retraction, arching through the back, and lower extremity extensor tone (Table 9.4). This posture may later interfere with the development of normal motor milestones, including rolling over, bringing their hands to midline, reaching for objects placed in front of them, sitting up, and getting into and out of sitting position. Positioning and handling techniques that inhibit this posture aim to help potential motor development, both the quality of movement and motor milestones achievement. Although these positioning and handling techniques attempt to keep the infant in flexion with shoulders forward, it is important that medical personnel and parents understand the importance of ensuring that an adequate airway be maintained (i.e., that the infant's neck is not held in too much flexion).

Extremity extensor tone may also be an isolated finding, and is always abnormal (i.e., normal extremity tone is predominantly flexor in preterm and term infants). Efforts should be made to position such infants in flexion (e.g., with swaddling).

Asymmetry

Asymmetries of posture, tone, and reflexes (Table 9.4) are more commonly found in preterm than in term infants. If they are single, isolated asymmetries, they are probably of no significance. Multiple, persistent asymmetries place the infant at increased risk of neuromotor dysfunction, and care should be taken to position the infant as symmetrically as possible in the bed. Most infants demonstrate a preference to turn their head to one side, usually to the right, but infants with a marked head preference should be placed on the nonpreferred side or positioned in their bed so that objects of interest (e.g., toys, the door people use to enter the room) are varied from side to side.

Hyperreflexia

Hyperreflexia is common in both fullterm newborns and preterm infants at term. Although unsustained (4+) clonus is common, asymmetric clonus and sustained (5+) clonus are worrisome findings. The infant with marked hyperreflexia and sustained clonus is often also jittery and irritable. In these cases, the infant often benefits from tight swaddling in a flexed position and decreasing environmental stimuli (e.g., placing the infant in a quiet, darkened room and disturbing him or her as little as possible).

Cranial Nerve and Oromotor Abnormalities

Many abnormalities of the cranial nerves (e.g., sunsetting of the eyes, marked disconjugate gaze, facial asymmetry, tongue fasciculations, marked tongue thrust, weak or absent suck, absent gag, hyperactive gag, and uncoordinated suck and swallow) are signs of central nervous system dysfunction. Physical, occupational, and speech therapists can help evaluate the infant with feeding problems; some infants may benefit from specific maneuvers (e.g., jaw support, positioning to inhibit extensor tone) that may improve the infant's ability to feed.

Sensory Abilities

Periodic observation of an infant's response to sensory stimuli can give clues to sensory impairment. Most preterm infants alert (move, demonstrate a change in heart or respiratory rate) to a bell or other loud sound shortly after birth (by 25 to 28 weeks gestation). They also blink in response to bright light, and they habituate to repetitive stimuli. Visual attention and visual acuity progressively improve with gestational age. Preterm infants at term and fullterm newborns should be able to fixate and follow briefly (30 to 60°); they have a fixed focal length of approximately 8 inches.

Infants with specific perinatal risk factors (see Chapter 12) should have more formal evaluations for possible hearing impairments. Some preterm infants are at risk for retinopathy of prematurity and should be evaluated by an experienced ophthalmologist at 6 weeks, then every 1 to 2 weeks until the retina is fully vascularized (see Chapter 8). This monitoring is important because, if the infant develops stage III+ ROP, cryotherapy should be performed as soon as possible.

Abnormal Behavior

Marked irritability, jitteriness, and lethargy are not only clues to central nervous system dysfunction, but also have implications as to management at home. An effort should be made to decrease sensory stimuli (e.g., dim lights, avoid noise, tightly swaddle) for the irritable, jittery infant. Parents of infants who are irritable, jittery, lethargic, easily disturbed, and/or difficult to console should be told about these observations regarding their infants' behaviors. Most parents feel that they are at fault if they have difficulty managing their infant at home. Discussing their infant's behavioral responses helps them to refocus from feelings of inadequacy to identifying more successful strategies.

DEVELOPMENTAL INTERVENTIONS

Whenever we care for high-risk neonates in the NICU, we are in some way "intervening" on their behalf. To most people, developmental interventions suggest specific (often fairly time-consuming and highly specialized) interventions designed to promote the infant's growth and development. A number of specific developmental interventions have been proposed, but few have been systematically evaluated. The few published studies evaluating infant stimulation and/or neurodevelopmental physical therapy have failed to consistently demonstrate beneficial effects on developmental outcome. Randomized control studies are difficult to do on this population because (*a*) they are expensive and time-consuming (i.e., follow-up for at least 1 year is necessary); (*b*) once an intervention is introduced, it is difficult to have a control group; and (*c*) the group being studied is so heterogeneous, with such a wide range of outcomes and a fairly low rate of disability, that a large sample size is needed.

Although few developmental interventions have been proven to reduce the incidence of developmental disability, common-sense interventions should be employed to avoid hindering developmental progress. Optimum strategies are those that are efficient, easily taught, and least invasive. The following section will discuss a number of intervention strategies, their rationale, and their limitations.

Social/Emotional Interventions

Many parents feel inadequate and redundant in their relationship to their NICU infant, and many resent their child's more "expert" caretakers. But the parents have the unique opportunity to be the only caretakers who have exclusively positive interactions with their infants: to talk to them in a soothing voice, to touch them gently, to hold and cuddle them. All other caretakers have some other job they must also perform, and this generally includes doing something unpleasant to the infant (e.g., suction, take temperature, listen with a cold stethoscope). What an infant really experiences is uncertain, but their reactions indicate that infants can feel pain and discomfort. To be able to counterbalance the day-to-day "torture" of the NICU infant with consistent, positive interactions with parents should benefit both the infant and his parents, by assigning to them an important role in care.

Scheduling Daily Cares

Even very immature fetuses and preterm infants have some sleep-wake cycles, although Prechtl and colleagues have pointed out that they do not have organized, well-defined states of alertness until approximately 36 weeks gestation. Fetal movements and fetal breathing movements demonstrate circadian rhythms. It makes sense to structure the preterm and fullterm infant's environment as much as possible. For the acutely ill infant, it is probably not safe to create day/night cycles by turning off or dimming the lights. However, it frequently is possible to shield the infant's eyes from intense room light without interfering with the caretakers' ability to care for and monitor the infant. Older, more stable infants benefit from placement in a quieter, less hectic room where the light can be adjusted and day/night cycles can be established.

Although it is not possible to avoid disturbing the sleep of both the acutely ill and recovering NICU infant with routine and necessary cares, it is usually possible to establish a regular schedule of these disturbances and to provide the infant with regular periods of undisturbed sleep. Nurses can establish a schedule of cares during which the child is fed after vital signs and routine bloods are obtained, and beds are changed, following which the infant is left undisturbed. Some have advocated that infants do much better (i.e., quicker recovery, shorter hospitalizations) when this schedule is determined by the child's own patterns of sleep and hunger and not by the staff.

Nonnutritive Sucking and Oromotor Stimulation

The ability to suck is well established by birth, even in the most immature preterm infant. However, it is not coordinated with swallow until about 32 to 36 weeks gestation. Several studies have demonstrated the importance of offering a preterm infant a pacifier to suck on, particularly while being gavage fed (nonnutritive sucking). These studies have shown that infants who were given the opportunity for nonnutritive sucking during gavage feedings had more rapid intestinal transit times, more rapid transition from gavage to bottle feedings, better weight gain (but not increased caloric intake), improved feeding behaviors during bottle feedings (e.g., longer period of sucking, less bottle jiggling, and fewer changes of position), and decreased length of hospital stays and hospital costs. This is one form of developmental intervention that makes sense developmentally, is easy and inexpensive, and is of probable benefit.

Delayed nipple feeding can be due to a number of causes, including exercise intolerance due to medical illness, poorly coordinated suck and swallow due to developmental delay or abnormalities, abnormal oromotor function (e.g., tongue thrust) generally due to central nervous system dysfunction, or choking and gagging with feeding due to abnormal swallowing or severe gastroesophageal reflux. It is helpful to observe the infant feeding. Specific interventions (e.g., jaw support, positioning the infant to break up his extensor tone) may be suggested by an occupational or physical therapist.

Some NICU infants have such severe oromotor or gastrointestinal abnormalities that they require feeding by gastrostomy or gavage indefinitely. Because of the risk of aspiration with a misplaced nasogastric or orogastric tube, gastrostomy should be considered in any child requiring prolonged gavage feedings. Gastrostomy feeding is safer, more efficient, easily taught to parents, and can be reversed by just pulling the tube when the child can feed by mouth. However, children who are exclusively fed via gastrostomy or gavage quickly lose the normal oromotor reflexes and develop a hypersensitivity to oral stimulation. Consequently, it is important to offer some oral feedings to those infants who can safely suck and swallow, and to offer oral stimulation (e.g., rub the infant's gums and lips with a washcloth or lemon swab) to those infants who may aspirate.

Positioning and Handling Techniques

Nurses and physicians generally position the critically ill neonate in ways that allow optimal monitoring and medical treatment (e.g., to allow ventilator use or stabilization of intravenous catheters). Some recommendations that are related to developmental concerns can be made for positioning even the critically ill infant; for example, avoid hyperextension of the infant's neck, place the infant in the lateral decubitus or prone position whenever possible, and position the infant as symmetrically as possible.

As a NICU infant recovers, it becomes increasingly possible to pay attention to positioning and handling techniques that are optimal for the infant's development. At approximately 32 to 34 weeks postmenstrual age, the preterm infant normally has somewhat stronger neck extensor than neck flexor tone. The neck flexors normally become much stronger by term. The term infant and the preterm infant (even by 30 weeks postmenstrual age) demonstrate the tonic labyrinthine primitive reflex (i.e., when the infant's head is extended, the shoulders retract, and the legs extend; and when the head is flexed, the shoulders come forward, and the legs flex). Positioning a neonate in the supine position enhances neck extension, shoulder retraction, and lower extremity extension (in its extreme, opisthotonus). These infants can retain this abnormal posture (almost as a learned posture), and it can interfere with development of gross motor (e.g., rolling over, sitting, getting into and out of the sitting position) and fine motor (e.g., playing with hands, reaching out for toys) abilities.

Positioning the recovering NICU infant in the prone or lateral decubitus position avoids enhancing this posture. In the prone position, the infant is not only safer (i.e., if reflux should occur, the airway is better protected) but has more opportunity to control movement of his or her head and upper body. An infant should be able to turn his or her head from side-to-side by term, to lift his or her head off the bed by one month, and later to be able to put weight on the arms, then weight shift over the arms. All these activities prepare the infant for later developmental tasks (e.g., sitting). Placing the infant in the lateral decubitus position, with some support behind the back, allows the infant to discover his or her hands and bring them to the mouth.

Neonates frequently demonstrate a preference to turn their head to one side. The asymmetric tonic neck reflex (i.e., extension of the limbs on the face side and flexion of the limbs on the occiput side when the head is turned to one side) can be elicited to some degree in all normal neonates. In addition, preterm infants often demonstrate some asymmetries of tone or reflexes. Thus, it is important to take care to position infants as symmetrically as possible and to be aware of any persistent asymmetries.

Most infants seem to enjoy the security of being swaddled, and this is especially true for irritable infants, infants with chronic lung disease, and infants withdrawing from drugs. Care should be taken to place the infant in flexion with the hips flexed and adducted (the normal extremity posture of term infants), to prevent tensor fasciae latae contractures in hypotonic infants. To encourage hand exploration, the infant's hands should be outside the blanket and therefore accessible.

Once the principles and techniques of handling and positioning the high-risk or handicapped infant are learned, the time and expense of integrating them into the regular care of the recovering and, in many cases even the acutely ill, NICU infant are negligible. When a nurse or parent is finished with the infant's cares, it takes no extra time to symmetrically position the infant in the prone or lateral decubitus position with extremity flexion and hip adduction. When picking up, holding, or carrying an infant, attention should be paid to keeping the head midline, the shoulders protracted, and the legs flexed.

Infant Stimulation

Whether or not high-risk preterm and term infants benefit from infant stimulation has been the subject of much debate, a number of studies, and a few reviews in recent years. Most now agree that bombarding NICU infants with all kinds of sensory stimuli is unlikely to be beneficial. Some feel that the preterm infant was not meant to be born yet, and sensory stimuli should be minimized. Others feel that the NICU environment provides the wrong kind of stimulation (e.g., not enough meaningful visual, vestibular, and kinesthetic stimulation).

TOUCHING AND HANDLING

Because most people experience pleasurable feelings from soft, sensitive touching, it makes sense to assume that touching may feel good to infants as well. Studies evaluating the effect of tactile and kinesthetic stimulation in preterm infants have reported better muscle tone and head control, consolability, activity, and weight gain; however, not all studies found the same things, especially with respect to activity level and weight gain. Some NICU infants (e.g., preterm infants with hyaline membrane disease, term infants with persistent pulmonary hypertension, infants with chronic lung disease) are extremely labile, and the slightest touch may trigger adverse reactions. Therefore, infants who may benefit from tactile and kinesthetic stimulation should be cautiously chosen. The personnel who do the stimulation should be able to recognize adverse effects.

AUDITORY/LANGUAGE STIMULATION

Even the most immature preterm infant can hear (i.e., has auditory brainstem responses), and by term, the infant can hear as well as adults. Recent data suggest that even the fetus in utero is subject to intense auditory stimulation. Consequently, many suggest that the infant be provided with more soothing, meaningful auditory stimulation, including music and language stimulation. Parents are encouraged to bring in a tape recorder with their favorite music (some insist it should be classical music!) and with recordings of their voices (e.g., reading a story). Caution should be exercised that the recordings are not played too loudly.

Infants begin very early to process the music of language (e.g., the inflections, rhythms, and flow) before they begin to learn individual words. At approximately 1 year of age, as the normal infant begins to learn one or two meaningful words, he or she begins to jargon, imitating the sounds of language in a very convincing manner. Several months later, the infant starts to insert some of the words that have been learned into this jargoning.

Consequently, it makes sense that, because the newborn can hear quite well, the most meaningful and developmentally appropriate auditory stimulation is the human voice. Parents should be encouraged to talk to their infants from birth on as much as possible. Initially, it does not matter what they say as long as the infant hears the sound of language. For example, it is not necessary to read stories, which may be time consuming, but the mother can talk about anything (the events of the day, her current concerns) as long as the infant gets to hear her voice.

VISUAL STIMULATION

An association between light intensity in a NICU and the incidence of retinopathy of prematurity has prompted most NICUs to reduce their overhead light intensity. In addition, the infant's eyes can be shielded (e.g., by covering the isolette top during sleep periods or by placing the infant in the prone position).

Preterm infants respond to visual stimuli by 30 weeks gestation and begin to express visual pattern preferences by 32 to 34 weeks gestation. Their visual acuity improves with age, and at term, their visual acuity is at least 20/200. They see black/white contrasts the best, and they express interest in patterns that resemble faces. Newborns have a fixed focal length of approximately 8 inches. These findings suggest that the strongest visual stimuli for the newborn is the parent's face when the infant is cradled in his or her arms.

PARENT TRAINING

There are a number of studies that have found that NICU infants do better when their parents have been involved in parent training programs that emphasize infant stimulation techniques. It is likely that the primary value of these programs is the fact that they encourage parental interaction with the child in the NICU and help them to conquer their natural inhibitions and fears. One possible danger to parent training programs is that, when the experts show the parents how to interact with their own child, parents may actually feel more inadequate and are inhibited from doing what comes naturally. Consequently, although all parents probably benefit from some encouragement and guidance, it should be accomplished with discretion and sensitivity and without much fanfare. Probably the most potent and successful infant stimulation techniques are those that are most natural—the human face and the human voice.

PARENT COUNSELING

Although discussions with parents regarding their child's current health status should occur on an ongoing basis in a NICU, a parent conference prior to the child's discharge from the NICU provides a unique opportunity to summarize the infant's NICU course, to give parents a chance to ask any questions, to discuss issues related to discharge, and to refocus from acute to long-term concerns (Table 9.5).

Review of Perinatal Course/Risk for Developmental Disability

A parent conference in preparation for discharge is an opportunity to review the child's progress and assess the parent's understanding of and commitment to the infant. It is helpful when reviewing the infant's NICU course to point out those perinatal risk factors that put the infant at risk for developmental disability and to put these risk factors into perspective

Table 9.5. Topics to Discuss in Parent Counseling Sessions Prior to NICU Discharge

Review perinatal course, answering any questions that arise
Discuss infant's risk for developmental disabilities in an honest but sensitive manner
Plan for discharge home
- Discharge teaching (well-baby care, CPR, use of equipment, e.g., monitors)
- Arrangements for necessary equipment (e.g., home apnea monitors, tracheostomy tubes, home oxygen systems)
- Medication (instructions on indications, dosage, and side effects; prescriptions; dispense syringes)
- Special interventions to be demonstrated regarding feeding, positioning, or handling

Discuss parents' feelings about infant's discharge: acknowledge and reassure them about feelings of ambivalence or fear
Recommend follow-up plans
- Pediatric primary care
- Developmental follow-up
- Ophthalmology follow-up
- Audiology follow-up
- Subspecialty follow-up (e.g., pulmonary, surgical, cardiology)
- Community supports and programs

(see Chapter 10). To neglect this discussion of the risk of disability is to do the parents a disservice. Whenever possible, parents should be reassured (e.g., if the neonatal neurodevelopmental examination is normal). If the child has an increased risk of developmental disability or of other complications, it is helpful to develop a specific plan for how the child will be followed, what the parents can do, and what community services are available. Very few conditions are associated with a 100% chance of handicap; therefore, it is important to emphasize that predictions are made based on experience with other children, that no one knows what the future holds for their child, and that it is not unrealistic to be hopeful as long as they understand what the concerns are.

Transition to the Community

Emphasizing the connection between the NICU and community resources helps parents to "let go" of the NICU and builds their confidence in their own abilities to care for their child by providing them with a support system that they can trust. The primary health care provider is the most important factor in this transition, and if possible, he or she should be a participant in discharge planning. In addition, the NICU staff and the primary care provider can work with the parents to find community support services that will be most helpful.

Part H of Public Law 99-457, passed by Congress in October 1986, encouraged states to provide a comprehensive, coordinated interagency system of early intervention services for handicapped infants and toddlers and their families. These services are available to infants who are developmentally delayed or who have conditions that typically result in developmental delay (e.g., Down's syndrome). Some states have also opted to provide these services to infants who are at risk for developmental delay.

These early intervention services include, for each child, a multidisciplinary assessment and an Individualized Family Service Plan (IFSP) developed by the multidisciplinary team and the parents. This plan would be designed to meet the child's identified developmental needs and would include those family services (e.g., drug counseling, home visits) that would enable the family to better meet the child's needs. An important component of

Table 9.6. Neurodevelopmental Care of the Recovering NICU Infant

Encourage family interactions with infant
Promote parental feelings of competency
Provide regular light/dark cycles when possible
Provide opportunities for nonnutritive sucking
Place infant in prone or decubitus position when possible
Measure head circumference and length once a week
Swaddle with arms and legs flexed, hips adducted, and hands exposed
Obtain head sonogram at 4 to 7 days, at 10 to 14 days, and prior to discharge in preterm infants <34 weeks gestation (or more frequently if abnormal or acute increase in head circumference); head CT scan prior to discharge in term asphyxiated infants
Perform neonatal neurodevelopmental examination for gestational age <33 weeks, intrauterine growth retardation, perinatal asphyxia, status/post extracorporeal membrane oxygenation, abnormal head ultrasound, etc.
Consult therapists for specific developmental interventions for infants with persistent feeding problems, neck extensor hypertonia, extremity extensor tone, marked hypotonia, or asymmetry
For infants at risk for visual and hearing impairment, arrange for specific tests (auditory brainstem responses, ophthalmology examination) and/or for follow-up
Meet with parents to review infant's perinatal course, to discuss risk of developmental disability, and to plan for NICU discharge
Complete discharge teaching
Encourage all parents to talk to their infants as much as possible; demonstrate appropriate positioning
Involve primary health care provider in discharge planning and schedule all follow-up appointments prior to discharge
Facilitate transition to the community by making parents aware of appropriate community programs

this process is the assignment of a case manager to each child in the program to help the family get the services they require.

Not all infants will qualify for this program at the time of NICU discharge, and most will never need these services. However, infants who are eligible should be referred before NICU discharge. Because the fact that a child required neonatal intensive care raises the risk of developmental delay to some degree, all parents should know about this program. The fear of handicap raises tremendous anxiety. To know that they are not alone and to have a plan helps parents to cope with the uncertainty of the future.

SUMMARY

As the NICU infant recovers from an acute illness, attention shifts from life-or-death matters to quality-of-life issues. This shift in focus is appropriate, and the health professional can do much to support the infant's family plan for discharge from the NICU and for the future. Some developmental interventions (e.g., family education and support) can begin prior to birth (during a high-risk pregnancy) and continue even during the infant's acute illness. Table 9.6 summarizes recommendations for the neurodevelopmental care and monitoring of high-risk, recovering NICU infants. The best strategy is to consider parents as partners and to provide them with as much knowledge and support as possible.

SUGGESTED READINGS

Allen MC, Capute AJ. The evolution of primitive reflexes in extremely premature infants. Pediatr Res 1986;20:1284–1289.

Allen MC, Capute AJ. Assessment of early auditory and visual abilities of extremely premature infants. Develop Med Child Neurol 1986;28:458–466.

Allen MC, Capute AJ. Neonatal neurodevelopmental examination as a predictor of neuromotor outcome in premature infants. Pediatrics 1989;83:498–506.

Allen MC, Capute AJ. Tone and reflex development before term. Pediatrics 1990;85(suppl):393–399.

Bernbaum JC, Pereira GR, Watkins JB, Peckham GJ. Nonnutritive sucking during gavage feeding enhances growth and maturation in premature infants. Pediatrics 1983;71:41–45.

Brown JV, LaRossa MM, Aylward GP, Davis DJ, Rutherford PK, Bakeman R. Nursery-based intervention with prematurely born babies and their mothers: are there effects? J Pediatr 1980;97(3):487–491.

Capute AJ, Palmer FB. A pediatric overview of the spectrum of developmental disabilities. Develop Behav Pediatr 1990;1(2):66–69.

Capute AJ, Palmer FB, Shapiro BK, Wachtel RC, Ross A, Accardo PJ. Primitive reflex profile: a quantitation of primitive reflexes in infancy. Develop Med Child Neurol 1984;26:375–383.

Capute AJ, Accardo PJ. Developmental disabilities in infancy and childhood. Baltimore: Paul H. Bookes, 1990.

Denhoff E. Current status of infant stimulation or enrichment programs for children with developmental disabilities. Pediatrics 1981;67:32–37.

Ferry PC. On growing new neurons: are early intervention programs effective? Pediatrics 1981;67:38–40.

Field T, Ignatoff E, Stringer S, et al. Nonnutritive sucking during tube feedings: effects on preterm neonates in an intensive care unit. Pediatrics 1982;70:381–384.

Field T, Schanberg SM, Scafidi F, et al. Tactile/kinesthetic stimulation effects on preterm neonates. Pediatrics 1986;77:654–658.

Glass P, Avery GB, Subramanian KNS, Keys MP, Sostek AM, Friendly DS. Effect of bright light in the hospital nursery on the incidence of retinopathy of prematurity. N Engl J Med 1985;313:401–404.

Goodman M, Rothberg AD, Houston-McMillan JE, Cooper PA, Cartwright JD, Van Der Velde MA. Effect of early neurodevelopmental therapy in normal and at-risk survivors of neonatal intensive care. Lancet 1985;2:1327–1330.

Leib SA, Benfield G, Guidubaldi J. Effects of early intervention and stimulation on the preterm infant. Pediatrics 1980;66:83–90.

Nijhuis JG, Prechtl HFR, Martin CB Jr, Bots RSGM. Are there behavioral states in the human fetus? Early Hum Develop 1982;6:177–195.

Piper MC, Kunos I, Willis DM, Mazer BL, Ramsay M, Silver KM. Early physical therapy effects on the high-risk infant: a randomized controlled trial. Pediatrics 1986;78:216–224.

Prechtl HFR, Fargel JW, Weinmann HM, Bakker HH. Postures, motility and respiration of low-risk preterm infants. Dev Med Child Neurol 1979;21:23–27.

Resnick MB, Fonda DE, Nelson RM, Eitzman DV, Bucciarelli RL. Developmental intervention for low birth weight infants: improved early developmental outcome. Pediatrics 1987;80:68–74.

Shapiro BK, Palmer FB, Capute AJ. Diagnosis and management of developmental disabilities. Comp Ther 1987;13:17–25.

Touwen BCL. The preterm infant in the extrauterine environment. Implications for neurology. Early Hum Develop 1980;4:287–300.

10

Assessment of Risk for Developmental Disability

Marilee C. Allen

As the shift in focus from acute care to long-term problems raises quality-of-life issues, the degree of uncertainty increases. Initially, the question is whether the infant will live or die. As the child's condition improves, questions regarding his or her outcome are raised. How is my child going to do? What kind of life will he or she have? The child's medical condition and subsequent growth and health problems are important components of the answers to these questions. However, how a child's central nervous system will develop is frequently the most difficult question to answer. It is not possible to say with certainty if a child will develop a handicap or to predict the type or severity. We can only discuss likelihood.

This question is important to answer as completely and honestly as possible. Parents need to begin preparing themselves and their child for the future. Children at high risk for developmental disability should have their development very closely monitored during infancy and childhood. Family support and early intervention programs can help parents and their children adapt and can minimize secondary complications. Appropriate feedback can help parents interpret what they perceive about their child's development and can help them to provide a nurturing, supportive environment. It is also important to be as reassuring as possible while emphasizing the need for continued follow-up.

This chapter will address the question of how to best determine, at the time of discharge from a NICU, a child's risk of developmental disability. A number of perinatal and demographic factors that increase an infant's risk of developmental disability have been identified. They can be used to help select high-risk infants in order to focus comprehensive follow-up and intervention efforts.

RELATIONSHIP OF RISK FACTORS TO CAUSATION

As stated previously, a large number of perinatal and demographic risk factors are associated with a higher incidence of developmental disability. However, it is important to remember that risk does not imply causation. There are very few conditions (e.g., anencephaly, some chromosomal disorders and dysmorphic syndromes) that lead inevitably to handicap. When a child is born prematurely, is small for gestational age, or is asphyxiated at birth, it is necessary to ask what other factors or conditions caused this to occur and whether these earlier, prenatal conditions could have either injured the central nervous system or made the fetus more vulnerable to injury or postnatal complications during the perinatal period.

It is generally difficult to measure the severity or duration of a perinatal insult (e.g., how limited was the maternal supply of nutrients to the fetus with intrauterine growth retardation, and for how long? How severe was the anoxic insult, and for how long?). Instead, the insult is defined by its effect on the newborn infant (e.g., size, Apgar scores, seizures). Because they are not a direct measure of causation, severity, or duration of the insult, these factors are generally not 100% predictive. The best predictors of developmental outcome are generally those that relate directly to cause (e.g., chromosomal disorders) or to the effect on the infant's central nervous system (e.g., periventricular echodensities on cranial ultrasound, abnormal neonatal neurodevelopmental examination).

Specific Risk Factors

One way to evaluate risk factors in relation to causation is to subgroup them according to the period of time in which they appear (Table 10.1).

DEMOGRAPHIC FACTORS

The demographic factors relate to the family's socioeconomic background (e.g., social class, maternal education, parental employment) and infant characteristics (e.g., gender, race). These factors tend to be associated with intelligence; for example, low social class is associated with a lower IQ. However, some of these demographic factors may also be related to access to health care. This may lead to a higher incidence of prenatal and perinatal complications and infant mortality and morbidity. Infant factors can relate to vulnerability to disease, such as the higher incidence of lung disease in white and male infants at a given gestational age. They are also associated with developmental problems; for example, boys are more likely to develop problems with language, attention, and learning.

PRENATAL FACTORS

Prenatal genetic conditions often have known risks of developmental disability. Some chromosomal disorders and dysmorphic syndromes have an incidence of mental retardation or motor impairment as high as 100%; in other syndromes, the occurrence of handicap is less certain. Some metabolic disorders are genetic and therefore prenatal in origin, but damage to the central nervous system occurs only after birth (e.g., phenylketonuria). If these conditions can be detected early enough, developmental sequelae can be prevented or minimized. This is the basis of the neonatal screening programs. It must also be remembered that intelligence is an inherited trait that is probably also influenced by environmental factors.

Other prenatal conditions that can have devastating effects on the fetal nervous system are congenital infections (e.g., cytomegalovirus, toxoplasmosis, rubella) and maternal ingestions (e.g., alcohol, phenytoin). Although alcohol and phenytoin have been shown to have teratogenic effects, causing congenital anomalies, characteristic dysmorphic features, and developmental disability, the effects of illicit drugs on the fetus have not been as well demonstrated. Heroin can cause intrauterine growth retardation, neonatal withdrawal syndrome, and behavioral effects (i.e., increased incidence of hyperactivity and behavioral problems). Maternal cocaine use has been associated with an increased incidence of abruptio placenta, prematurity, anomalies (primarily genitourinary), neonatal withdrawal syndrome, and cerebral infarction in the infant. A number of maternal illnesses such as severe hy-

Table 10.1. Perinatal and Demographic Risk Factors

- Demographic
  - Socioeconomic/educational background
    - Social class
    - Maternal education
    - Parental employment
    - Method of payment for health care
  - Infant characteristics
    - Gender
    - Race
- Prenatal
  - Genetic
    - Chromosomal disorders
    - Dysmorphic syndromes
    - Inborn errors of metabolism
    - Inheritance of intellect
  - Maternal conditions
    - Congenital infections (toxoplasmosis, rubella, cytomegalovirus, syphilis, HIV)
    - Ingestions (alcohol, phenytoin, heroin, cocaine)
    - Illness (severe hypertension, diabetes, lung disease, connective tissue diseases)
  - Intrauterine growth retardation
- Obstetrical
  - Pregnancy-induced hypertension
  - Abruptio placenta
  - Placenta previa
  - Prolapsed cord
  - Malpresentation
  - Birth injury
  - Prematurity
- Neonatal
  - Hypoxic-ischemic encephalopathy
  - Seizures
  - Hypoglycemia
  - Polycythemia
  - Chronic lung disease
  - Infection
  - Poor nutrition/growth
  - Abnormal cranial ultrasound/CT scan/MRI
  - Abnormal neurodevelopmental examination

pertension, diabetes, lung disease, or connective tissue diseases can compromise nutrient and oxygen supply to the infant and thereby increase the infant's risk of intrauterine growth retardation, premature delivery, and/or poor developmental outcome.

OBSTETRICAL FACTORS

A number of obstetrical factors that are associated with infant mortality and morbidity have been identified. However, these obstetrical factors generally have not been highly associated with developmental disability in the infant. This is primarily because, in general, they have a relatively low prevalence, and when they do occur, a good outcome for the infant is still likely.

For example, abruptio placenta can lead to severe maternal and fetal blood loss, shock, and asphyxia, which subsequently results in severe damage to the infant's central nervous system. However, the abruption is frequently small and/or the infant can be promptly delivered and blood volume replaced, with no long-term effects on either the mother or the infant. The abruption may be causal or may be caused by something else (e.g., preeclampsia or cocaine abuse), but it may only be related to poor fetal outcome if the fetus is compromised. Factors related to the condition of the fetus (e.g., severe asphyxia, cerebral infarction) are more likely to be associated with poor developmental outcome.

Both prematurity and intrauterine growth retardation are heterogeneous conditions, with a variety of causes, complications, and outcomes. The cause of the growth retardation (e.g., chromosomal disorder, congenital infection, pregnancy-induced hypertension) or premature delivery (e.g., infection, fetal distress, abruption) and the subsequent complications (e.g., hypoglycemia, asphyxia, chronic lung disease, intraventricular hemorrhage) are the most important considerations when evaluating the risk of developmental disability for a small-for-gestational-age or preterm infant.

NEONATAL FACTORS

Neonatal complications (e.g., hypoxic-ischemic encephalopathy, seizures) are often measures of the effect of the insult on the infant. The more severely the infant is affected (e.g., Sarnat stage 3 of hypoxic-ischemic encephalopathy scale or severe, persistent seizures), the worse the outcome. Many physiological aberrations such as hypoglycemia or polycythemia are associated with later developmental disability primarily if the infant is symptomatic. Neonatal complications are most common in infants who are already at risk (e.g., hypoglycemia in preterm, small-for-gestational-age, or asphyxiated infants). The neonatal factors that are most predictive of later developmental disability are those that are indicators of central nervous system structure (e.g., abnormalities on cranial ultrasound or CT scan) or function (e.g., neonatal seizures, abnormal neonatal neurodevelopmental examination).

DEGREES OF RISK

Not all perinatal and demographic factors are equally predictive of developmental outcome. An extremely preterm infant with chronic lung disease has a greater risk of developmental disability than a fullterm newborn with an Apgar score of 3 at 5 minutes. Even within categories of risk factors (e.g., infection, abnormal cranial ultrasounds), the degree of risk can vary with the type of problem identified or its severity. A newborn with congenital cytomegalovirus infection is far more likely to develop cerebral palsy, mental retardation, or hearing and visual impairment if he or she is symptomatic at birth. A preterm infant with a large intraparenchymal hemorrhage has a much greater risk of cerebral palsy and/or mental retardation than a preterm infant with only a small germinal matrix hemorrhage.

The risk of later developmental disability increases with multiple risk factors, and the effects may be more than additive. There are demonstrable but generally small effects of prematurity or intrauterine growth retardation on IQ, but these effects are far more pronounced in children of lower socioeconomic classes. Preterm, small-for-gestational-age infants have a higher risk of developmental disability than either fullterm, small-for-gestational-age infants or preterm, appropriate-for-gestational-age infants.

Perinatal Factors Associated with Mildly Increased Risk

Table 10.2 lists a number of risk factors in terms of their relative degrees of risk for developmental disability. Factors that carry a mildly increased risk have been shown to be associated with a higher incidence of developmental disabilities in large population studies,

Table 10.2. Perinatal Predictors of Neurodevelopmental Outcome

Mildly increased risk
Socioeconomic status
Prematurity
Intrauterine growth retardation of unknown etiology
Apgar scores
Asymptomatic congenital infection
Asymptomatic hypoglycemia
Asymptomatic polycythemia
Obstetrical factors
Grades 1 and 2 periventricular/intraventricular hemorrhage
Moderate risk
Mild to moderate hypoxic-ischemic encephalopathy
Neonatal seizures
Congenital anomalies
Chronic lung disease
Sepsis or meningitis
Maternal ingestions
Symptomatic hypoglycemia
Symptomatic polycythemia
High risk
Known dysmorphic syndromes
Symptomatic congenital infections
Microcephaly, poor postnatal head growth
Severe hypoxic-ischemic encephalopathy
Abnormal cranial ultrasound/CT scan/MRI
Abnormal neonatal neurodevelopmental examination

but for individual infants, they are not very helpful in predicting outcome. Very low birth weight preterm infants (birth weight <1500 grams) have a higher risk of cerebral palsy and mental retardation than the general population, but the majority of infants are free of these major handicaps. In addition, the risk of major handicap does not appear to be related to birth weight or gestational age, except perhaps at the lowest extreme (i.e., birth weight <750 grams).

Apgar scores correlate with developmental outcome, but they are poorly predictive of individual outcome. Nelson and Ellenberg, using the data from the National Collaborative Perinatal Project, showed that even very low Apgar scores of 0 to 3 are not very predictive of later cerebral palsy unless they extend out to 10 to 20 minutes after birth. Infants with an Apgar score of 0 to 3 at 10 minutes had a very high mortality rate (69%), but as many as 80% of survivors were normal at age 7 years.

Asymptomatic infants with hypoglycemia, polycythemia, or congenital infection may have a slightly higher risk of handicap than infants without those conditions. As noted above, obstetrical factors, prematurity, and intrauterine growth retardation are risk factors, but associated complications are far better individual predictors of outcome. Germinal matrix and intraventricular hemorrhages without ventricular dilation (grades 1 and 2) appear to be associated with a mildly increased risk of developmental disability in preterm infants, although the significance of this risk is still somewhat controversial.

Perinatal Factors Associated with Moderate Risk

Perinatal factors that carry a moderate risk for developmental disability are listed in Table 10.2. Most are relatively uncommon, but when they occur, they carry a definite risk of developmental disability. These infants should be monitored during infancy and childhood. Sarnat and Sarnat developed a scoring system (Table 10.3) for severity of hypoxic-ischemic encephalopathy that includes neonatal symptoms, seizures, and EEG characteristics. Although stage 3 carries a uniformly poor prognosis (either death or handicap), stage 2 is associated with a moderate risk of handicap, and stage 1 is more benign. Neonatal seizures carry an increased risk of cerebral palsy, mental retardation, and epilepsy, but the degree of risk relates to their etiology. For example, recognized and treated hypocalcemia or subarachnoid hemorrhage has a good prognosis; meningitis or hypoxic ischemic encephalopathy has a moderate risk of handicaps; and developmental brain anomalies show an extremely poor prognosis. The presence of congenital anomalies, even without an identified syndrome, carries a higher risk of developmental disability.

Table 10.3. Components of Staging System for Hypoxic-Ischemic Encephalopathy[a]

	Stage 1	Stage 2	Stage 3
Level of consciousness	Hyperalert	Lethargic or obtunded	Stuporous
Neuromuscular control			
Muscle tone	Normal	Mild hypotonia	Flaccid
Posture	Mild distal flexion	Strong distal flexion	Intermittent decerebration
Stretch reflexes	Overactive	Overactive	Decreased or absent
Segmental myoclonus	Present	Present	Absent
Complex reflexes			
Suck	Weak	Weak or absent	Absent
Moro	Strong, low threshold	Weak; incomplete; high threshold	Absent
Oculovestibular	Normal	Overactive	Weak or absent
Tonic neck	Slight	Strong	Absent
Autonomic function	Generalized sympathetic	Generalized parasympathetic	Both systems decreased
Pupils	Mydriasis	Miosis	Variable, often unequal; poor light reflex
Heart rate	Tachycardia	Bradycardia	Variable
Bronchial and salivary secretions	Sparse	Profuse	Variable
Gastrointestinal motility	Normal or decreased	Increased diarrhea	Variable
Seizures	None	Common, focal, or multifocal	Uncommon (excluding decerebration)
Electroencephalogram findings	Normal (awake)	Early: low-voltage continuous delta and theta Later: periodic pattern (awake) Seizures, focal	Early: periodic pattern with isopotential phases Later: totally isopotential
Duration	<24 hrs	2 to 14 days	Hours to weeks

[a]Reprinted with permission from Sarnat HB, Sarnat MS. Neonatal encephalopathy following fetal distress. Arch Neurol 1976; 33:696–705. Copyright 1976, American Medical Association.

Perinatal Factors Associated with High Risk

Many chromosomal disorders and dysmorphic syndromes (e.g., Down's syndrome, Cornelia de Lange syndrome, Prader-Willi syndrome) have as one of their manifestations mental retardation and/or motor impairment with abnormalities of tone (generally, hypotonia with mild motor delay). Symptomatic toxoplasmosis, rubella, cytomegalovirus, and herpes infections are associated with very high mortality and handicap rates. Infants born with microcephaly and infants who manifest poor postnatal head growth have a high incidence of developmental disability, and this incidence is extremely high in infants who manifest both microcephaly and poor postnatal head growth. Severe hypoxic-ischemic encephalopathy (stage 3 of Sarnat's scoring system) is also associated with a high incidence of developmental disability.

Cranial imaging techniques and the neonatal neurodevelopmental examination are two excellent methods of determining an individual infant's degree of risk for developmental disability. Although there are very few findings that indicate certain handicap, a number of findings are associated with a very high risk for developmental disability. These findings indicate the need for careful, comprehensive developmental follow-up and may be indications for referral for early intervention services. Each of these methods is discussed in the following two sections.

Abnormalities of Cranial Ultrasound/CT Scan/MRI

Cranial ultrasound, computerized tomography, and magnetic resonance imaging are the most useful technologies for assessing intracranial structure in neonates, and each has its strengths and weaknesses. Computerized tomography requires exposure to radiation. Cranial ultrasounds are portable and can be performed in a NICU. Moving and effectively monitoring a sick, unstable infant is frequently an issue with computerized tomography and magnetic resonance imaging; of the two, computerized tomography allows better access to the infant.

Cranial ultrasound is the initial study of choice for diagnosing subependymal-intraventricular hemorrhage. Periventricular leukomalacia can often be detected by cranial ultrasound in the first week of life; it appears as a diffuse, somewhat ill-defined area of increased echogenicity. This then evolves over the next several weeks into cystic areas (decreased echogenicity). Periventricular leukomalacia may be either hemorrhagic or nonhemorrhagic, and only computerized tomography can distinguish between the two. However, in the early stages, computerized tomography may be normal.

Cranial ultrasound is less sensitive for detecting lesions close to the internal table of the skull, low in the brain, and in the posterior fossa. It is limited to infants with an open anterior fontanelle. Magnetic resonance imaging and computerized tomography are both effective for evaluating morphological and structural abnormalities and can be performed on older children. Magnetic resonance imaging is best able to detect abnormalities of and delay in patterns of myelination. It can also evaluate periventricular leukomalacia better than computerized tomography.

The preterm infant's brain is more vulnerable to certain types of injuries than that of the term infant, and the areas that are damaged are also often different. Tables 10.4 and 10.5 list the various findings on neuroimaging studies for preterm and term infants, respectively. Major findings can be viewed in relation to infarction, hemorrhage, and/or abnormal parenchymal density.

Table 10.4. Abnormalities on Cranial Ultrasound/CT Scan/MRI in Preterm Infants

Intracranial hemorrhage
- Subependymal or germinal matrix hemorrhage (grade 1)
- Intraventricular hemorrhage without ventricular dilation (grade 2) or with ventricular dilation (grade 3)
- Intraparenchymal (grade 4) hemorrhage

Ventricular dilation
Hydrocephalus
Periventricular leukomalacia
- Unilateral vs. bilateral
- Large vs. small
- Persistent vs. transient

Cortical atrophy
Porencephaly

Table 10.5. Abnormalities on Cranial Ultrasound/CT Scan/MRI in Fullterm Newborns

Infarctions
Hemorrhage
- Intraventricular
- Intraparenchymal
- Subarachnoid
- Subdural
- Intracerebellar

Encephalomalacia
Cortical atrophy
Porencephaly
Calcifications

Cortical atrophy, porencephaly, and intracranial calcifications can occur in either preterm or term infants. They generally signify a serious insult to the central nervous system and, therefore, a poor prognosis. Cortical atrophy results from diffuse brain injury and results in loss of brain tissue. Porencephaly is usually a result of a discrete infarction with subsequent loss of brain tissue adjacent to one of the lateral ventricles. Intracranial calcifications are seen in infants with congenital infections (e.g., toxoplasmosis, cytomegalovirus) or are late sequelae of hemorrhages. Cortical atrophy, porencephaly, and calcifications are usually signs of earlier damage, and if seen within days after birth, they suggest a prenatal insult.

NEUROIMAGING ABNORMALITIES IN PRETERM INFANTS

The major abnormalities seen in preterm infants are periventricular, intraventricular, or intraparenchymal hemorrhage; ventricular dilation or hydrocephalus; and periventricular leukomalacia or echodensities. These are best detected initially by cranial ultrasound, which is also easiest to use in the sick preterm infant. Computerized tomography and magnetic resonance imaging are both effective for evaluating the evolution of hydrocephalus and periventricular leukomalacia.

Periventricular/Intraventricular Hemorrhage (PVH/IVH)

Approximately 32 to 55% of preterm infants with birth weights <1500 grams develop PVH/IVH. Preterm infants above 32 weeks gestation who suffer hypoxia and/or respiratory distress are also vulnerable. A head ultrasound performed at 4 to 7 days will detect 90 to 96% of all hemorrhages in preterm infants. Mild hemorrhages clear sooner than severe ones, but most are resolved by 3 months.

Many use the grading system of Papile et al. In this system, grade 1 is a subependymal or germinal matrix hemorrhage; grade 2 is blood in the ventricles without ventricular dilation; grade 3 is blood in the ventricles with ventricular dilation; and grade 4 is intraparenchymal hemorrhage. Others describe the presence and severity of the hemorrhage separately from the degree of ventricular dilation. The grade 4 intraparenchymal hemorrhage is really a hemorrhagic infarction of the brain parenchyma just lateral to the lateral ventricle. Many feel that the hemorrhage is not intrinsically damaging to the brain; rather, it is a marker of brain insult, especially in the case of hemorrhagic intraparenchymal infarction.

Initial studies did not show an increased incidence of major handicaps in preterm infants with grade 1 or 2 hemorrhages. However, in larger sample sizes or with better or later testing, there might be a slightly increased risk of developmental problems in preterm infants with grade 1 or 2 hemorrhages in comparison to those without hemorrhages. Infants with grade 3 intraventricular hemorrhages have up to a 30% incidence of cerebral palsy and/or mental retardation and a 50% incidence of some developmental disability. Infants with grade 4 intraparenchymal hemorrhage are at even higher risk; they have approximately a 70% incidence of cerebral palsy and/or mental retardation and a 90% incidence of some developmental disability. The most common type of cerebral palsy seen in preterm infants with IVH is spastic diplegia. This is due to the location of the pyramidal tracts traveling through the internal capsule from the motor cortex to the limbs. Because the fibers to the lower extremities are medial to the fibers to the upper extremities and the fibers nearest to the ventricle are most likely to be damaged, the legs are affected much more than the arms.

Ventricular Dilation/Hydrocephalus

The occipital horn is generally the first part of the ventricle to enlarge after an intraventricular hemorrhage. Ventricular hemorrhage has been defined as an occipital horn greater than 1.6 cm in diameter. There is, however, significant interobserver and interstudy variability with respect to this measurement. Enlargement of the ventricles may be due to increased intracranial pressure or to necrosis and absorption of surrounding brain tissue. A number of studies have shown that preterm infants have an increased incidence of developmental disabilities with increased ventricular size, regardless of the presence of intraventricular hemorrhage.

Posthemorrhagic hydrocephalus occurs when intracranial hemorrhage causes arachnoiditis and/or obstruction to CSF outflow, resulting in ventricular dilation and compression of brain tissue. Infants with hydrocephalus have a high incidence of developmental disability (approximately 50 to 70%). If they are handicapped, they are more likely to be multiply handicapped than preterm infants with a similar hemorrhage and no hydrocephalus.

Periventricular Leukomalacia/Echodensities

Periventricular leukomalacia is an ischemic lesion of the periventricular white matter superolateral to the lateral ventricle; it may or may not be hemorrhagic. On cranial ultrasound, it initially appears as intraparenchymal echodensities, then becomes cystic over time. If the cysts are small, focal, and unilateral, there appears to be up to a 50 to 80% chance of developmental problems, especially cerebral palsy. If the cysts are bilateral, large, and diffuse, the risk of developmental disability (cerebral palsy and/or mental retardation) is extremely high (90 to 100%).

NEUROIMAGING ABNORMALITIES IN FULLTERM NEWBORNS

Major imaging abnormalities observed in fullterm newborns include infarctions; intraventricular, intraparenchymal, or subarachnoid hemorrhages; and diffuse encephalomalacia. Focal cerebral infarctions have a vascular distribution and typically have a wedge shape. In the first 2 to 3 days, computerized tomography may not detect an acute infarction. Infarctions may be seen with in utero exposure to cocaine, hypoxic-ischemic insults, and following treatment with extracorporeal membrane oxygenation (ECMO). The infant who develops a cerebral infarction is certainly at risk for developmental disability, depending on the size and location of the infarction. Nevertheless, newborns have a tremendous ability to compensate, and many with localized infarctions do well, with absent or mild motor impairment or mild cognitive impairments (e.g., learning disabilities).

The fullterm infant who suffers a hypoxic ischemic insult or birth trauma and/or is treated with ECMO can develop an intraventricular, intraparenchymal, or subarachnoid hemorrhage. Intraventricular hemorrhages in fullterm infants often derive from the choroid plexus. Subarachnoid hemorrhages are characterized by blood in the basal and pontine cisterns and cisterna magna. Severe hemorrhage may present as an acute syndrome with rapid deterioration to coma, brainstem dysfunction, seizures, and decerebrate posturing. Alternatively, it may present with subacute or even intermittent symptoms. The prognosis is related mainly to the location and degree of intraparenchymal involvement. Most infants with subarachnoid hemorrhage alone do well. Subdural and intracerebellar hemorrhages are generally related to birth trauma or perinatal asphyxia. They are relatively uncommon, but if severe, they may lead to death or later handicap.

An hypoxic-ischemic insult can result in a diffuse encephalomalacia. This abnormality in the densities of the brain parenchyma can best be detected by computerized tomography and correlates well with developmental outcome. The more extensive and diffuse the abnormalities, the worse the outcome.

The Neonatal Neurodevelopmental Examination

The neonatal neurodevelopmental examination, which is described in Chapter 9, has been used to assess preterm and term infants at risk for developmental disability. Fullterm, asphyxiated infants with abnormalities of tone, especially initial hypotonia followed by extensor hypertonia, have a high incidence of handicap, including severe multiple handicaps. High-risk preterm infants with an abnormal neurodevelopmental examination also have a high incidence of later developmental disability (primarily cerebral palsy and minor neuromotor dysfunction). In both fullterm and preterm infants, the more abnormal the examination, the higher the likelihood of developmental disability. Certain components of the examination (e.g., neck extensor hypertonia) are more predictive than others. In preterm infants, the examination is less predictive when it is performed prior to 36 weeks postmenstrual age than when it is performed near term (40 weeks postmenstrual age).

Like other risk factors, an abnormal neonatal neurodevelopmental examination is not 100% predictive of developmental disability. It can only be used to select a group of infants who need careful developmental follow-up and to guide intervention efforts (see Chapter

9). A normal neonatal examination can be reassuring; the vast majority of neonates (90 to 97%) with normal examinations do not develop a major handicap.

CONCLUSION

Perinatal and demographic risk factors should be assessed in both fullterm and preterm NICU infants prior to their discharge home. These risk factors cannot predict with certainty an individual infant's developmental outcome, but they are useful in guiding discharge planning. Reviewing them helps parents and staff to provide an overview of the child's prenatal, perinatal, and neonatal course. The absence of significant risk factors can be reassuring, although even fullterm infants with no risk factors still have a risk of developmental disability (albeit a small one). All infants should receive well-baby care that includes an assessment of developmental progress. However, NICU infants with perinatal risk factors, especially if they have multiple factors, require specific developmental follow-up that focuses on sequential developmental assessments, early diagnosis of developmental disabilities, and appropriate referral for early intervention services.

SUGGESTED READINGS

Allen MC. Developmental outcome and followup of the small for gestational age infant. Semin Perinatol 1984; 8:123–156.

Allen MC. Prematurity. In: Capute AJ, Accardo PJ, eds. Developmental disabilities in infancy and childhood. Baltimore: Paul H. Brookes, 1990.

Allen MC, Capute AJ. Neonatal neurodevelopmental examination as a predictor of neuromotor outcome in premature infants. Pediatrics 1989; 83:498–506.

Allen MC, Jones MD Jr. Medical complications of prematurity. Obstet Gynecol 1986; 67:427–437.

Bierman-van Eendenburg MEC, Jurgens-van der Zee AD, Olinga AA, et al. Predictive value of neonatal neurological examination: a follow-up study at 18 months. Develop Med Child Neurol 1981; 23:296–305.

Brown JK, Purvis RJ, Forfar JO, Cockburn P. Neurological aspects of perinatal asphyxia. Develop Med Child Neurol 1974; 16:567–580.

Cooke RWI. Early and late cranial ultrasonographic appearances and outcome in very low birthweight infants. Arch Dis Child 1987; 62:931–937.

Costello AM, Hamilton PA, Baudin J, et al. Prediction of neurodevelopmental impairment at four years from brain ultrasound appearance of very preterm infants. Develop Med Child Neurol 1988; 30:711–722.

Dubowitz LMS, Dubowitz V, Palmer PG, et al. Correlation of neurologic assessment in the preterm newborn infant with outcome at 1 year. J Pediatr 1984; 105:452–456.

Dykes FD, Dunbar B, Lazarra A, Ahmann PA. Posthemorrhagic hydrocephalus in high-risk preterm infants: natural history, management, and long-term outcome. J Pediatr 1989; 114:611–618.

Fitzhardinge PM, Flodmark O, Fitz CR, Ashby S. The prognostic value of computed tomography as an adjunct to assessment of the term infant with postasphyxial encephalopathy. J Pediatr 1981; 99:777–781.

Graziani LJ, Pasto M, Stanley C, et al. Neonatal neurosonographic correlates of cerebral palsy in preterm infants. Pediatrics 1986; 78:88–94.

Guzzetta F, Shackelford GD, Volpe S, et al. Periventricular intraparenchymal echodensities in the premature newborn: critical determinant of neurologic outcome. Pediatrics 1986; 78:995–1006.

Hadders-Algra M, Touwen BCL, Huisjes HJ. Neurologically deviant newborns: neurological and behavioural development at the age of six years. Develop Med Child Neurol 1986; 28:569–578.

Holden KR, Mellits ED, Freeman JM. Neonatal seizures. I. Correlation of prenatal and perinatal events with outcomes. Pediatrics 1982; 70:165–176.

Nelson KB, Ellenberg JH. Apgar scores as predictors of chronic neurologic disability. Pediatrics 1981; 68:36–44.

Palmer P, Dubowtiz LMS, Levine MI, Dubowitz V. Developmental and neurological progress of preterm infants with intraventricular haemorrhage and ventricular dilatation. Arch Dis Child 1982; 57:748–753.

Papile L-U, Munsich-Bruno G, Schaefer A. Relationship of cerebral intraventricular hemorrhage and early childhood neurologic handicaps. J Pediatr 1983; 103:273–277.

Papile L-U, Burstein J, Burstein R, Koffler H. Incidence and evolution of subependymal and intraventricular hemorrhage: a study of infants with birth weights less than 1,500 gms. J Pediatr 1978; 92:529–534.

Pena IC, Teberg AJ, Finello KM. The premature small-for-gestational-age infant during the first year of life: comparison by birth weight and gestational age. J Pediatr 1988; 113:1066–1073.

Robertson C, Finer N. Term infants with hypoxic-ischemic encephalopathy: outcome at 3–5 years. Develop Med Child Neurol 1985; 27:473–484.

Sarnat HB, Sarnat MS. Neonatal encephalopathy following fetal distress. Arch Neurol 1976; 33:696–705.

Sran SK, Baumann RJ. Outcome of neonatal strokes. Am J Dis Child 1988; 142:1086–1088.

Stevenson DK, Sunshine P. Fetal and neonatal brain injury. Philadelphia: Decker, 1989.

Volpe JJ. Neurology of the newborn. 2nd ed. Philadelphia: Saunders, 1987.

Volpe JJ, Herschovitch P, Perlman JM, Raichle ME. Positron emission tomography in the newborn: extensive impairment of regional cerebral blood flow with intraventricular hemorrhage and hemorrhagic intracerebral involvement. Pediatrics 1983; 72:589–601.

11

The Thyroid

Emily L. Germain-Lee and Leslie P. Plotnick

"Immunizations aside, the number of brilliant successes to be claimed by preventive medicine is not huge, but neonatal screening for hypothyroidism is certainly a shining one."

—Dr. Richard Goldbloom
in *Pediatric Notes, Vol 14, No 4, Jan. 25, 1990*

Thyroid hormones play a major role in the development of the neonate. By affecting basic cellular functions such as cell growth and differentiation, oxidative metabolism, protein synthesis, and carbohydrate and lipid metabolism, thyroid hormones influence numerous diverse processes, such as somatic and skeletal growth, nervous system development, erythropoiesis, and epidermal maturation. As a result, the multisystem problems seen in an infant in the neonatal intensive care unit may be due to or may be compounded by problems with the thyroid. Thus, it is of utmost importance that thyroid function be evaluated in these infants, not only while the infant is in the NICU, but also following discharge in order to ensure the infant's normal neurological development and somatic growth.

THYROID HORMONES AND THEIR REGULATION

The production of thyroid hormones is regulated by thyrotropin-releasing hormone (TRH) made by the hypothalamus. TRH stimulates the anterior pituitary gland to secrete thyroid-stimulating hormone (TSH), which in turn stimulates the thyroid gland to produce mainly thyroxine (T_4). T_4 is made from the coupling of two molecules of diiodotyrosine. Thyroxine is converted by deiodination to triiodothyronine (T_3) in the kidney, liver, and other peripheral tissues. T_3 is the metabolically active form of thyroid hormone. Reverse T_3 (rT_3) is synthesized from T_4 by a deiodinase distinct from the one that produces T_3 from T_4. rT_3 is less potent than T_3, and its levels are elevated during fetal life and during illness. High circulating T_4 and T_3 levels exert a negative feedback effect on the pituitary gland to suppress the further release of TSH.

T_4 exists both bound to carrier proteins and free in the circulation. Normally, 99.8% of the total thyroxine pool exists in the bound form, with 75% bound to thyroxine-binding globulin (TBG), 20% to thyroxine-binding prealbumin, and 5% to albumin. Only 0.2% of the total thyroxine exists as free T_4. T_3 concentrations in the blood are approximately 2% that of T_4 levels.

LABORATORY EVALUATION

All evaluations of thyroid function should begin with a determination of thyroid hormone levels present in the circulation. Levels of thyroid hormones can be directly measured by radioimmunoassay (RIA). RIAs for total T_4 and T_3 and for free T_4 and T_3 are available. While direct measurement of TBG by RIA is also available, most laboratories use an indirect measurement called the T_3 resin uptake (T_3RU) to assess the number of available protein binding sites not occupied by T_4. In this assay, radiolabeled T_3 added to the patient's serum binds to the available TBG binding sites that are not occupied by T_4; a resin that binds T_3 is then added to adsorb the unbound, radiolabeled T_3. Therefore, the fewer TBG binding sites available, the more T_3 binds to the resin and the higher the T_3RU. The free thyroxine index (FTI) is a commonly used method to correct the T_4 for protein binding by multiplying the T_4 by the T_3RU.

In order to interpret abnormal thyroid hormone levels, it is usually necessary to obtain TSH levels, which are currently most commonly measured by RIA. If TSH levels are high in the presence of a low T_4, the patient has an intrinsic thyroid abnormality (primary hypothyroidism). In its early phase, primary hypothyroidism may be manifested initially by an elevation of TSH alone. However, if the TSH is low in the presence of a low free T_4, a TRH stimulation test is necessary. Normally, when TRH is infused intravenously (7 μg/kg), there is at first a rapid rise in the serum TSH, followed by a slow decline back to the normal range. Both the rate and magnitude of the TSH response after TRH infusion are useful in distinguishing primary thyroid dysfunction from pituitary or hypothalamic dysfunction (central hypothyroidism).

Radiological studies in the neonate that utilize radioisotopes for the localization of ectopic thyroid tissue or for the evaluation of dyshormonogenesis are helpful, but limited. Radiological studies are usually not performed in neonates because of logistical problems in administering the test. For example, a common problem is the regurgitation of orally-administered radiographical trace by the infant, resulting in areas on the skin that can be falsely interpreted as thyroid tissue. In addition, these studies require that the infant be transported for radiological evaluation, which may be difficult for the severely ill patient in the NICU.

THYROID DEVELOPMENT

The thyroid gland first appears by approximately 4 weeks gestation and then migrates to its normal position by 7 weeks. At 8 to 10 weeks gestation, the fetal thyroid traps iodide, and by 10 to 12 weeks, both the thyroid and pituitary glands are well-formed, although inactive. By the end of the first trimester, the fetal thyroid can couple iodotyrosines to form thyroxine and triiodothyronine and can release thyroid hormones into the circulation. These do not cross the placenta. During the last trimester, serum total and free T_4 levels progressively increase with an accompanying gradual increase in TBG levels. These changes occur despite a constant TSH level. Before 30 weeks gestation, there is a preferential conversion of T_4 to rT_3 rather than to T_3, leading to relatively high rT_3 levels and low T_3

Table 11.1. Normal Values of Thyroid Function Tests vs. Age[a]

Age	T_4 (μg/dl)	T_3 (ng/dl)	TBG (mg/dl)	TSH (μU/ml)
Cord blood	10.8 (6.6–17.5)[b]	50 (14–86)	2.7 (0.7–4.7)	9.0 (<2.5–17.4)
1 to 3 days	16.5 (11.0–21.5)	240 (100–380)		8.0 (<2.5–13.3)
1 to 4 weeks	12.9 (8.2–16.6)	176 (99–310)	2.5 (0.5–4.5)	4.0 (0.6–10.0)
1 to 12 months	11.2 (7.2–15.6)	175 (102–264)	2.6 (1.6–3.6)	2.1 (0.6–6.3)
1 to 5 years	10.5 (7.3–15.0)	168 (105–269)	2.1 (1.3–2.8)	2.0 (0.6–6.3)
6 to 10 years	9.3 (6.4–13.3)	150 (94–241)	2.0 (1.4–2.6)	2.0 (0.6–6.3)
11 to 15 years	8.1 (5.6–11.7)	133 (83–213)	2.0 (1.4–2.6)	1.9 (0.6–6.3)
16 to 20 years	8.0 (4.2–11.8)	130 (80–210)	2.0 (1.4–2.6)	1.8 (0.2–7.6)
21 to 50 years	7.3 (4.3–12.5)	123 (70–204)	1.8 (1.2–2.4)	1.8 (0.2–7.6)

[a]From Donohoue PA. The thyroid gland. In: Oski FA, DeAngelis CD, Feigin RD, Warshaw JB, eds. Principles and practice of pediatrics. Philadelphia: Lippincott, 1990:1817. Data are adapted from Fisher DA. The thyroid. In: Kaplan SA, ed. Clinical pediatric endocrinology. Philadelphia: Saunders, 1990: 95; and LaFranchi S. Hypothyroidism, congenital and acquired. In: Kaplan SA, ed. Clinical pediatric and adolescent endocrinology. Philadelphia: Saunders, 1982:87.
[b]Range (±2 S.D. from the mean)

levels. During the last 5 to 10 weeks of gestation, this pattern is reversed, leading to progressively increasing T_3 levels and decreasing rT_3 levels.

NEONATAL THYROID FUNCTION: FULLTERM VS. PREMATURE

As shown in Table 11.1, normal values for thyroid function tests vary as a function of postnatal age in the fullterm infant and are markedly different from those in an adult. TSH levels increase within 30 minutes after birth, rapidly decrease in the first 24 hours of life, and then slowly decrease over the next 2 days, returning to near baseline levels by 48 to 96 hours of age. Total T_4 and free T_4 levels peak at 24 hours and remain higher than baseline for 2 to 3 weeks after birth before decreasing slowly over the next few weeks of life. T_3 levels show a rise in the first 3 to 6 hours after birth, followed by a secondary rise at 24 to 72 hours and then a return to baseline levels by approximately 1 week of age. TBG levels remain relatively constant throughout this period.

This pattern of T_4 and TSH levels in the first 5 days of life is also seen in premature infants. However, as shown in Figure 11.1, the early rises of T_4 and TSH levels are lower in premature infants than in fullterm infants. The blunting of the elevation of these hormone levels is more severe in lower birth weight premature infants. As shown in Figure 11.2, there is a direct correlation between the decrease in T_4 levels at birth and the gestational age of the infant; i.e., the younger the gestational age, the lower the T_4. This gap is maintained even as the postnatal age of the infant increases. The normal ranges of thyroxine levels for premature versus term infants at various postnatal ages are summarized in Tables 11.2A and 11.2B. T_3 levels are also low in the premature infant as a result of a preferential conversion

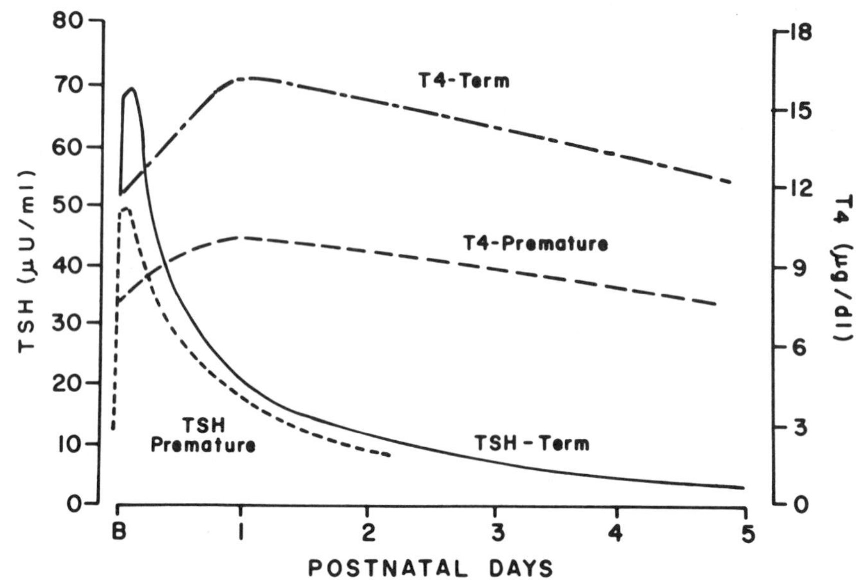

Figure 11.1. Changes in serum TSH and T_4 concentrations in fullterm and premature infants during the first 5 days of life. (From Fisher DA, Klein AH. Thyroid development and disorders of thyroid function in the newborn. Reprinted with permission of N Engl J Med 1981;304:706.)

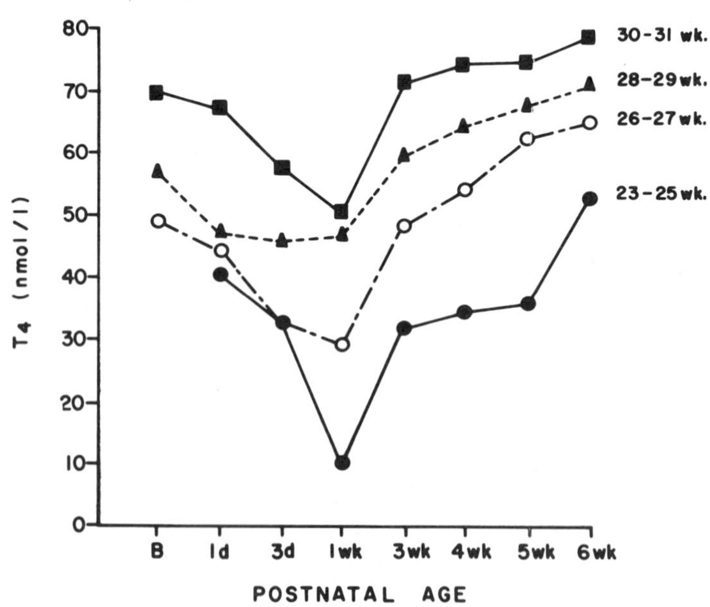

Figure 11.2. Mean T_4 values in four gestational age groups vs. postnatal age. (Reprinted with permission from Mercado M, Yu VYH, Francis I, Szymonowicz W, Gold H. Thyroid function in very preterm infants. Early Hum Dev 1988;16:134.)

Table 11.2A. Serum T_4 Levels in Premature Infants vs. Age[a]

	Estimated Gestational Age (weeks)				
	30 to 31	32 to 33	34 to 35	36 to 37	Term
Cord	6.5±1.0[b]	7.5±2.1	6.7±1.2	7.5±2.8	8.2±1.8
12 to 72 hours	11.5±2.1	12.3±3.2	12.4±3.1	15.5±2.6	19.0±2.1
3 to 10 days	7.7±1.8	8.5±1.9	10.0±2.4	12.7±2.5	15.9±3.0
11 to 20 days	7.5±1.8	8.3±1.6	10.5±1.8	11.2±2.9	12.2±2.0
21 to 45 days	7.8±1.5	8.0±1.7	9.3±1.3	11.4±4.2	12.1±1.5
		30 to 37 weeks			Term
46 to 90 days		9.6±1.7			10.2±1.9

[a]Reprinted with permission from Cuestas RA. Thyroid function in healthy premature infants. J Pediatr 1978;92:964.
[b]Serum T_4 (μg/dl); mean ± 1 SD

Table 11.2B. T_4 and Free T_4 (FT_4) Levels in Sera From Premature and Fullterm Newborns (Cord Blood), 2-Month-Old Infants, and Adults[a]

Age	T_4 (μg/dl)[b]	FT_4 (ng/dl)[b]
Cord samples:		
26 to 29 weeks	6.7 (5.9–7.7) n=18	1.25 (1.12–1.39) n=18
30 to 31 weeks	7.8 (7.0–8.7) n=23	1.41 (1.28–1.55) n=23
32 to 33 weeks	8.9 (8.1–9.7) n=31	1.59 (1.49–1.70) n=31
≥34 weeks	10.4 (9.9–11.0) n=88	1.67 (1.61–1.74) n=88
2-month-old infants	11.2 (9.6–13.1) n=9	2.08 (1.88–2.30) n=9
Adults	7.6 (6.9–8.3)	1.30 (1.20–1.42)

[a]Reprinted with permission from Klein AH, Oddie TH, Parslow M, Foley TP Jr, Fisher DA. Developmental changes in pituitary-thyroid function in the human fetus and newborn. Early Hum Dev 1982;6:324.
[b]Geometric mean with 95% confidence limits of the mean in parentheses.

to rT_3, but these levels gradually normalize. Similarly, TBG levels are lower in infants less than 34 weeks gestation. They increase slightly and then remain relatively steady with time.

MASS POPULATION SCREENING

Mass population screening was started in 1974 and has permitted much earlier detection of hypothyroidism in both fullterm and premature infants. Currently, infants in all states are screened within the first 3 to 7 days of life with an initial T_4 determination, except in Illinois where infants are initially screened with a TSH measurement. Several of the states that screen with an initial T_4 do a TSH measurement concurrently or in the 5 to 11% of infants with the lowest T_4s. The initial screen should not be done until at least the third day of life, after the normal postdelivery T_4 elevation and TSH surge have returned to baseline. Seven states require a second screen to be done between the second and sixth

Table 11.3. Congenital Hypothyroxinemia

		Initial Screen		Follow-up Screen (2 to 6 weeks of age)			
Etiology	Prevalence	T_4	TSH	T_4	Free T_4	T_3RU	TSH
Transient hypothyroxinemia	1:200 (overall) 1:1–5 (premature)	Low	Nl	Nl	Nl	Nl/High	Nl
Transient primary hypothyroidism	1:40,000 (fullterm) (U.S.A.) 1:100–600 (fullterm) (iodine-deficient areas) Common (prematures)	Low	High	Nl	Nl	Nl	Nl
Permanent primary hypothyroidism							
Thyroid dysgenesis	1:4,000	Low	High	Low	Low	Low	High
Thyroid dyshormonogenesis	1:30,000						
Central hypothyroidism	1:100,000	Low	Low/Nl	Low	Low	Low	Low/Nl
TBG deficiency	1:5,400–13,000	Low	Nl	Low	Nl	High	Nl

weeks of life. For the acutely ill premature infant, where obtaining samples for the initial neonatal screen may be problematic, the current recommendation is that the first specimen be received within the first 14 days of life. Preferably, this should be done before a blood transfusion because a transfusion can cause a false elevation of T_4 and a false depression of TSH by mixing with adult blood. If this is unavoidable, one should wait at least 3 days before obtaining the specimen. The second screen should be done prior to discharge. There have been unfortunate cases in which hypothyroidism was missed in the acutely ill NICU infant because a neonatal screen was not obtained.

ETIOLOGIES OF HYPOTHYROXINEMIA

Hypothyroxinemia (low serum T_4 levels) in the neonate can result from a variety of conditions. The overall prevalence and the patterns of thyroid function tests typically seen in each of these conditions are summarized in Table 11.3.

Transient Hypothyroxinemia

Premature infants, as well as small-for-gestational-age and ill infants, often exhibit a condition known as transient hypothyroxinemia. This is manifested by low serum T_4 levels without an accompanying elevation in TSH levels and with normal T_4 and TSH responses to TRH. These infants also appear to have slightly lower TBG levels and slightly lower T_4 affinities for TBG, which can thus result in normal free T_4 levels in some of these infants. Transient hypothyroxinemia is quite common and, in a study by Mercado et al. in 1988, has been observed at least once during the first 6 weeks of life in 100% of 23 to 25 week gestation infants, 40% of 26 to 27 week gestation infants, 33% of 28 to 29 week gestation infants, and 17% of 30 to 31 week gestation infants. This condition is believed to be representative of tertiary hypothyroidism resulting from immaturity of the hypothalamic-pituitary-thyroid axis. Transient hypothyroxinemia usually resolves spontaneously by approximately 34 weeks gestation and does not require treatment. Although the majority of the low T_4 levels seen in premature infants can be attributed to transient hypothyroxinemia, it is important to measure TSH levels in order to rule out actual primary hypothyroidism.

Hypothyroidism

Hypothyroidism can result from a problem within the thyroid gland itself (primary hypothyroidism), from lack of pituitary stimulation of the thyroid gland (secondary hypothyroidism), or from a lack of hypothalamic stimulation (tertiary hypothyroidism). Secondary and tertiary hypothyroidism are also referred to as central hypothyroidism.

Clinical signs of hypothyroidism are mostly seen with primary hypothyroidism and include dry, coarse, and cool skin often with cutis marmorata, large fontanels, large tongue, umbilical hernia, poor feeding, weak cry, anemia, prolonged physiological jaundice, delayed stooling, bradycardia, lethargy, depressed nasal bridge, and puffiness of the eyelids. Because these symptons may be subtle or may appear late, one must often rely on laboratory evaluation to detect impaired thyroid function.

TRANSIENT PRIMARY HYPOTHYROIDISM

Transient primary hypothyroidism encompasses those conditions with low T_4 levels, elevated TSH levels, and markedly increased TSH response to TRH. Transient hypothyroidism can be caused by iodine deficiency or excess, or by antithyroid medications or immunoglobulins passed transplacentally to the fetus. Although this condition occurs in 1 in 40,000 fullterm infants, premature infants are at a much increased risk for this condition.

Iodine Deficiency

Transient primary hypothyroidism resulting from iodine deficiency is commonly seen in countries with inadequate iodine supplies. For example, the incidence of transient hypothyroidism in fullterm infants in Belgium and Central Germany is 1:600 and 1:100, respectively. Similarly, in endemic goiter areas in Africa, the incidence has been found to be as high as 1 in 10 live births. This condition is rarely seen in North America, where iodine deficiency is not a problem. Premature infants are at a higher risk for transient primary hypothyroidism caused by iodine deficiency because they require higher iodine intake levels than term infants to maintain a positive iodine balance. In one study, conducted in Belgium by Delange et al. in 1984, approximately 20% of premature infants developed transient primary hypothyroidism from iodine deficiency, and the incidence decreased with increasing gestational age. Typically, the initial TSH levels in these infants are within normal limits, and hypothyroidism develops subsequently during the first 1 to 2 weeks of extrauterine life.

Iodine Excess

Iodine-induced hypothyroidism is a much more common cause of transient hypothyroidism in the premature infant in this country, representing, in fact, the most common cause of transient primary hypothyroidism in the NICU population. Excess iodine is believed to have an inhibitory effect on thyroid hormone synthesis and release (Wolff-Chaikoff effect) and thereby causes hypothyroidism. An excess iodine load can result from even the most apparently routine procedures, such as repeated blooddrawing or painting of the umbilical stump. Povodine and betadine, which is composed of 10% povodine-iodine and has an available iodine content of 1%, have both been shown to result in excess iodine loads from skin absorption. Indeed, a recent Australian study by Smerdely et al. in 1989 examined thyroid function tests in low birth weight infants treated either with topical iodinated antiseptics or with chlorhexidine. Within 14 days, 25% of the infants exposed to iodine had elevated TSH and diminished T_4 levels and elevated urinary excretion of iodine; in contrast, in the non-iodine-exposed control patients, no transient neonatal hypothyroidism was observed. Of note is that the greater the iodine exposure, the more profound the hypothyroidism.

Premature infants are particularly susceptible to iodine-induced hypothyroidism for several reasons. First, premature infants absorb greater amounts of iodine through their skin than do term infants as a result of the paucity of subcutaneous tissue. Second, the ability of the thyroid cell to regulate iodine transport matures near term. Thus, premature infants with high plasma iodine levels will have greater uptake of iodine into thyroid cells. Finally, premature infants are at a greater risk of iodine exposure given their increased stay in the hospital, multiple invasive procedures, and increased risk of undergoing surgical procedures, including abdominal procedures in which there is peritoneal absorption of iodine, and cardiac catheterizations.

In Utero Exposure

Iodine exposure can also occur in utero because iodine can readily cross the placenta. For example, radiographical contrast material given to the mother during pregnancy can result in fetal iodine intoxication. Similarly, medications containing iodine, such as certain aminophylline preparations and sinus medications, that are given to the mother during pregnancy can also lead to iodine intoxication in the infant.

Finally, transient hypothyroidism in both fullterm and preterm infants can result from transplacental passage of other substances capable of suppressing the infant's own thyroid function. One example is the use of antithyroid drugs like propylthiouracil or methimazole for maternal hyperthyroidism. Less common examples include TSH receptor blocking antibodies and the antimicrosomal and antithyroglobulin autoantibodies found in maternal autoimmune thyroid disease. These autoantibody effects can persist for up to several months in the infant. Transient congenital hypothyroidism resulting from iodine exposure or maternal use of antithyroid drugs and iodine-containing drugs leads much more frequently to goiter formation than do other causes of hypothyroidism.

PERMANENT PRIMARY HYPOTHYROIDISM

Permanent primary hypothyroidism refers to congenital thyroid dysfunction resulting from developmental abnormalities of the thyroid gland. Permanent hypothyroidism occurs in approximately 1 out of 4000 live births with equal frequencies in preterm and fullterm infants. The incidence varies with race, occurring more frequently in Asian and Hispanic infants (1:2,000), less frequently in white infants (1:5,000), and least frequently in black infants (1:32,000). Overall, there is a 2:1 female-to-male preponderance. Patients with permanent primary hypothyroidism have low T_4 and elevated TSH levels.

Permanent primary hypothyroidism most commonly results from abnormal migration of thyroid tissue during fetal development, which leads to the formation of an ectopic thyroid gland that does not produce adequate amounts of thyroid hormone. Thyroid aplasia and hypoplasia are the second most common cause of permanent primary hypothyroidism. The third most common cause is dyshormonogenesis due to abnormalities of thyroid hormone synthesis and secretion, such as defects in iodine-trapping, organification, coupling, or deiodinase activity. Rarely, radioactive iodine given to a woman who is unsuspectingly pregnant for treatment of hyperthyroidism or cancer of the thyroid can cause damage of the fetal thyroid and result in permanent congenital hypothyroidism. All of these conditions require lifelong treatment with l-thyroxine and can lead to profound mental retardation and neurological dysfunction if not treated promptly and adequately.

Management

All infants with primary hypothyroidism should undergo replacement therapy to avoid the possibility of irreversible brain damage. As soon as the diagnosis is made in the newborn, treatment should be started with l-thyroxine at a dose of 8 to 10 μg/kg/day, except in infants with underlying cardiac disease in whom congestive heart failure could be precipitated. In these infants, one should begin with a lower dose and build up to the recommended regimen over a 1 to 2 week time span. Generic brands of l-thyroxine may have variable absorption; therefore, it may be more difficult to maintain a therapeutic range. Each tablet can be softened in formula immediately prior to its use and then administered with a plastic dropper directly into the infant's mouth. Soy-based formulas may result in excessive fecal loss of l-thyroxine and necessitate higher doses. The goal of treatment in all cases should be to maintain T_4 levels in the upper half of the normal range for age.

The duration of treatment depends on the etiology of the hypothyroidism and on whether the hypothyroidism is transient or permanent. If, for example, the hypothyroidism is thought to be secondary to iodine toxicity, the iodine exposure should be discontinued as soon as possible with close monitoring of thyroid function tests. Then, l-thyroxine therapy can be tapered, usually over 1 month after the iodine exposure has been removed. In other cases of hypothyroidism believed to be transient, such as exposure to antithyroid drugs, it is advisable to continue replacement therapy and to monitor thyroid function closely. In general, continued treatment with l-thyroxine is recommended either until the patient appears to be maintaining normal thyroid function on a dose that has obviously been outgrown, or until the patient reaches 3 years of age, by which time a significant portion of thyroid-dependent brain development has already been completed. In either case, thyroid function tests should initially be followed every few weeks until normal levels are observed.

Patients with permanent primary hypothyroidism should be maintained on l-thyroxine replacment therapy throughout their lives. Infants from 6 to 12 months of age usually require a dose of 5 to 8 μg/kg/day; children from 1 to 3 years of age require 3 to 6 μg/kg/day; and children over the age of 3 years require about 3 to 4 μg/kg/day, increasing to adult doses of 100-200 μg/kg/day. Thyroid function tests should be checked at least every few weeks during the first several months of life and every 3 months in the early years thereafter to ensure adequate treatment. Height and weight should also be monitored. In addition, neurological development should be followed. Several months of treatment may be necessary before TSH levels return to the normal range, and one should not attempt to normalize the TSH level by continuing to increase T_4 levels. Rarely, the pituitary set-point in these patients may be increased, thus causing the TSH to remain elevated in spite of normal thyroxine levels.

Outcome

If primary hypothyroidism is not treated promptly, the infant is at risk for profound mental retardation. Therapy should be started as early as possible, preferably within the first few weeks of life. In a recent study by the New England Congenital Hypothyroidism Collaborative, 72 children whose treatments for congenital hypothyroidism were started at an average of 24 days of age were followed for several years, along with age and sex-matched controls, including siblings. No differences in IQ between the patients and controls were found. Other studies have shown that if treatment is not started until 6 weeks to 3 months of age, the average IQ decreases by approximately 5%, whereas if treatment is not initiated until 6 months of age, the average IQ is less than or equal to 55. This decrease in IQ is irreversible. In addition, other neurological disorders, including speech and hearing defects, attention deficit disorder, and ataxia, may develop.

CENTRAL HYPOTHYROIDISM

Central hypothyroidism refers to inadequate thyroid function resulting either from a lack of TSH stimulation (secondary hypothyroidism) or from a lack of TRF stimulation (tertiary hypothyroidism). Both of these forms of hypothyroidism are much less prevalent (1:100,000) than primary hypothyroidism. Central hypothyroidism can be distinguished from primary hypothyroidism on the basis of the pattern of thyroid function tests. Total and free T_4 levels are low in both, but TSH levels are not elevated and are often low in central hypothyroidism. The serum T_4 is usually not as low in central hypothyroidism as in primary disease. As a result, the clinical symptoms are usually not as severe in central hypothyroidism.

Patients with central hypothyroidism should be tested for other possible pituitary hormonal deficiencies, especially to rule out ACTH deficiency, which could be life-threatening. Clues to panhypopituitarism include hypoglycemia, midline defects of the head (such as cleft lip, cleft palate, or septo-optic dysplasia), optic nerve hypoplasia, abnormal eye movements such as new onset nystagmus or esotropia, severe CNS malformations, and micropenis in the male infant. If central hypothyroidism is suspected, l-thyroxine therapy should not be initiated until the adrenal axis has been evaluated and treatment started if necessary because the initiation of thyroid replacement may cause an increased clearance of cortisol and precipitate adrenal crisis. Once the adrenal axis is evaluated, l-thyroxine therapy should be started at the same doses as in primary hypothyroidism. The neurological outcome of infants with central hypothyroidism is difficult to assess because many of these children already have associated central nervous system abnormalities. However, the clinical symptoms overall are usually less pronounced compared to those of primary hypothyroidism, including the degree of intellectual impairment.

Thyroxine-Binding Globulin (TBG) Deficiency

TBG deficiency is a common cause of newborn hypothyroxinemia, representing 10% of fullterm males whose initial thyroid screens reveal low T_4 levels. The disorder is inherited as an X-linked trait and occurs at a frequency of 1:5,400 to 13,000. Male infants with TBG deficiency have normal free T_4 and TSH levels and, therefore, normal thyroid function. However, they have anomalously low total T_4 and T_3 levels with high T_3RU values. Heterozygous females have intermediate levels of TBG and resultant low-normal T_4 levels and high-normal T_3RU levels. Family members should be made aware of the inheritance pattern of this trait. Although TBG deficiency does not require treatment, it is important in the NICU infant to consider other disease processes, such as protein malnutrition, protein-losing enteropathy, hepatic cirrhosis, and nephrotic syndrome, that can lower TBG levels by lowering the total protein levels.

MATERNAL HYPOTHYROIDISM

Mothers who have untreated hypothyroidism during pregnancy should be treated with l-thyroxine as soon as possible. These mothers have increased numbers of stillbirths, abortions, and premature deliveries. The infant makes thyroid hormones independently of the mother, and only minimal transplacental passage of thyroxine from the maternal to fetal circulation occurs. As a result, the infant's thyroid function should be preserved.

Infants born to mothers being treated with l-thyroxine are not affected by this medication because l-thyroxine crosses the placenta in only minimal amounts. In addition, only minimal amounts of l-thyroxine pass into breast milk; therefore, it is not a contraindication to breastfeeding.

(Also, see Transient Primary Hypothyroidism, In Utero Exposure.)

OTHER THYROID ABNORMALITIES IN THE PREMATURE AND ILL INFANT

Transient Hyperthyrotropinemia

Although rare, premature infants have a higher incidence of transient hyperthyrotropinemia, which is marked by elevated serum levels of TSH with normal serum levels of total and free T_4. The TSH elevation is usually transient, lasting a few days to several months. It is important to monitor thyroid function tests to ensure that the TSH elevation subsides and that the infant does not suffer from early primary hypothyroidism, in which TSH levels can rise before T_4 levels drop. Rarely, the apparent TSH elevation may result from artifacts in TSH assays such as interference by maternal immunoglobulins or by components of parenteral nutrition, such as lipid emulsions.

Low T_3 Syndrome

Premature infants and infants with nonthyroidal illnesses are particularly susceptible to the low T_3 syndrome, which is also known as the euthyroid sick syndrome. This syndrome is characterized by low T_3 levels, normal or low T_4 levels, and normal TSH levels. Low T_3 syndrome is believed to result from a decreased rate of conversion of T_4 to T_3 in nonthyroidal tissues and preferential conversion to reverse T_3. This inhibition of T_4-to-T_3 conversion in turn is believed to result from prematurity and from various stressors, such as respiratory distress syndrome, hypoxia, hypoglycemia, malnutrition, and infection. These infants may also exhibit low total T_4 levels because of the decreased ability of the premature infant's pituitary to secrete TSH. In some patients, however, the free T_4 levels may be normal due to low TBG levels or to the presence of a circulating inhibitor of thyroxine that binds to TBG. As the infant recovers from the underlying problem, the TSH levels usually rise, and the T_3 and T_4 levels return to normal. Thyroid function tests should be followed to make sure that the rise in TSH levels is not accompanied by a further fall in thyroxine levels, which is characteristic of primary hypothyroidism. Treatment for the low T_3 syndrome is not recommended; the decreased T_4 and T_3 levels are believed to serve a protective function by slowing down metabolic processes in the premature and/or ill infant. In a study of 39 premature infants with low T_3 syndrome, Fisher et al. showed normal neurological development up to 1 year of age without treatment.

Respiratory Distress Syndrome

Because thyroxine is thought to aid in the induction of surfactant production by type II pneumocytes in the lung, it has been speculated that thyroxine deficiency could make an infant more prone to respiratory distress syndrome (RDS). While this theory is still somewhat controversial, several studies have shown T_4 and T_3 levels in infants with RDS to be significantly lower than those in healthy preterm infants for several weeks after birth. Whether the reduced thyroxine levels in these patients precipitated the RDS or vice versa remains to be determined. Nevertheless, it is important to monitor TSH levels in these patients because of their additional increased risk for transient primary hypothyroidism secondary to prematurity and/or iodine exposure.

Medications

Certain medications commonly given to infants in the NICU and following discharge can cause abnormalities of thyroid function. Glucocorticoids can cause transient increases in TSH levels and decreases in total and free T_4 and T_3 levels by enhancing hormonal clearance rates. Phenytoin can also decrease total and free T_4 even into the hypothyroid range by inhibiting the binding of T_4 and T_3 to TBG and therefore increasing the cellular uptake and degradation of T_4. Phenobarbital can decrease T_4 and T_3 levels by enhancing the hepatic degradation and metabolic clearance of T_4. Finally, certain medications, like betamethasone or ritodrine, and general anesthesia, administered to the mothers of premature infants prior to delivery, can also lead to low T_4 levels in the infant. Hypothyroxinemia resulting from the use of any of these medications may necessitate treatment with l-thyroxine.

Neonatal Hyperthyroidism

Unlike neonatal hypothyroidism, congenital hyperthyroidism is rare, accounting for less than 5% of all cases of hyperthyroidism. However, when it occurs, neonatal hyperthyroidism (also known as neonatal thyrotoxicosis) may require that the infant be monitored in the neonatal intensive care unit. Symptoms and signs include jitteriness and irritability, tachycardia, tachypnea, cardiac failure, diarrhea, failure-to-thrive, proptosis, hepatomegaly, jaundice, and thrombocytopenia. In addition, these infants often have goiters, which can even be significant enough to cause respiratory distress.

Neonatal thyrotoxicosis occurs almost exclusively in infants of mothers with Graves' disease, with 1 in 70 such infants being afflicted. It may be initially masked by hypothyroidism caused by the placental passage of antithyroid drugs such as propylthiouracil (PTU) or methimazole that are administered to the mother during pregnancy. For this reason, it is recommended that the mother's dose be tapered to the lowest that adequately controls her hyperthyroidism. In addition, PTU is preferable to methimazole during pregnancy because PTU crosses the placenta to a much lesser extent. PTU is also preferable in the postpartum period if the mother is breastfeeding because of its significantly decreased ability to pass into the milk. These antithyroid drugs are usually cleared from the infant's circulation within 2 to 4 weeks after birth, and thyroid function studies return to normal within 4 to 6 weeks after birth. The hyperthyroidism that can develop in the neonate is believed to be secondary to transplacental passage of maternal thyroid-stimulating immunoglobulins (TSI). Laboratory evaluation typically shows elevated total and free T_4 and T_3 levels with undetectable TSH levels. In some cases, T_4 levels can be normal; therefore, T_3 levels must be measured. The effect of the maternal immunoglobulins may persist for several months. Very rarely, the infant may produce the TSI from his or her own lymphocytes, in which case the hyperthyroidism may persist for a longer period of time.

MANAGEMENT

Treatment is indicated if the infant exhibits symptoms of hyperthyroidism. If tachycardia is a predominant symptom, propranolol should be started at 2 mg/kg/day orally and can be gradually increased. If other symptoms are also present, therapy includes Lugol's solution (5% iodine and 10% potassium iodide), 1 drop every 8 hours, and propylthiouracil (PTU), 5 to 10 mg/kg/day. Before starting PTU, a baseline white count with differential should be obtained because PTU can cause granulocytopenia. In some cases, dexamethasone is also helpful. If there is no improvement within 24 hours, the Lugol's and PTU doses should be increased by 50%. Thyroid function tests need to be followed carefully. Sequelae of neonatal thyrotoxicosis, even in patients who have been treated immediately upon symptom detection, include premature craniosynostosis and neurodevelopmental delay.

Thyroxine-Binding Globulin Excess

This X-linked dominant trait, occurring with an approximate prevalence of 1:40,000, is harmless, but it can result in an elevated T_4 level on the newborn screen. This is associated with a normal TSH and free T_4 and a decreased T_3RU. The patients are, therefore, euthyroid. Family members should be made aware of the inheritance pattern of this trait.

CONCLUSION

A variety of factors contribute to the increased risk of thyroid abnormalities for the infant in the neonatal intensive care unit. These risk factors include prematurity itself as well as concurrent illnesses, medications, and iodine exposure. As a result, one must always maintain a high index of suspicion for the development of hypothyroidism, especially in patients exposed to iodine during invasive procedures. It is important to monitor thyroid function tests in all infants in the NICU so that any necessary treatment can be initiated promptly. Delaying treatment may put the infant at additional risk for severe neurological and somatic developmental delay.

Thyroid abnormalities diagnosed while the patient is in the NICU may persist for many months or, in the case of permanent primary hypothyroidism, can last a lifetime. In addition, the propensity in these infants for developmental delay and failure-to-thrive may be compounded by abnormalities in thyroid function if not adequately and promptly treated. Therefore, the necessity for continuing to assess thyroid function in those infants with abnormal thyroid function tests following their discharge from the NICU is extremely important.

SUGGESTED READINGS

Abbassi V, Merchant K, Abramson D. Postnatal triiodothyronine concentrations in healthy preterm infants and in infants with respiratory distress syndrome. Pediatr Res 1977; 11:802–804.

Benson RC. Medical and surgical complications during pregnancy. In: Benson RC, ed. Current obstetric and gynecologic diagnosis and treatment. Los Altos: Lange Medical Publications, 1982:851.

Borges M, Lanes R, Moret LA, Balochi D, Gonzalez S. Effect of asphyxia on free thyroid hormone levels in full term newborns. Pediatr Res 1985; 19:1305–1307.

Chabrolle JP, Rossier A. Goitre and hypothyroidism in the newborn after cutaneous absorption of iodine. Arch Dis Child 1978; 53:495–498.

Coakley JC, Francis I, Gold H, Mathur K, Connelly JF. Transient primary hypothyroidism in the newborn: experience of the Victorian neonatal thyroid screening programme. Aust Paediatr J 1989; 25:25–30.

Cuestas RA. Thyroid function in healthy premature infants. J Pediatr 1978; 92:963–967.

Cuestas RA, Engel RR. Thyroid function in preterm infants with respiratory distress syndrome. J Pediatr 1979; 94:643–646.

Cuestas RA, Lindall A, Engel RR. Low thyroid hormones and respiratory-distress syndrome of the newborn. N Engl J Med 1976; 295:297–302.

Delange F, Bourdoux P, Ermans A-M. Transient disorders of thyroid function and regulation in preterm infants. In: Delange F, Fisher DA, Malvaux P, eds. Pediatric thyroidology. Basel, Switzerland: S. Karger AG, 1985:369–393.

Delange F, Dalhem A, Bourdaux P, et al. Increased risk of primary hypothyroidism in preterm infants. J Pediatr 1984; 105:462–469.

Delange F, Dodion J, Wolter R, et al. Transient hypothyroidism in the newborn infant. J Pediatr 1978; 92:974–976.

Diamond FB, Parks JS, Tenore A, Marino JM, Bongiovanni AM. Hypothyroxinemia in sick and well preterm infants. Clin Pediatr 1979; 18:555–561.

DiGeorge AM. Disorders of the thyroid gland. In: Nelson WE, Behrman RE, Vaughan VC, eds. Nelson textbook of pediatrics. Philadelphia: Saunders, 1987:1193–1201.

Donohoue PA. The thyroid gland. In: Oski FA, DeAngelis CD, Feigin RD, Warshaw JB, eds. Principles and practices of pediatrics. Philadelphia: Lippincott, 1990:1816–1824.

Fisher DA. The thyroid. In: Kaplan SA, ed. Clinical pediatric endocrinology. Philadelphia: Saunders, 1990:87–126.

Fisher DA, Foley BL. Early treatment of congenital hypothyroidism. Pediatrics 1989; 83:785–789.

Fisher DA, Klein AH. Thyroid development and disorders of thyroid function in the newborn. N Engl J Med 1981; 304:702–712.

Fisher DA, Klein AH, Hadeed A. Normal and abnormal thyroid function in premature infants: the low T_3 syndrome. In: Hesch R-D, ed. The "low T_3 syndrome". London: Academic Press, 1981:225–231.

Franklin RC, Carpenter LM, O'Grady CM. Neonatal thyroid function: influence of perinatal factors. Arch Dis Child 1985; 60:141–144.

Franklin RC, O'Grady CM. Neonatal thyroid function: effects of nonthyroidal illness. J Pediatr 1985; 107:599–602.

Franklin RC, Purdie GL, O'Grady CM. Neonatal thyroid function: prematurity, prenatal steroids, and respiratory distress syndrome. Arch Dis Child 1986; 61:589–592.

Hadeed AJ, Asay LD, Lein AH, Fisher DA. Significance of transient postnatal hypothyroxinemia in premature infants with and without respiratory distress syndrome. Pediatrics 1981; 68:494–498.

Hirano T, Singh J, Srinivasan G, Pildes R. Postnatal thyroid function in low birth weight infants: a longitudinal assessment of free thyroxine and thyroid hormone binding globulin. Acta Endocrinol 1985; 110:56–60.

Ingbar SH. The thyroid gland. In: Wilson JD, Foster DW, eds. Williams textbook of endocrinology. Philadelphia: Saunders, 1985:707 and 725.

Job JC. The pituitary. In: Job JC, Pierson M, eds. Pediatric endocrinology. New York: Wiley, 1981:122–123.

John R, Bamforth FJ. Serum free thyroxine and free triiodothyronine concentrations in healthy fullterm, preterm and sick preterm neonates. Ann Clin Biochem 1987; 24:461–465.

Jospe N, Berkovitz GD, Corcoran LE, Humphrey RL. Factitious transient neonatal hyperthyrotropinemia. J Endocrinol Invest 1988; 11:129–132.

Kanarek KS, Villaveces C, Duckett G, Root A. Serum concentrations of growth hormone, insulin, free thyroxine, thyrotropin, and cortisol in very-low-birth-weight infants receiving total parenteral nutrition. Am J Dis Child 1988; 142:993–995.

Klein AH, Oddie TH, Parslow M, Foley TP Jr, Fisher DA. Developmental changes in pituitary-thyroid function in the human fetus and newborn. Early Hum Dev 1982; 6:321–330.

Kling S, ed. Newborn screening—an overview of newborn screening programs in the U.S. and Canada. Illinois Department of Public Health, 1988. Personal communication.

Kotoyan M. Aspects of perinatal endocrinology. Pediatr Clin North Am 1977; 24:529–531.

l'Allemand D, Gruters A, Beyer P, Weber B. Iodine in contrast agents and skin disinfectants is the major cause for hypothyroidism in premature infants during intensive care. Horm Res 1987; 28:42–49.

l'Allemand D, Gruters A, Heidemann MD, Schurnbrand P. Iodine-induced alterations of thyroid function in newborn infants after prenatal and perinatal exposure to povodine iodine. J Pediatr 1983; 102(6):935–938.

Lanes R, Borges M, Moret LA, Febres F. Evaluation of the pituitary-thyroidal axis in newborns undergoing exchange transfusion. Eur J Pediatr 1986; 145:70–72.

Mercado M, Yu VYH, Francis I, Szymonowicz W, Gold H. Thyroid function in very preterm infants. Early Hum Dev 1988; 16:131–141.

Nagashima K, Onoda K, Suzuki S, Sakaguchi M, Kuroume T. Reevaluation of thyroid function in low birth weight infants based on free triiodothyronine and triiodothyronine. Biol Neonate 1985; 48:341–345.

Nagashima K, Shimano S, Yagi H, Yunoki H, Noji T, Kuroume T. Thyrotropin measured by the immunoradiometric assay in low birth weight infants. Horm Metab Res 1988; 20:758–760.

New England Congenital Hypothyroidism Collaborative. Elementary school performance of children with congenital hypothyroidism. J Pediatr 1990; 116:27–32.

Panny SR. Division of Hereditary Disorders, State of Maryland, Department of Health and Mental Hygiene. Personal Communication from Kling S, ed. Newborn screening—an overview of newborn screening programs in the U.S. and Canada, Illinois Department of Public Health, 1988.

Shenkman L, Mitsuma T, Penna M, et al. Evidence for hypothyroidism in endemic cretinism in Brazil. Lancet 1973; 2:67–69.

Smerdely P, Boyages SC, Wu D, et al. Topical iodine-containing antiseptics and neonatal hypothyroidism in very-low-birthweight infants. Lancet 1989; 2:661–664.

Sobel EH, Saenger P. Hypothyroidism in the newborn. Pediatr Rev 1989; 11:15–20.

Styne DM. The thyroid gland. In: Pediatric endocrinology for the house officer. Baltimore: Williams & Wilkins, 1988:92–101.

Theodoropoulos T, Braverman LE, Vagenakis AG. Iodide-induced hypothyroidism: a potential hazard during perinatal life. Science 1979; 205:502–503.

Uhrmann S, Marks K, Maisels MJ, et al. Thyroid function in the preterm infant: a longitudinal assessment. J Pediatr 1978; 92:495–598.

Wilson DM, Hopper AO, McDougall IR, et al. Serum free thyroxine values in term, premature and sick infants. J Pediatr 1982; 101:113–117.

12

Screening for Hearing Loss

Jacob K. Felix

The first 3 years of life are the most important for acquisition of speech and language. This requires the presence of an intact auditory system, i.e., normal hearing. Therefore, early identification of the hearing impaired is necessary so that they can benefit from amplification of their residual hearing and begin other forms of habilitation. Infant hearing screening efforts were initiated in the 1950s because few of the prelingually hearing impaired received habilitation before the age of 3 years. As recently as 1987, the average age at identification of hearing loss was 19 months. This delay resulted in the loss of a significant portion of the critical language learning period. Early behavioral screening techniques lacked the sensitivity and specificity necessary to make them clinically useful when applied to large groups of infants. Nevertheless, screening efforts continued, ultimately leading to acceptance of the Auditory Brainstem Response (ABR) technique, a modification of the standard electroencephalogram, as a hearing screening method. Because of its reliability and high sensitivity, the American Speech, Language and Hearing Association (ASHA) recently accepted it as the preferred methodology for infant hearing screening.

The overall incidence of severe-to-profound hearing loss in the United States is 1:1000 live births. Groups at a significantly higher risk for hearing loss have been identified, the Neonatal Intensive Care Unit (NICU) graduate being one of them. Studies have reported the incidence of confirmed hearing loss in NICU graduates to be between 2 and 10%, making this group the focus of intensive hearing screening efforts for the past 15 years.

To give an overview of the current status of infant hearing screening, this chapter will review the rationale for infant screening, the groups at high risk for hearing loss, the recommended screening methodology, the best time to perform infant hearing screening, and the importance of appropriate referral and follow-up.

RATIONALE

We are well aware of the benefits of early identification and intervention. Diseases such as congenital hypothyroidism, phenylketonuria, and galactosemia lead to mental retardation or death if not detected early. Congenital cataracts and glaucoma will cause blindness if not diagnosed and treated early. Basic research on animals investigating synaptogenesis and maturation of the visual system has shown the existence of critical periods of activity-dependent plasticity, which are limited to the first few months of life. According to Kalil, "As the brain develops, existing synapses between nerve cells are refined, and new connections are made. The changes are not automatic; they depend in part on the young neurons generating impulses." Similarly, prelingual hearing loss will greatly handicap those affected if untreated early in life. The critical period for acquisition of speech and language skills is birth to 3 years. Thereafter, evidence suggests that auditory plasticity of the brain becomes limited. Stimulation of the inner ear early in life appears to be necessary for normal maturation of the auditory system. This includes perception at the cerebral level, a prerequisite for the ability to learn language.

Intervention

The earlier hearing loss is recognized, the earlier habilitation can be started. Audiologists now fit hearing aids to infants as young as 4 months and, in some cases, even earlier. Other aspects of habilitation should also begin as soon as the hearing loss is recognized, even if the exact threshold of the deficit cannot be confirmed. This intervention might include aural, speech, and language training; manual communication (sign language); parental training; and counseling.

To the degree that the effects of hearing loss can be minimized, the future potential of affected infants will be maximized. Currently, the prelingually deaf rarely are able to read beyond the fourth grade level, their academic achievements are limited, and they earn 18% less than the general population. Most of this discrepancy is attributed to the tardiness of their diagnosis and subsequent habilitation. Intervention at a much earlier age can only help to decrease this difference.

HIGH-RISK GROUPS

Various investigators and organizations have labored to identify at-risk or high-risk groups in order to provide them with early identification and follow-up. In 1982, the American Academy of Pediatrics, the American Speech, Language and Hearing Association, the American Nurses Association, and the Academy of Otolaryngology, Head and Neck Surgery published an updated Joint Committee Position Statement on infant hearing screening in which they identify seven high-risk groups for hearing loss (Table 12.1). A second update of the Joint Committee Position Statement is in preparation. It will be printed in AAP News and published in *Pediatrics* in 1991 or early 1992.

Table 12.1. Risk Criteria for Hearing Impairment[a]

Family history of childhood hearing impairment
Congenital perinatal infection (e.g., cytomegalovirus, rubella, herpes, toxoplasmosis, syphilis)
Anatomical malformations involving the head and neck (e.g., dysmorphic appearance, including syndromal and nonsyndromal abnormalities; overt or submucous cleft palate; morphological abnormalities of the pinna)
Birth weight <1500 grams
Hyperbilirubinemia at level exceeding indications for exchange transfusion
Bacterial meningitis, especially *Hemophilus influenzae*
Severe asphyxia, which may include infants with Apgar scores of 0 to 3 or who fail to institute spontaneous respiration by 10 minutes and those with hypotonia persisting to 2 hours of age

[a]American Academy of Pediatrics Joint Committee on Infant Hearing. Position Statement 1982. Pediatrics 1982; 70:496. Reproduced by permission of Pediatrics.

Family History

Families with a history of hereditary childhood hearing impairment constitute the largest risk group. Over 130 different forms of hereditary hearing loss are known. Eighty to 85% are caused by autosomal recessive gene defects, 15 to 20% are autosomal dominant, and 1 to 3% are X-linked. Gene defects account for 50 to 60% of all cases of congenital hearing loss.

Congenital Perinatal Infections

The second largest high-risk group is composed of infants with documented congenital infection. Cytomegalovirus, the major offender, is excreted in the urine of 1 to 3% of all newborn infants. A large percentage will have active disease. Up to one-third with active disease will develop sensorineural hearing loss due to the infection. Some are born deaf; others acquire the hearing loss in the first years of life. The hearing loss can be unilateral or bilateral, and it can range from mild to profound. Other congenital infections are also associated with hearing loss. Congenital toxoplasmosis affects 1:1000 life births. A follow-up study of infants with untreated congenital toxoplasmosis reports a high incidence of hearing loss. Congenital syphilis is on the rise again, but if properly treated, most infected infants will have normal hearing. Congenital Rubella Syndrome was the first intrauterine infection recognized to cause hearing loss. The introduction of rubella vaccine in 1969 has all but eliminated the disease from the United States. Although hearing related data on congenital herpes simplex, human immunodeficiency virus, enterovirus, and parvovirus B19 infection are too scant to give risk figures for each disease, we nevertheless recommend all infants with documented congenital infections be screened for possible hearing loss.

Anatomical Malformations

A third high-risk group includes infants with craniofacial malformations affecting the head and neck. These include major malformations such as cleft lip and palate, minor malformations including ear pits and ear tags, and syndromes such as Apert's, Treacher-Collins', and Goldenhar's. Many of these infants are found to have conductive as well as sensorineural hearing loss.

Birth Weight Less Than 1500 Grams

The very-low-birth-weight infant (<1500 grams) constitutes the fourth major risk group. These infants are at risk for hearing loss because of complications associated with their prematurity, including hypoxemia, hypotension, ischemia, intraventricular hemorrhage, systemic infections, and exposure to numerous pharmacological drugs, including aminoglycosides and furosemide, during their hospitalization. Up to 5% of this group are found to have confirmed sensorineural hearing loss.

Hyperbilirubinemia Exceeding Exchange Indications

Excessive hyperbilirubinemia is a known cause of sensorineural hearing loss. The Joint Committee recommends screening infants in whom the hyperbilirubinemia exceeds a level at which exchange blood transfusion is indicated. Studies have shown reversible effects of hyperbilirubinemia on the ABR. In many of the reported cases, an abnormal ABR response was obtained when the bilirubin levels were elevated, but the response improved after exchange transfusion.

Bacterial Meningitis

Infants with bacterial meningitis make up a sixth at-risk population. Although *Hemophilus influenzae* was the first organism recognized to cause meningitis-associated hearing loss, other bacteria, including β-hemolytic group B streptococcus, are known to cause hearing loss.

Severe Asphyxia

Infants experiencing severe asphyxia comprise the seventh group recognized to be at risk for hearing loss. They may suffer brain damage affecting the brainstem nuclei, including the inferior colliculi and the Organ of Corti. Many are left with multiple handicaps, which might include sensorineural hearing loss.

NICU Patients

In addition to the groups recommended for screening by the Joint Committee, we and other researchers have studied NICU patients because they represent a captive population and include many of the at-risk infants discussed above. Follow-up studies of NICU graduates have found a 2 to 10% incidence of confirmed sensorineural hearing loss, making this a valuable group to undergo screening. Taken together, these eight groups include up to 50 to 75% of all infants with prelingual hearing loss.

METHODOLOGY

Auditory Brainstem Response

Infant hearing screening should be performed according to the 1989 ASHA guidelines, although we take exception to their recommendation for bilateral screening, as will be discussed further in the text. The recommended ABR is an objective electrophysiological procedure that does not require patient cooperation and can be used in many different clinical settings. It utilizes earphones or inserts to provide the infant with a sound stimulus that is time-locked to recording electrodes attached to the scalp. The normal ABR response consists of five waves, which appear as the sound stimulus travels through the auditory system (Fig. 12.1). Wave I is thought to arise from the auditory nerve, wave V from the region of the inferior colliculus, and waves II, III, and IV from the auditory fibers and nuclei in between. If both ears are to be screened, each one is tested separately. The sound stimulus is repeated 2000 times, allowing the averaged response to emerge from background brain wave activity. The sound stimulus should contain energy throughout the speech frequency spectrum. Clicks are the signal type most widely used, although tone pips or bursts could be used. Stimulus rate, duration, and polarity are other variables that must be carefully controlled.

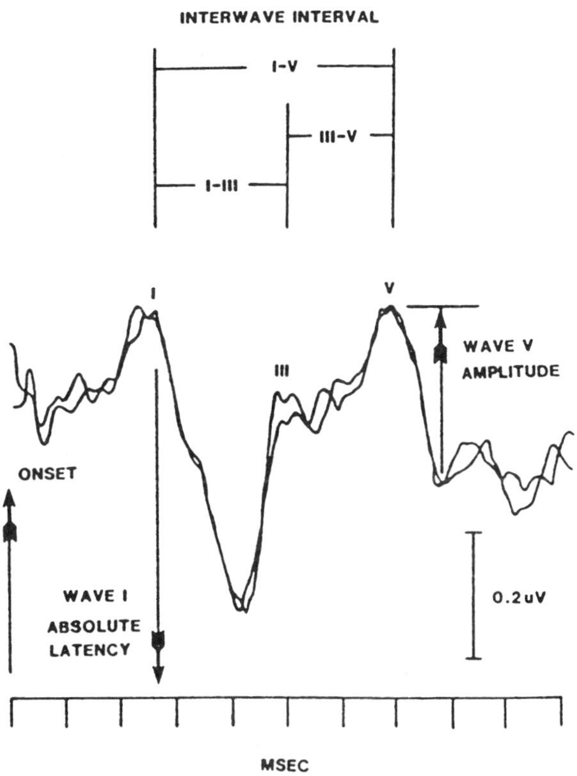

Figure 12.1. Newborn auditory brainstem response illustrating the latency, amplitude, and interwave interval measurement characteristics of 2 sequential tracings. The ABR screen is performed twice to assure reproducibility of the response. Each trace represents the sum of 2000 trials. (Reprinted with permission from Jacobson JT, Hyde ML. The auditory brainstem response in neonatal hearing screening. In: Swigart ET, ed. Neonatal hearing screening. San Diego: College-Hill Press, 1986.)

When analyzing the infant's response to the ABR, the most essential component is the presence of wave V (Figure 12.1), which indicates the sound stimulus has reached the level of the inferior colliculus. The absence or delayed appearance of wave V is indicative of a hearing problem. It is recommended that a 40 dB normal hearing level (nHL) intensity be utilized as the threshold for pass/fail.

Although the equipment itself is expensive and bulky, the ABR can usually be performed in the Special Care Nursery setting and requires 30 to 45 minutes for unilateral screening. Most infants can be successfully screened 15 to 30 minutes after feeding. The advantages of the ABR include its ability to screen young infants whether awake or asleep (even unconscious patients can be tested) and the fact that it is unaffected by medication they may be receiving. The only patient cooperation required is that they remain quiet during the test to avoid muscle artifact. Sedation is rarely required. Disadvantages are the length of time required for each screening test to be completed and the requirement that the screen be performed by someone experienced in the ABR technique.

Although the 1989 ASHA guidelines recommend bilateral newborn hearing screening of all high-risk infants, it is our practice to perform only unilateral screening if a normal response is obtained on the first ear screened and the child is free of craniofacial malformations, which could cause a unilateral hearing loss. A 40 dB pass/fail criteria is used.

Only if and when mass screeners become available might routine bilateral screening become practical.

In the future, it is likely that the ABR technique will be simplified, requiring less time for completion and enabling less experienced personnel to perform the screen. Such advances will help decrease the cost of screening, which is now $50 to $250 for the screening procedure and interpretation of the report. At this time, several mass-screening devices are being marketed for use on at-risk infants. If they prove to be reliable with acceptable sensitivity and specificity, they will greatly expand the opportunities for screening by making it possible for hospitals with limited resources to perform the procedure.

Crib-O-Gram

Numerous behavioral screening methodologies have been tried and abandoned, except for the Crib-O-Gram, which is used in a small number of nurseries as an initial screening method. The Crib-O-Gram is a semiautomated screening device that exposes the infant to a 92 dB sound stimulus and records any change in movement or activity following the stimulus via a pressure-sensitive transducer placed under the infant's mattress. Because of the low specificity of the Crib-O-Gram, when a failure is noted, the infant must be rescreened using the ABR to determine if a hearing deficit is actually present. In addition, the extent of the deficit must be determined because the Crib-O-Gram uses a 92 dB stimulus intensity for screening. Therefore, infants with mild-to-moderate or unilateral hearing loss cannot be identified with this technique.

WHEN TO SCREEN

The 1982 Joint Committee Position Statement recommends that "the hearing of infants who manifest any item on the list of risk criteria should be screened, preferably under the supervision of an audiologist, optimally by 3 months of age, but no later than 6 months of age." It is strongly recommended that infants be screened prior to leaving the hospital because compliance with screening after discharge is far from satisfactory. If possible, it is best to wait until the infant is near 40 weeks gestational age and stable in a Special Care-type setting. Screening prior to 35 weeks gestational age may not yield an easily interpretable result because of amplitude and latency differences due to prematurity. It is difficult to screen in the NICU setting because of electrical interference. In our experience, screening 5 to 10 days prior to scheduled discharge is ideal. This gives the physician time to review and explain the screening results to the parents, especially if an abnormality is detected, and to arrange for hearing screening follow-up.

IDENTIFICATION AND FOLLOW-UP

To be successful, any hospital-based hearing screening program should be designed to allow for the identification of all at-risk infants (not just the NICU patient), to have reliable ABR screening capability, and to provide intervention and follow-up. This requires the involvement of numerous professionals in the identification process. At a minimum, a multidisciplinary team consisting of pediatrics and audiology is required. In many hospitals, ABR screening is performed by personnel from neurology. Otolaryngology services also should be available, at least on a consultative basis. Administrative and secretarial support

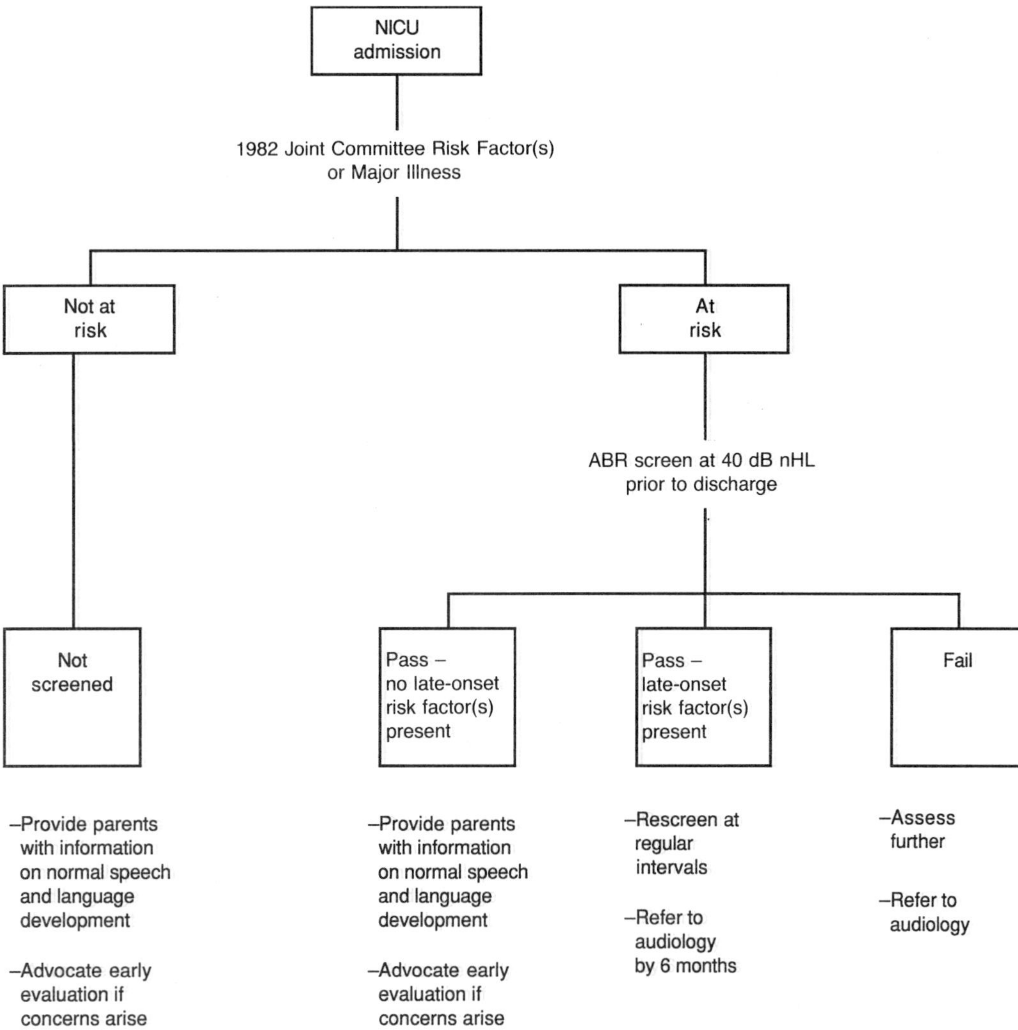

Figure 12.2. Hearing Screening Algorithm

is essential to assure a timely flow of information between the hearing screening team members and the primary care provider. The ultimate success of the program will depend upon the participation and cooperation of the nursery staff for the timely identification and screening of at-risk patients; communication with the parents, primary care pediatricians, and audiologist; and arranging for the follow-up of infants with suspected or confirmed hearing loss.

A logical movement of NICU infants through the hearing screening process is shown in Figure 12.2. Although admitted to the NICU, some infants will have neither a major illness (requiring NICU care for >2 days and more than observational care) nor a high-risk factor as identified by the 1982 Joint Committee. These infants do not require ABR screening. However, information on normal speech and language development should be given to the patients.

If a high-risk factor or major illness is present, screening should be performed prior to discharge. Infants who pass at 40 dB do not require special audiological follow-up if they are free of risk criteria for late-onset hearing loss.

Late-onset risk factors include a documented perinatal infection, especially cytomegalovirus, a family history of progressive hearing impairment, or a history of persistent pulmonary hypertension of the newborn (PPHN). Recent studies have shown a 10 to 50% incidence of late-onset (3 to 24 months) hearing loss in patients treated for PPHN. These infants should be rescreened at 3- to 6-month intervals and be referred to audiology by 6 months for follow-up until 2 years of age.

Infants who fail the screen at 40 dB should receive an examination of the head and neck to look for physical defects that might have been overlooked initially. The infant should be screened for CMV infection if this has not previously been done. If possible, they should undergo otoscopy to assess the status of the middle ear. It is not uncommon to find fluid in the middle ear, especially in infants who have required prolonged gavage feeding or endotracheal intubation. In reality, otoscopy is extremely difficult in these small infants, and in the absence of signs of infection, it is probably best deferred until the infant is bigger. Many will have a unilateral hearing loss with a threshold of 45 to 60 dB that resolves within several weeks to months (Felix JK, Shannon DA, Krumholz A, Beanland C. Unpublished data). In our experience, those with a bilateral hearing deficit and thresholds above 50 to 60 dB on the initial screen generally have a permanent loss. These infants should be referred to audiology as early as possible and undergo a repeat ABR 4 to 8 weeks after the initial screen to help determine if early intervention will be needed. Amplification is usually recommended if the thresholds are consistently above 45 to 50 dB. Sedation is sometimes required to perform the ABR in these older infants.

One problem with ABR screening that has not yet been overcome is the large number of transient positives obtained on the initial screening. While the sensitivity of the ABR approaches 100%, the specificity is only 80 to 85% for confirmed hearing loss in NICU graduates. Therefore, the positive predictive value of the ABR is only about 10 to 20% in a population where the prevalence of confirmed hearing loss is 2 to 5%. Most of these transient positives occur in infants who required prolonged intubation, diuretic therapy, and/or gavage feedings. On the initial screen, they may have a unilateral hearing loss with 45 to 60 dB thresholds. Whether these represent false-positives or merely transient positives is still unclear. However, when counseling parents of these infants, one can express optimism that the child's ultimate hearing status may be normal. In contrast, the infant whose initial screen reveals a bilateral loss with thresholds >60 dB is more likely to have a permanent loss. In all cases, confirmatory testing by an audiologist should be completed by 6 months developmental age as recommended by the Academy of Pediatrics in the 1982 Joint Position Statement.

Sixteen states have hearing screening programs in place. Five more are in the planning or pending stage (Table 12.2). If located in a state or region with an active hearing screening program, the hospital staff should coordinate their efforts with the existing program to assure maximum efficiency in the identification and screening of at-risk infants and to avoid a duplication of effort. Not all hearing screening programs utilize the same risk criteria, and financial support varies considerably from state to state.

Acknowledgment

The author wishes to recognize the excellent secretarial assistance of Deborah L. Birckhead in the preparation of this chapter.

Table 12.2. States with Screening Programs—Active or Planned/Pending[a]

States with Active Infant Hearing Screening Programs[b]		
Arizona	Kentucky	Rhode Island
Colorado	Maryland	Tennessee
Connecticut	Massachusetts	Utah
Florida	New Jersey	Virginia
Georgia	Ohio	
Illinois	Oklahoma	
States with Programs Planned or Pending		
Alabama	California	Wisconsin
Alaska	Kansas	

[a]Source: Legislative Information Office, ASHA, 1989
[b]Some programs are mandated, others are voluntary. Different high-risk registers are used in different states—some tied in with other programs.

SUGGESTED READINGS

Abrams IF. Nongenetic hearing loss. In: Joffe BF, ed. Hearing loss in children. Baltimore: University Park Press, 1977.

Allen T. Patterns of academic achievement among hearing impaired students: 1974 and 1983. In: Schildroth A, Karchmer M, eds. Deaf children in America. San Diego: College-Hill Press, 1986:161–206.

American Academy of Pediatrics Joint Committee on Infant Hearing. Position Statement 1982. Pediatrics 1982; 70:496-497.

Bergstrom L, Hemenway WG, Downs MP. A high risk registry to find congenital deafness. Otolaryngol Clin North Am 1971; 4:369–399.

Cevette MS. Auditory brainstem response testing in the intensive care unit. Semin Hearing 1984; 5:57 69.

Chin KC, Taylor MJ, Perlman M. Improvement in auditory and visual evoked potentials in jaundiced preterm infants after exchange transfusion. Arch Dis Child 1985; 60:714–717.

Committee on Infant Hearing. Audiologic screening of newborn infants who are at risk for hearing impairment. ASHA 1989; 31:89–92.

D'Souza SW, McCartney E, Nolan M, Taylor IG. Hearing, speech and language in survivors of severe perinatal asphyxia. Arch Dis Child 1981; 56:245–252.

Duara S, Suter CM, Bessard KK, Gutberlet RL. Neonatal screening with auditory brainstem responses: results of follow-up audiometry and risk factor evaluation. J Pediatr 1986; 108:276–281.

Elssmann SF, Matkin ND, Sabo MP. Early identification of congenital sensorineural hearing impairment. Hear J 1987; 40:13–17.

Galambos R, Hicks GE, Wilson MJ. The auditory brainstem response reliably predicts hearing loss in graduates of a tertiary intensive care nursery. Ear Hear 1984; 5:254–260.

Hendricks-Munoz KD, Walton JP. Hearing loss in infants with persistent fetal circulation. Pediatrics 1988; 81:650–656.

Jacobson JT, Hyde ML. The auditory brainstem response in neonatal hearing screening. In: Swigart ET, ed. Neonatal hearing screening. San Diego: College-Hill Press, 1986:67–98.

Kalil RE. Synapse formation in the developing brain. Sci Am 1989; 261:76–85.

Konigsmark B, Gorlin R. Genetic and metabolic deafness. Philadelphia: Saunders, 1976.

Kramer SJ, Vertes DR, Condon M. Auditory brainstem responses and clinical follow-up of high risk infants. Pediatrics 1989; 83:385–392.

Kuriyawa M, Tomiwa K, Konishi Y, Mikawa H. Improvement in auditory brainstem response of hyperbilirubinemic infants after exchange transfusion. Pediatr Neurol 1986; 2(3):127–132.

McKusick VA. Mendelian inheritance in man. 8th ed. Baltimore: The Johns Hopkins University Press, 1989.

Naulty CM, Weiss IP, Herer GR. Progressive sensorieural hearing loss in survivors of persistent fetal circulation. Ear Hear 1986; 7:74–77.

Rose SP, Conneally PM, Nance WE. Genetic analysis of childhood deafness. In: Bess FH, ed. Childhood deafness. New York: Grune and Stratton, 1977:19–35.

Ruben RJ, Rapin I. Plasticity of the developing auditory system. Ann Otol Rhinol Laryngol 1980; 89:303–311.

Saigal S, Lunyk O, Bryce Larke RP, Chernesky MA. The outcome in children with congenital cytomegalovirus infection. Am J Dis Child 1982; 136:896–901.

Salomy A, Eldredge L, Tooley WH. Neonatal status and hearing loss in high risk infants. J Pediatr 1989; 114:847–852.

Schein JD, Delk MT. The deaf population of the United States. Silver Spring, MD: National Association of the Deaf, 1974.

Shannon DA, Felix JK, Krumholz A, Goldstein P, Harris KC. Hearing screening of high risk newborns with brainstem auditory evoked potentials: a follow-up study. Pediatrics 1984; 73:22–26.

Shimizu H, Walters RJ, Kennedy DW, Allen MC, Markowitz RK, Luebkert FR. Crib-O-Gram versus auditory brainstem response for infant hearing screening. Laryngoscope 1985; 95:806–810.

Simmons FB, McFarland WH, Jones FR. An automated hearing screening technique for newborns. Acta Otolaryngol 1979; 87:1–8.

Swigart ET, ed. Neonatal hearing screening. San Diego: College-Hill Press, 1986.[a]

Wald ER, Bergman I, Taylor HG, Chiponis D, Porter C, Kubek K. Long-term outcome of group B streptococcal meningitis. Pediatrics 1986; 77:217–221.

[a]Swigart (1986) in particular is a good general reference.

13

Surgical Management

L.R. Scherer, III

Even though sophisticated intensive care has made it possible for pediatric surgeons and neonatologists to manage many congenital and acquired neonatal surgical problems, some neonates require extended postoperative management and long-term follow-up. This chapter will discuss management of some common surgical problems in the recovering NICU infant, including tracheoesophageal fistula, congenital abdominal wall defects, inguinal hernia, undescended testes; the indications for and management of gastrostomies, ileostomies, and colostomies; follow-up of nonoperatively managed necrotizing enterocolitis; and the use of ventricular drains in the management of hydrocephalus.

ESOPHAGEAL ATRESIA

Esophageal atresia occurs in approximately 1 in 4000 live births. Over 85% of patients have a distal tracheoesophageal fistula. Advances in pediatric anesthesia, pediatric surgical care, and neonatal intensive care have led to 95% survival. Patients with poor outcome include those with very low birth weight, severe pneumonia, or severe associated anomalies. Fortunately, esophageal and respiratory problems are of major importance in only a few patients. The majority develop into healthy, active children.

Postoperative Complications

Postoperatively, these infants may demonstrate a variety of difficulties. Feeding difficulties include pooling of secretions in the posterior pharynx, coughing and gagging with feedings, dysphagia, and gastroesophageal reflux. Respiratory difficulties include stridor, a persistent, "barking" cough, and in some patients, aspiration. In some instances, such symptoms are caused by a recurrent or missed tracheoesophageal fistula or a stricture at the esophageal anastomosis, but more commonly, they represent esophageal dysmotility and/or a distended proximal esophageal pouch. Tracheomalacia, particularly at the site of the fistula, is the usual cause of stridor and the characteristic barking cough. However, one must also consider the possibility that the cause is compression of the trachea by the aortic arch.

Diagnostic Approaches

Barium through the gastrostomy and a barium esophagram will demonstrate the size of the proximal pouch and identify an esophageal stricture. The esophagram will detect gastroesophageal reflux or direct aspiration. Bronchoscopic evaluation of the airway is necessary to identify a laryngotracheoesophageal cleft or to determine the extent of tracheomalacia.

Recurrent Tracheoesophageal Fistula

Coughing or cyanosis during feeding should alert the physician to the possibility of a persistent or recurrent tracheoesophageal fistula. If a barium swallow is not diagnostic or better delineation of the position of a fistula is required, bronchoscopy and esophagoscopy should be performed under general anesthesia using a ventilating bronchoscope. Fistulae will not close spontaneously, and operative correction is required.

Esophageal Stricture

Anastomotic strictures are the most common late postoperative complication. A stricture may appear at the site of a previous leak, or it may be the result of ischemic injury at the time of surgery. Persistent gastroesophageal reflux may also cause late stricture. Strictures generally respond to repetitive dilation during the first year of life. Rarely, they require local injection of triamcinolone (a corticosteroid with marked anti-inflammatory effects) or resection.

Esophageal Dysmotility and Gastroesophageal Reflux

Infants with esophageal atresia suffer from abnormal motility of the distal segment and from altered anatomy of both the distal esophagus and the angle of His. These contribute to the 20 to 30% incidence of significant gastroesophageal reflux. Significant reflux causes esophagitis with or without a secondary stricture, failure to thrive, cough, apnea, and recurrent pneumonia. The presence of reflux is confirmed by a barium swallow. The severity can be assessed by pH probe monitoring or esophageal biopsy. If the reflux cannot be controlled by prone and head-up positioning, thickened feedings, or administration of histamine antagonists or metoclopramide, fundoplication is necessary. Due to the poor motility of the distal esophagus, it is imperative that the surgeon perform the plication loosely around the distal esophagus.

Poor pharyngeal coordination and altered esophageal motility with poorly coordinated peristalsis lead to long-term esophageal dysfunction. This can be documented by manometric studies and by cineesophagrams. Many such patients have a hacking cough. The etiology of the cough is unknown, but it may be secondary to recurrent aspiration. Such infants may suffer from lower respiratory tract infections more frequently than normal children.

Tracheomalacia

Tracheomalacia is most commonly due to poor support of the trachea posteriorly and occasionally to compression by the aortic arch anteriorly. Aortopexy is useful in some patients with tracheomalacia.

CONGENITAL ABDOMINAL WALL DEFECTS (OMPHALOCELE AND GASTROSCHISIS)

Congenital abdominal wall defects occur in 1/2500 to 1/5000 live births. Infants with these disorders frequently have a protracted hospital course. Although mortality is over 80% in the 30% of infants in whom omphalocele is accompanied by another major anomaly, mortality with isolated omphalocele or gastroschisis is currently <10%. Improved survival is largely due to the recognition and treatment of the hypothermia, hypotension, and hypoxia that can accompany these conditions.

Prolonged Intestinal Dysfunction

Prolonged intestinal dysfunction occurs frequently with gastroschisis or a ruptured omphalocele and is attributable to a full-thickness injury of the bowel that results from prolonged prenatal exposure to amniotic fluid. Prior to 1970, such infants often died of malnutrition, but since the development of total parenteral nutrition, they can be supported until intestinal function returns. A secondary anomaly of gastroschisis, jejunoileal atresia, is due to an intrauterine vascular accident.

Treatment of intestinal dysfunction may require a gastrostomy to decompress the gastrointestinal tract early in the postoperative course. As intestinal function returns, the gastrostomy may be used to slowly and progressively infuse enteral feedings. One should bear in mind that, in patients with gastroschisis or ruptured omphalocele, intestinal dysfunction may not resolve for 3 to 4 months.

Other Problems

Because of abnormal prenatal anatomy, abdominal wall defects are associated with two postnatal conditions. First, the liver may retain its globular shape and remain in a midline position just inferior to the xiphoid rather than returning to the usual subcostal position. It is therefore subject to injury from blunt trauma. In such instances, parents must be cautioned that the child should avoid body contact sports.

Second, due to the increased abdominal pressure generated during closure of the abdominal wall defect, inguinal hernias are frequently encountered. Increased intra-abdominal pressure dilates the inguinal ring, and if the processus vaginalis is patent, an inguinal hernia will evolve. The hernia should be repaired in the usual manner without delay.

Long-Term Follow-up

Long-term follow-up studies have shown that intestinal dysfunction and malabsorption eventually resolve and infants progress to normal diets and normal gastrointestinal function. Intellectual impairment, if present, appears to be related to prematurity, intrauterine growth retardation, or nongastrointestinal neonatal complications.

One might anticipate that these infants would suffer from late bowel obstruction. Intestinal malrotation is common, and adhesions, either from surgical manipulation or, in infants with gastroschisis or ruptured omphalocele, from the inflammatory response to amniotic fluid, occur frequently. However, intestinal obstruction is fortunately rarely seen, but the families of all patients and later, the patients themselves, must be made aware of the possibility and of the presenting signs and symptoms.

INGUINAL HERNIA AND UNDESCENDED TESTES

It is not uncommon for a premature infant to develop an inguinal hernia while recovering in the neonatal intensive care unit. In infants with birth weights <2000 grams, the incidence is 13%, and the incidence is 30% in those weighing <1000 grams at birth. In both males and females, 60% of inguinal hernias are right-sided; only 10% are bilateral. The risk of incarceration in the first few months of life is close to 30%.

Embryologically, the testis begins its descent from the retroperitoneum in the seventh month of gestation, and 95% of the testes are within the scrotum by the ninth month. For reasons that are not clear, premature birth adversely affects descent of the testes and closure of the processus vaginalis. As a result, the incidence of undescended testes and inguinal hernia is markedly increased. Embryologically, the hernia in females develops similarly with descent of the peritoneal diverticulum of Nuck and the round ligament into the labia majora.

The incidence of inguinal hernia in female children is only 1%, but in newborn infants, the incidence of inguinal hernia is similar in males and females. The risk of incarceration in females is higher than in males. Also of significance is the fact that females require surgical reduction of an incarcerated hernia more often than males. The organs most often involved in the incarcerated hernia in females are the ovary and the Fallopian tube. At the time of surgery, a palpable gonad within the labia or the inguinal canal should be inspected for testicular tissue. If an abnormal gonad is encountered, small wedge biopsies should be taken to determine histological type.

The principal risk of early hernia repair is postoperative apnea. The risk of apnea appears to be the same for the premature neonate with a history of apnea as it is for the fullterm infant without such a history. The risk of postanesthetic apnea is increased until 52 to 60 weeks postconception. The cause of apnea is not known. It may result from a combination of factors, including immaturity of the diaphragmatic and intercostal muscles, alveolar hypoventilation, abnormal responses to hypoxia and hypercarbia, and depression of brainstem ventilatory control mechanisms by anesthetic agents. Because the risk of postanesthetic apnea is high, infants who are <52 weeks postconceptual age and require general anesthesia must be admitted to the hospital and monitored for 24 hours following surgery.

The following recommendations are offered as guidelines for the treatment of inguinal hernias in preterm infants and seriously ill neonates. First, hernias should be examined frequently for reducibility. The reducible hernia is generally repaired about a week prior to discharge, depending on the infant's general health and associated diseases. Second, if a reducible hernia develops after discharge, early herniorraphy is recommended because of the high risk of incarceration. As mentioned, the infant must be monitored postoperatively in the hospital for 24 hours.

In premature infants with undescended testes, 26% of the testes will not have descended by 40 weeks postconception. However, by 1 year of age, only 6% of testes will remain undescended. If the testes fail to descend, orchiopexy should be performed before 2 years of age. If neither testis is palpable at birth, chromosomal analysis should be performed to determine if an intersexual abnormality is present.

GASTROSTOMY

Gastrostomy may be required for management of the newborn with either neurological, esophageal, or intestinal dysfunction. The most common type of gastrostomy is the "temporary" gastrostomy. This type of gastrostomy is easily created, is unlikely to leak, and closes spontaneously once the tube is removed.

There are many advantages to a gastrostomy over the prolonged use of orogastric or nasogastric tubes. In the latter case, the tubing is small and tends to become obstructed. It can also become dislodged, leading to pulmonary aspiration. It provides unpredictable decompression of the gastrointestinal tract, and it can also obstruct the Eustachian tube. A gastrostomy allows for effective decompression, facilitates enteral feeding, and avoids upper airway obstruction.

Indications

A gastrostomy is placed most commonly for decompression of the gastrointestinal tract in association with esophageal atresia with distal tracheoesophageal fistula, intestinal atresia, meconium ileus, or congenital abdominal wall defects. As the infant recovers, the gastrostomy can be used to introduce and advance enteral feedings. Approximately 20% of infants with esophageal atresia will require dilation of their anastomoses. The gastrostomy allows the passage of a string, allowing the dilator to be guided through the lumen of the esophagus in an antegrade or retrograde fashion.

If a gastrostomy is to be used primarily for long-term feeding in a neurologically impaired infant, the infant must first be evaluated for gastroesophageal reflux with radiographic contrast studies, milk scintiscan, pH probe analysis, and/or esophageal biopsy.

Complications

The most serious, but fortunately the least frequent, complication of a gastrostomy is separation of the stomach from the anterior abdominal wall. This usually occurs from early dislodgment of the gastrostomy tube. Therefore, the gastrostomy tube must be adequately secured to the abdominal wall. If the tube becomes dislodged within the first 3 weeks after placement, it should be reinserted with gentle manipulation and fluoroscopic confirmation of gastric placement. A Foley catheter should be used for this purpose. The balloon should be inflated and pulled up against the abdominal wall until the gastrostomy has "matured."

The most common complication following gastrostomy is leakage of gastric contents. This indicates either that the flange or balloon of the tube has migrated away from the abdominal wall or that the tube has not been secured to the abdominal wall, allowing erosion to enlarge the hole. Both can be prevented by pulling the flange or balloon of the catheter firmly against the anterior abdominal wall. This requires that the catheter be secured exteriorly. One method employs a rubber nursing nipple as an exterior stent for the tube. If the gastrostomy site has enlarged, the tube may be removed for 8 to 24 hours, and a smaller tube reinserted.

Upper gastrointestinal obstruction is occasionally seen due to migration of a gastrostomy tube. These children present with vomiting. Migration is confirmed by contrast radiographs, and the catheter is repositioned. Recently, a short-flanged catheter has been developed to avoid many of the above complications.

ILEOSTOMY AND COLOSTOMY

Fortunately, most enterostomies in newborns are temporary, remaining in place only until the disease is controlled or a definitive procedure is performed. Congenital and acquired diseases of the newborn requiring enterostomy include atresias, imperforate anus, Hirschsprung's disease, meconium ileus, necrotizing enterocolitis, and midgut volvulus.

Indications

Bowel anastomosis may be difficult to perform if an atresia is complicated by perforation and purulent peritonitis or if there is a large difference in size between dilated proximal bowel and unused distal bowel. An enterostomy is placed until peritoneal inflammation resolves or until the lumens are of more equal size.

Newborns presenting with a high imperforate anus will require a diverting colostomy until they are old enough for a definitive anorectoplasty. The colostomy should completely divert the fecal stream to avoid contamination of a fistulized urinary tract. The distal mucous fistula must be periodically irrigated and cleansed.

When Hirschsprung's disease presents in the neonatal period, a colostomy is required to decompress the obstructed colon and prevent enterocolitis. The colostomy is formed above the transition zone (between the lower aganglionic colon and proximal normal ganglionic colon) if a transition is located at surgery by the histological examination of frozen sections. Otherwise, a blind right transverse loop colostomy is formed. The colostomy is taken down at the time of the definitive pull-through or shortly afterwards.

The thick, inspissated meconium of cystic fibrosis of the pancreas may present with intestinal obstruction that cannot be relieved either medically, using N-acetylcysteine or Gastrograffin, or surgically. In that case, an enterostomy is formed proximal to the obstruction. Postoperatively, the distal loop is irrigated to liquefy the inspissated meconium.

Necrotizing enterocolitis requires operative intervention and bowel resection in approximately one-third of cases. A primary anastomosis is almost always impossible because of peritoneal soilage, and an enterostomy is required. The enterostomy can be closed once the peritoneal inflammation has resolved. Closure is usually performed prior to discharge, thus decreasing the risks of nutritional and growth complications associated with enterostomies in the small intestine. Midgut volvulus is frequently accompanied by ischemic injury to the bowel, which necessitates resection. A primary anastomosis may not be warranted until vascular integrity is confirmed. Therefore, a jejunostomy is often created.

Complications

The more proximal the enterostomy, the greater the skin irritation from intestinal contents. Fluid from a proximal enterostomy is very alkaline and contains a large quantity of pancreatic juice and thus is very corrosive. The contents of an ileostomy are still liquid, but less irritating. The colostomy is the easiest to manage because stool is formed and soilage is minimal. Enterostomies are best managed with stoma bags with a Karaya gum ring and Stomadhesive surrounding the enterostomy. These procedures help keep corrosive intestinal contents away from the skin. Excoriated skin requires meticulous care. This involves proper cleansing, removal of all adhesive and intestinal contamination, use of a topical preparation to protect the skin, and drying of the area with mild heat from a hair dryer prior to application of a new appliance.

Infants with proximal enterostomies are also more prone to fluid and electrolyte disorders. Intravenous fluid replacement and parenteral nutrition may be required. The enterostomy should be closed as soon as the peritoneal inflammation has resolved and the infant is medically stable.

Other complications include prolapse, dehiscence, necrosis, and retraction of the ostomy, as well as stricture, intestinal fistula, incisional hernia, and intestinal obstruction. Prolapse most often complicates a loop enterostomy and develops from the distal segment. It rarely presents a functional problem, but if vascular compromise or obstruction results, the stoma must be revised to an end enterostomy. Dehiscence, incisional hernia, and intestinal obstruction result from inadequate closure of the fascia around the stoma due to technical problems, infection, or poor nutrition. Treatment requires reexploration of the wound, revision of the stoma, or closure of the enterostomy. Necrosis and retraction, stricture, and intestinal fistula are usually secondary to ischemic injury or infection. If an enterostomy is formed using a loop of intestine under tension or damaged bowel as in necrotizing enterocolitis, the bowel may become necrotic and retract or form a stricture. Retraction below the skin level or strictures that cannot be dilated require operative revision. A proximal fistula within the stoma is due either to a distal stricture or to a fascial suture placed through-and-through the lumen. An externally draining fistula requires no further treatment.

Several nutritional complications may develop with an enterostomy. The greater complications occur with the more proximal enterostomies such as a proximal ileostomy or jejunostomy. The first complication occurs due to loss of the majority of the ileum. The ileum is responsible for the absorption of vitamin B_{12}, folate, and bile salts. Therefore, B_{12} deficiency develops, and due to the loss of the bile salt pool, deficiencies of long-chain fatty acids and fat-soluble vitamins (D, A, E, K) are seen. Also, the absorption of fluid, zinc, and magnesium are affected with major resections of the ileum. These children often present with steatorrhea. Due to mucosal injury at the level of the ileostomy, there may be occult blood loss, resulting in the development of iron deficiency. Most of these infants have a significant intestinal adaptive capability. With the use of prolonged total parenteral nutrition and gradual introduction of modular enteral feedings, infants with <40 cm of intestine who lack an ileocecal valve have adapted to total enteral feeding. The caloric requirements of these infants are often increased due to their underlying surgical illness, the adaptability and growth requirements of their intestinal mucosa, and increased nitrogen losses from intestinal output. These children often require a period of total parenteral nutrition with a goal of 2.5 to 4.0 g/kg/day of protein as amino acids, 2 to 4 g/kg/day as fat, and a total calorie requirement of 120 to 160 kcal/kg/day. Total parenteral nutrition also requires supplementation with fat- and water-soluble vitamins, iron, folic acid, and trace minerals, including further supplementation with selenium, zinc, calcium, and phosphorus. As the infant recovers from surgery and intestinal function returns, small volumes of continuous feeding may be started, initially providing 3 to 5 kcal/kg/day of hyposmolar elemental solution. As feeding tolerance progresses, as measured by intestinal output (less than 30% of the enteral feeding), the enteral feedings are increased in caloric increments of 5 to 10 kcal/kg/day. Infants who do not have their entire small intestine to use as an absorptive surface most often require an elemental formula such as Pregestimil. Those children who have all of their small intestine or who have a colostomy may tolerate a standard formula. When the infant is able to tolerate 75% of calories by enteral feedings, it is important to evaluate for the presence of malabsorption of vitamin B_{12}, fat-soluble vitamins, zinc, iron, folate, and calcium. Initially, a nutritional assessment should be done every week to determine if appropriate parenteral nutrition is being prescribed, and as these infants begin to tolerate their enteral feedings, nutritional assessments are required bimonthly to document their intestinal adaptation. This nutritional assessment should include CBC with differential, total protein, albumin, transferrin, prealbumin, electrolytes, liver functions, magnesium, calcium, phosphorus, zinc, and selenium.

FOLLOW-UP OF MEDICALLY MANAGED NECROTIZING ENTEROCOLITIS

Although the incidence of necrotizing enterocolitis (NEC) in high-risk neonatal populations may be as high as 10%, only about one-third of these infants require surgery during the acute illness for intestinal perforation or extensive bowel necrosis. The remainder are managed nonoperatively; feedings are stopped, and antibiotics, intravenous fluids, and bowel decompression are started. Resolution of the necrotizing process is assessed by physical examination (presence of bowel sounds, decreasing abdominal distention, lack of abdominal tenderness to palpation, absence of blood in stools), radiographs (resolution of pneumatosis and bowel dilation), and laboratory findings (stable platelet and white blood cell counts, normal acid-base balance). Feedings are initiated cautiously and advanced slowly using a hyposmolar elemental formula such as one-quarter strength Pregestimil. At this stage in the management of NEC, the most common complication is intestinal dysfunction. This may present as feeding intolerance, malabsorption, overgrowth of intestinal flora, or the presence of blood in stools. Causes of post-NEC intestinal dysfunction include poor intestinal motility, intestinal strictures, and mucosal abnormalities, including enzyme deficiencies and poor absorptive capabilities. Strictures occur in 10 to 30% of infants who have had NEC and are usually located in the terminal ileum or colon. They may cause partial or complete obstruction. Partial obstruction may allow the infant to advance to nearly complete enteral nutrition, only to develop signs of obstruction when a critical volume is reached. Contrast enema will identify most strictures in infants and should be done in all post-NEC infants who develop signs or symptoms of intestinal obstruction. Most strictures require surgical resection. Management of post-NEC intestinal dysfunction *not* due to strictures usually requires patience because most of such infants eventually recover with normal intestinal function. There is, however, a small but significant risk of recurrence of NEC in these high-risk patients. Therefore, patience must be combined with a high index of suspicion for recurrent NEC.

HYDROCEPHALUS

The leading cause of hydrocephalus in high-risk neonatal patients is intraventricular hemorrhage. Ventricular dilation may occur either early or late. Early dilation is thought to be due to blockage of the cerebrospinal fluid (CSF) pathways by clotted blood. Late dilation is due to obliterative arachnoiditis. Less common causes of hydrocephalus in the newborn include congenital malformations such as aqueductal stenosis, Dandy-Walker syndrome, or Arnold-Chiari malformation; infections of the ependyma or meninges; or vascular malformations and trauma.

Decisions regarding timing and method of treatment are complicated by the fact that hydrocephalus spontaneously arrests in up to 50% of cases. Therefore, close surveillance of ventricular size by ultrasonography is warranted. If there is continued ventricular enlargement, there are a variety of techniques that may allow the clinician to delay surgery while awaiting spontaneous arrest/resolution or an increase in infant size. These include repetitive lumbar or ventricular punctures and/or drugs that decrease CSF production such as acetazolamide (Diamox), furosemide, or ethacrynic acid. However, surgical decompression is necessary for the treatment of sustained ventricular dilation. The most commonly employed surgical treatment of hydrocephalus involves shunting of CSF from the ventricle to the peritoneal cavity.

A unique slit-valve catheter has become the most widely used. The slit valve at the peritoneal end of the catheter opens at a predetermined pressure. This protects the catheter tip from being invaded by fibrous tissue or omentum. The catheter also has a pump with a one-way valve mounted on the skull that allows the catheter to be flushed or tested for proper function.

The most significant complication of the ventriculoperitoneal shunt is obstruction by cellular debris, choroid plexus, omentum, or fibrous tissue. The incidence of infection is reported to be as low as 5%. The use of ventriculoatrial shunts has been abandoned due to a high rate of infection and an incidence of vascular thrombosis that may be as high as 20%.

The outlook for the infant who develops hydrocephalus has dramatically improved, primarily because of more sophisticated diagnostic techniques and improved technological innovations in treatment modalities. With follow-up of larger populations of neonates who have been successfully shunted, additional complications are being recognized. Better understanding of CSF physiology and biochemistry offers hope for future improvements in the treatment of hydrocephalus.

SUGGESTED READINGS

Berseth CL, Malachowski N, Cohn R, et al. Longitudinal growth and late morbidity of survivors of gastroschisis and omphalocele. J Pediatr Gastro Nutr 1982; 1:375.

Campbell JR, Sasaki TM. Gastrostomy in infants and children: an analysis of complications and techniques. Am Surg 1974; 9:505.

Dudley NE, Phelan PD. Respiratory complications in longterm survival of esophageal atresia. Arch Dis Child 1976; 51:279.

Ein SH. Divided loop colostomy that does not prolapse. Am J Surg 1984; 147:250.

Filler RM, Eraklis AJ, Das JB, et al. Total intravenous nutrition, an adjunct to the management of infants with a ruptured omphalocele. Am J Surg 1971; 121:454.

Filler RM, Rosello PJ, Lebowitz RL. Life threatening anoxic spells caused by tracheal compression after repair of esophageal atresia: correction by surgery. J Pediatr Surg 1976; 11:739.

Fonkalsrud EW. The undescended testis. Curr Prob Surg 1978; 15:5.

Gierup J, Olsen K, Sundkirst A. Aspects on the treatment of omphalocele and gastroschisis. Twenty years clinical experience. Z Kinderchirurgie 1982; 35:3.

Greenwood RD, Rosenthal A, Nadas AS. Cardiovascular malformations associated with omphalocele. J Pediatr 1974; 85:818.

Grosfeld JL, Cooney DE. Care of the child with a colostomy. Pediatrics 1977; 59:469.

Holder TM, Leape LL, Ashcraft KW. Gastrostomy: its use and dangers in pediatric patients. N Engl J Med 1972; 286:1345.

Holt PJ, Allan WC. The natural history of ventricular dilation in neonatal intraventricular hemorrhage and its therapeutic implications. Ann Neurol 1981; 10:293.

Jolley SG, Johnson DG, Roberts CC, et al. Patterns of gastroesophageal reflux in children following repair of esophageal atresia and distal tracheoesophageal fistula. J Pediatr Surg 1980; 15:857.

Levene MI, Starte DR. A longitudinal study of post-hemorrhagic ventricular dilation in the newborn. Arch Dis Child 1981; 56:905.

Levene MI, Wigglesworth JS, Dubowitz V. Cerebral structure and intraventricular hemorrhage in the neonate: a real-time ultrasound study. Arch Dis Child 1981; 56:416.

McComb JG, Ramos AD, Platzker ACG, et al. Management of hydrocephalus secondary to intraventricular hemorrhage in the preterm infant with a subcutaneous ventricular catheter and reservoir. Neurosurgery 1983; 13:295.

Nixon HH. Pediatric problems associated with stomas. Clin Gastroenterol 1982; 11:351.

Rescorla FJ, Grosfeld JL. Inguinal hernia repair in the perinatal period and early infancy: clinical considerations. J Pediatr Surg 1984; 19:832.

Rowe MI, Clatworthy HW. Incarcerated and strangulated hernias in children. Arch Surg 1970; 101:136.

Rowe MI, Copelson LW, Clatworthy HW. The patent processus vaginalis and the inguinal hernia. J Pediatr Surg 1969; 4:102.

Schwartz MZ, Richardson CJ, Hayden CK, et al. Intestinal stenosis following successful management of necrotizing enterocolitis. J Pediatr Surg 1980; 15:890.

Werlin SL, Dods WJ, Hogan WJ, et al. Esophageal function in esophageal atresia. Dig Dis Sci 1981; 26:796.

14

Dermatology

Bernard A. Cohen

The skin of the newborn differs from that of the adult in several ways (Table 14.1). It is less hairy, has less sweat and sebaceous gland secretions, is thinner, has fewer intercellular attachments, and fewer melanosomes. These differences are magnified in the preterm neonate. Consequently, preterm newborns are poorly equipped to handle thermal stress and sunlight. They have increased transepidermal water loss and increased transepidermal penetration of toxic substances and medications, and they are more likely to develop blisters or erosions in response to heat, chemical irritants, mechanical trauma, and inflammatory skin conditions.

BARRIER PROPERTIES AND USE OF TOPICAL AGENTS

The barrier properties of the skin reside primarily in the stratum corneum, the compact layer of flattened keratinocytes that cover the surface. Although keratinization begins at 24 weeks, it is not complete until close to term. Although transepidermal water loss and drug absorption through the epidermis in fullterm infants is similar to that in older children and adults and maturation of skin barrier properties is complete by several days of age in 36-week infants, maturation may be delayed for up to several weeks in more premature infants. Maturation is further delayed by epidermal injury, inflammation, or hyperemia. Finally, any infant, especially a premature infant, has a higher surface area-to-volume ratio than an older child or adult. This automatically exaggerates transcutaneous absorption of topical agents.

Percutaneous absorption of toxic substances in preterm infants and in term infants with disruption of barrier function has been well documented. Aniline dyes used to mark diapers have caused methemoglobinemia. Topical steroids can produce systemic effects and adrenal suppression. Accidental exposure to pentachlorophenol in nursery linens has caused poisoning. Topical application of povidone iodine has resulted in elevated plasma iodine levels and thyroid dysfunction. Isopropyl alcohol, ethyl and methyl alcohol, chlorhexidine, and other substances are also readily absorbed and may produce toxic reactions.

It is generally best not to use topical agents in newborns and infants unless the agent is nontoxic when administered systemically. Antiseptic agents should be used with great caution and applied with swabs to limited areas of the skin, particularly during the first several weeks of life in premature infants under 30 weeks gestation. Injury to the skin induced by tape, monitor skin electrodes, adhesives, and cleansing agents should be kept

Table 14.1. Structural and Functional Differences of Adult, Term, and Preterm Infant Skin

	Adult	Term	Preterm (30 wks)	Significance
Epidermal thickness	50 μm	50 μm	27.4 μm	↑ Permeability to topical agents ↑ Transepidermal water loss
Cell attachments (desmosomes, hemidesmosomes)	Normal	Normal	Fewer	↑ Tendency to blister
Dermis	Normal	↓ Collagen and elastic fibers	↓ ↓ Collagen and elastic fibers	↓ Elasticity ↑ Blistering
Melanosomes	Normal	Fewer	1/3 term infant	↑ Photosensitivity
Eccrine glands	Normal	Delayed activity for 1–7 days ↓ Neurologic control for 2–3 years	Total anhidrosis	↓ Response to thermal stress
Sebaceous	Normal	Normal	Normal	Barrier properties? Lubricant? Antibacterial?
Hair	Normal	↓ Terminal hair	Persistent lanugo	Helpful in assessing gestational age

to a minimum. When lubrication is necessary, small amounts of petrolatum or other fragrance-free, bland emollients should be used.

At birth, the skin is covered with a greasy, white material with a pH of 6.7 to 7.4. Although the function of this vernix caseosa is unknown, it may have lubricating and antibacterial properties. Beneath the vernix, the skin has a pH of 5.5 to 6.0. Overwashing, particularly with harsh soaps, may result in irritation, alkaline pH, and a decrease in normal barrier function. Consequently, bathing should be done gently with tap water. Mild soaps should be restricted to the umbilicus, diaper area, neck, axillae, and other areas where cutaneous bacteria are most numerous. In ill newborns, bathing may be limited to saline compresses to areas of irritated, macerated skin.

THERMOREGULATION

Cold stress is a major risk to naked preterm infants. Decreased epidermal and dermal thickness results in increased heat loss from radiation and conduction. Minimal subcutaneous fat and an immature nervous system further decrease the premature infant's ability to respond to cooling. Heat loss may be minimized by increasing ambient humidity and temperature and by covering the child with a plastic bubble, but the maintenance of normal body temperature is associated primarily with increasing postnatal age and weight approaching 2000 grams.

In bigger premature infants, hyperthermia may be a problem in the presence of phototherapy or insulated clothing. Although sweat glands are anatomically complete at 28 weeks gestation, they may not be fully functional until 42 to 44 weeks.

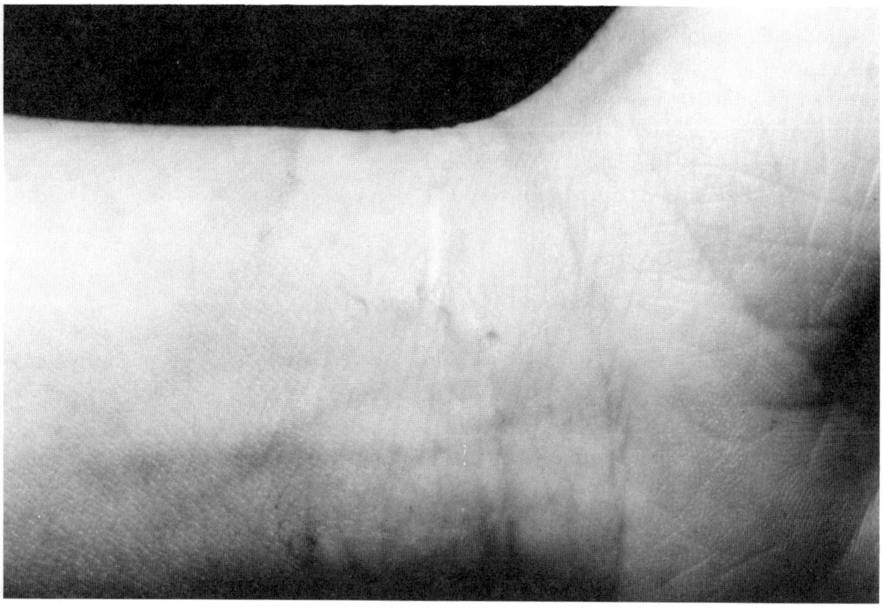

Figure 14.1. A linear scar and sinus tract from an intravenous cut-down site and suture persist on the wrist of a 4-year-old girl.

CUTANEOUS COMPLICATIONS OF THE INTENSIVE CARE NURSERY

Damage to the skin, sometimes resulting in a scar, is an inevitable complication of nursery care and monitoring. Careful management of the skin in the nursery and after discharge will minimize the risk of functional impairment and cosmetic disfigurement. Parents should be instructed in the natural course and care of these lesions.

Surgical Scars

Small wounds, such as those from the percutaneous insertion of arterial or venous catheters, generally heal with barely noticeable scars. Even more obvious scars usually fade over the first 2 years of life, particularly if the wounds conform to the normal skin lines. Dimpling may result from sutures used to keep the catheters in place (Fig. 14.1). Scarring and dimpling may be minimized by gentle massage of the affected area.

Large surgical wounds tend to heal with extensive scarring that may eventually require plastic surgical revision. Although some of these scars may become more subtle with increasing age, others grow with the child.

Chest tubes are frequently inserted in situations that allow little time to select the optimal site. Placement that avoids breast tissue will eliminate one type of damage that will require later surgical repair. Gentle massage after removal may prevent the formation of adhesions and dimpling at the insertion site. Fortunately, as with other surgical scars, these lesions tend to become less obvious over the first several years of life.

Arterial Catheters

Cutdown incisions always carry the risk of local scarring (Fig. 14.1). However, arterial catheterization may also be associated with much more extensive, serious tissue damage. Extensive ischemia and necrosis of the genital and buttock skin is an unusual complication of umbilical artery catheterization. Ensuing ulcerations may take months to heal and often require surgical repair. Radial artery catheterization has rarely been associated with necrosis of the fingers. More subtle findings, such as a discrepancy in hand size, may not be evident for months or years.

Chemical and Thermal Burns

Infiltration of soft tissue by intravenous fluids often produces cutaneous inflammation and necrosis (Fig. 14.2). Hypertonic fluids such as glucose and calcium may result in full-thickness sloughing of the skin and contractures. These lesions usually heal over weeks to months, but they may require splinting, physical therapy, and surgical repair, particularly if they are located over joints.

Removal of adhesives used to secure dressings, endotracheal and nasotracheal tubes, and monitor leads can result in extensive trauma. Although full-thickness sloughs are rare, postinflammatory hyperpigmentation and hypopigmentation are common. Pigmentary changes may persist for years in dark pigmented individuals. Fortunately, it is more usual for these changes to disappear within the first year of life.

Accidental thermal burns have been reported following exposure to heated water beds, radiant warmers, transcutaneous oxygen monitors, and heated humidified air.

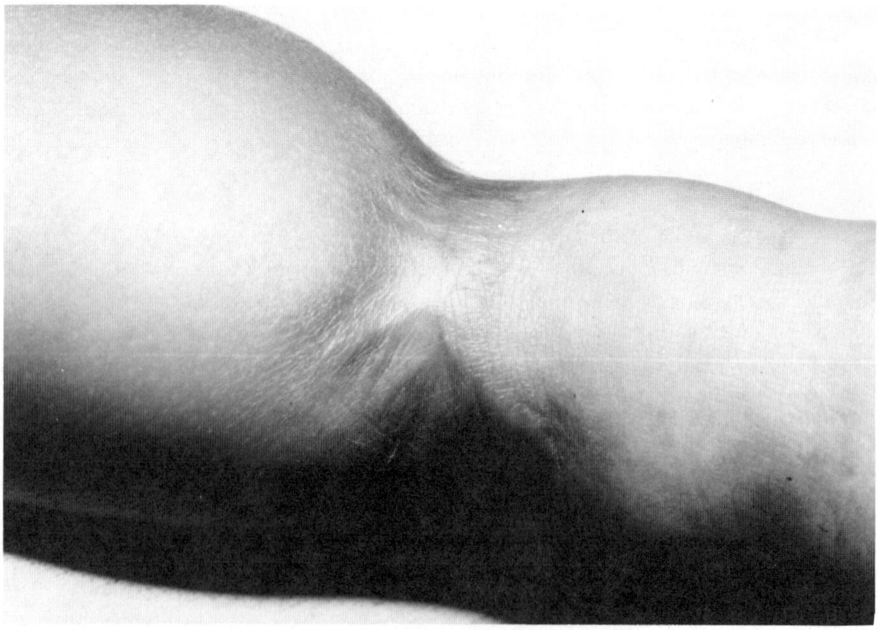

Figure 14.2. Scar on the leg of a 3-year-old child resulted from the infiltration of hyperalimentation solution.

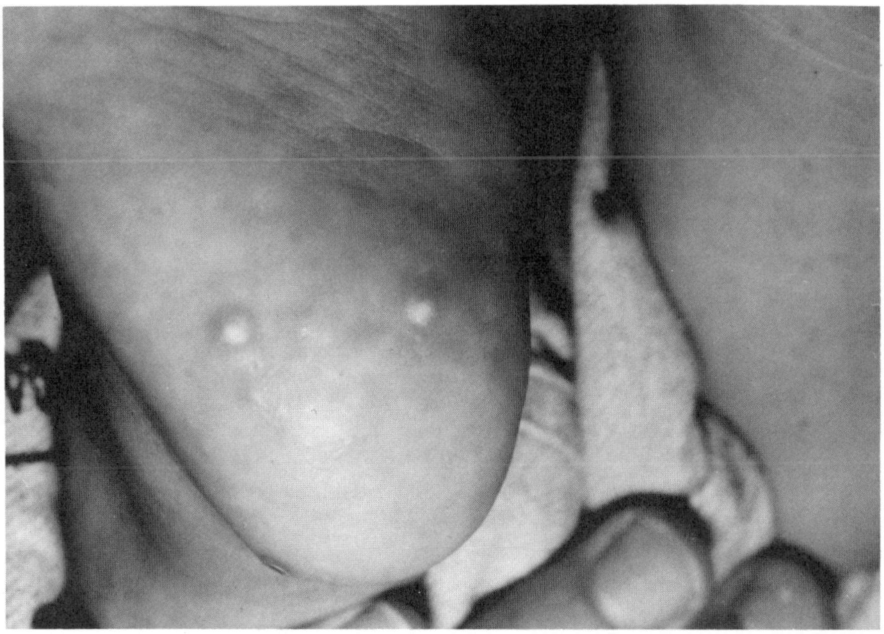

Figure 14.3. Calcified nodules on the heel of a 14-month-old child.

Heel Stick Nodules

Repeated blood sampling from the heel leads to the formation of 3 to 5 mm, deep-seated papules and nodules in many NICU graduates (Fig. 14.3). Although the lesions are most prominent in children who have had frequent heel sticks, they are occasionally seen in infants who have had only a few. Nodules and papules may be palpable at the time of discharge from the nursery. Over a period of several months, they generally become more superficial and resemble milia. Papules typically calcify over the ensuing months and resolve spontaneously in 18 to 30 months. Parents should be advised of the innocent nature of the lesions. During this time, the infants are asymptomatic, and walking is not delayed.

EVALUATION OF NEWBORN SKIN

Although skin eruptions in infancy are often transient and innocent, some herald the onset of devastating disease. Consequently, all practitioners who provide care for high-risk newborns should develop a systematic approach to evaluating rashes in this setting.

Historical Data

Initially, the clinician must have a detailed picture of skin symptoms, including date of onset, inciting factors, evolution of lesions, and evidence of pruritus (scratching). Recent maternal and neonatal infections, drug or toxic exposures, and dietary changes may be important. The family history may suggest a hereditary or infectious disorder, and the clinician may need to interview and examine family members with similar complaints.

Skin Examination

Examination of the skin must be performed in a well-lighted room and must include hair, nails, scalp, and mucous membranes. If cold stress is a risk, care must be taken to expose only a small portion of the body surface at a time. Although no special equipment is required, a hand lens may aid in the assessment of skin texture and small, poorly defined lesions.

Skin Assessment

A systematic approach to the evaluation of cutaneous findings leads to a reasonable differential diagnosis. The distribution and pattern of lesions should be noted. For example, is the rash symmetric and widespread or localized to one part of the body? Do lesions involve intertriginous areas or acral and periorificial areas?

Next, the organization of lesions should be assessed. Are they scattered or grouped? If the lesions are grouped, are they herpetiform, zosteriform, or linear? Finally, the morphology of the primary and secondary lesions should be determined. Primary lesions include macules, papules, plaques, vesicles, bullae, nodules, and tumors. Secondary lesions such as pustules, excoriations, crusts, and scars either evolve spontaneously from a primary lesion or develop after patient manipulation.

TRANSIENT SKIN DISORDERS OF THE NEWBORN

A number of innocent skin conditions occur in newborns. Although they are often transient, they may be dramatic. Early recognition is important to distinguish them from more serious disorders.

Transient Vascular Phenomena

ACROCYANOSIS AND CUTIS MARMORATA

During the first 2 to 4 weeks of life, cold stress may be associated with acrocyanosis and cutis marmorata. In acrocyanosis, the hands and feet become variably and symmetrically blue in color without edema or other cutaneous changes. Cutis marmorata is identified by the characteristic reticulated cyanosis or marbling of the skin that symmetrically involves the trunk and extremities. Both patterns usually resolve with warming of the skin, and recurrence is unusual after 1 month of age. Acrocyanosis is readily differentiated from persistent central cyanosis, which occurs in association with pulmonary or cardiac disease. Cutis marmorata that persists beyond the neonatal period may be a marker for trisomy 18, Down's syndrome, Cornelia de Lange syndrome, and hypothyroidism. Cutis marmorata telangiectatica congenita (congenital phlebectasia) may mimic cutis marmorata, but lesions are persistent and often asymmetrical. Congenital phlebectasia may be either an isolated finding or may occur in association with other mesodermal and neuroectodermal anomalies.

HARLEQUIN COLOR CHANGE

The harlequin color change is noted when the infant is in the lateral decubitus position. The dependent half of the body turns bright red and contrasts with the pale upper half. The color reverses when the infant is rolled from side to side. This phenomenon lasts from seconds to 20 minutes, and recurrences are common until 3 to 4 weeks of life. The cause is unknown, and it is not associated with serious underlying disease.

Benign Pustular Dermatoses

Several innocent pustular eruptions must be differentiated from potentially serious infectious dermatoses.

ERYTHEMA TOXICUM NEONATORUM

Erythema toxicum neonatorum (ETN) is the most common pustular rash and occurs in up to 70% of fullterm infants. Lesions usually appear on the second or third day of life, but onset may be as early as prior to delivery or as late as 2 to 3 weeks of age. ETN typically begins with 2 to 3 mm erythematous, blotchy macules and papules. These evolve over several hours into pustules on a broad, erythematous base, giving affected infants a "flea-bitten" appearance. Lesions may be isolated or clustered on the face, trunk, and proximal extremities. They usually fade over 5 to 7 days. Recurrences, however, may occur for several weeks. A Wright's stain of the pustule contents reveals sheets of eosinophils and occasional neutrophils, and 15 to 20% of patients will have a circulating eosinophilia.

TRANSIENT NEONATAL PUSTULAR MELANOSIS

Transient neonatal pustular melanosis occurs in 4% of newborns, particularly in black male infants. Unlike ETN, lesions are usually present at birth. The disorder characteristically appears as 2 to 5 mm pustules on a nonerythematous base on the chin, neck, upper chest, sacrum, abdomen, and thighs. Over several days, lesions develop a central crust, which then desquamates, leaving a hyperpigmented macule with a collarette of fine scale. Lesions in different stages of development are usually present simultaneously. Often, the only manifestation of the eruption is the presence of brown macules with a rim of scale. A Wright's stain of the pustular smear shows numerous neutrophils and rare eosinophils.

ACROPUSTULOSIS OF INFANCY

Acropustulosis of infancy is a chronic, recurrent, pustular eruption that appears on the palms and soles but may also involve the scalp, trunk, buttocks, and extremities. Onset may occur during the newborn period or early infancy, and episodes typically last from 1 to 3 weeks with intervening remissions for 1 to 3 weeks. Disease-free periods tend to lengthen until the rash resolves by 2 to 3 years of age. During flares, infants are usually fussy. Pruritus is severe. Histopathology of the lesions reveals sterile intraepidermal pustules. A Wright's stain shows numerous neutrophils and occasional eosinophils. Although oral Dapsone (1 to 3 mg/kg/day) will suppress lesions and symptoms in 24 to 48 hours, brief courses of moderate- or high-potency topical steroids to the palms and soles may provide safe, temporary relief.

SEBACEOUS GLAND HYPERPLASIA

Sebaceous gland hyperplasia is common over the nose and cheeks of term infants. Lesions consist of multiple, 1 to 2 mm, yellow papules that result from maternal or endogenous androgenic stimulation of sebaceous gland growth. Parents should be counseled that the eruption resolves within 4 to 6 months.

MILIARIA

Miliaria results from obstruction to the flow of sweat and rupture of the eccrine sweat duct. In miliaria crystalline, superficial, 1 to 2 mm vesicles appear on noninflamed skin when the duct is blocked by keratinous debris just beneath the stratum corneum. Small papules and pustules are typical of miliaria rubra (prickly heat), in which the obstruction occurs in the midepidermis. Deep-seated papulopustular lesions of miliaria profunda, which occur when the duct ruptures at the dermal-epidermal junction, occur only rarely in infancy.

Miliaria occurs frequently in term and preterm infants after the first week of life in response to thermal stress. Lesions erupt in crops in the intertriginous areas, scalp, face, and trunk. Cooling the skin and loosening clothing results in prompt resolution of the rash.

MILIA

Milia appear as pearly yellow, 1 to 3 mm papules on the face, chin, and forehead of 50% of newborns. Although milia usually resolve without treatment during the first month of life, they may persist for several months. Histology demonstrates miniature epidermal inclusion cysts, which arise from the pilosebaceous apparatus of vellus hairs. Large numbers of lesions distributed over a wide area and persistence beyond several months of age should suggest the possibility of the oral-facial-digital syndrome or trichodysplasia. Increasing numbers of lesions, particularly in areas of normal trauma such as the hands, knees, and feet, may occur in patients with mild variants of scarring epidermolysis bullosa where blistering is subtle.

NEONATAL ACNE

Neonatal acne develops in up to 20% of newborns. Lesions may be present at birth or appear in early infancy. Closed comedones (whiteheads) predominate, although open comedones (blackheads), red papules, pustules, and rarely, cysts may also occur. As in sebaceous hyperplasia, maternal and endogenous androgens probably play a role in the pathogenesis of neonatal acne. Treatment is usually unnecessary because lesions involute spontaneously within 1 to 3 months. The risk of acne in adolescence does not seem to be increased.

DIFFERENTIAL DIAGNOSIS

Benign pustular dermatoses may be differentiated from herpes simplex infection by the absence of multinucleated giant cells on Wright's stained smears of pustular contents. Negative Gram stain and potassium hydroxide preparations exclude bacterial and candidal infection. However, in seriously ill infants, viral and bacterial cultures may be required to confirm the clinical impression. Serological studies for syphilis and scrapings for ectoparasites will exclude syphilis and scabies in children with acropustulosis.

SUBCUTANEOUS FAT NECROSIS OF THE NEWBORN

Fat necrosis is a benign, self-limited process that usually occurs in otherwise healthy infants. Discrete red or hemorrhagic nodules and plaques up to 3 cm in diameter appear most commonly over areas exposed to trauma, such as the cheeks, back, buttocks, arms, and thighs, during the first few weeks of life. Lesions are usually painless, but marked tenderness may be present. Although the cause is unknown, difficult deliveries, hypothermia, perinatal asphyxia, and maternal diabetes predispose to the development of fat necrosis.

Parents should be advised that most nodules resolve without scarring in 1 to 2 months. However, lesions occasionally become fluctuant, drain, and heal with atrophy. When calcification occurs, infants should be evaluated for primary hyperparathyroidism, and calcium levels must be monitored.

THE SCALY NEWBORN

Included in this category are the icthyoses. The reader is referred to standard texts for a complete discussion of these disorders.

Diaper Dermatitis and Related Disorders

These disorders are characterized by acute changes (erythema, edema, and vesiculation) and/or chronic changes (scale, lichenification, and increased and decreased pigmentation) in the skin. Microscopically, these disorders show infiltration of the dermis with inflammatory cells, variable thickening of the epidermis, and scale.

Diaper dermatitis is one of the most common skin disorders of infancy. In its most common form, it represents an *irritant contact dermatitis*. The diaper area is a prime target for an irritant dermatitis because it is bathed in urine and feces and is often occluded by plastic diaper covers. Although ammonia from urine was first thought to play a leading role in the pathogenesis of diaper dermatitis, recent evidence points to feces as the principal culprit. Once the epidermal barrier is disrupted, the skin may become sensitive to other irritants such as soap, powder, and detergents. Watery stools, particularly after antibiotic exposure or vial infections, often trigger severe dermatitis that is recalcitrant to conservative measures.

Irritant reactions are usually confined to convex surfaces of the perineum, lower abdomen, buttocks, and proximal thighs. The intertriginous areas are invariably spared. Gentle, thorough cleansing of the area and the application of lubricants (e.g., petrolatum) and barrier pastes (e.g., zinc oxide) usually result in clearing of the dermatitis. A tapering course of low-potency topical steroid ointment (e.g., hydrocortisone) in severe cases may speed resolution of symptoms and clinical findings.

Although less common than irritant dermatitis, *allergic contact dermatitis* may account for occasional diaper rashes. Fragrance, preservatives, and emulsifiers in topical baby products may be associated with allergic reactions in the diaper area as well as on the face, trunk, and extremities. Avoidance of the offending agent, aggressive use of emollients, and judicious use of topical steroids will clear these reactions within several days.

Persistent diaper dermatitis may be due to other disorders such as candidiasis and seborrheic dermatitis. *Candidiasis* appears as a brilliant red eruption with sharp borders, satellite red papules, and pustules. Lesions typically involve the skin creases. Candidiasis is a common complication of systemic antibiotic therapy and chronic irritant dermatitis. Examination of material from a pustule by Gram stain or potassium hydroxide preparation reveals pseudohyphae. Diaper candidiasis may be accompanied by oral thrush, candida paronychia of the fingers or toes, and candidiasis of other intertriginous areas. Diaper candidiasis responds rapidly to topical antifungals such as nystatin, cyclopirax, ketoconazole, and the imidazoles (micronazole, clotrimazole, econazole). Although a brief course of topical steroids may speed clinical improvement, high-potency agents may produce skin atrophy in a short period of time and should be avoided. Several studies demonstrate that a new broad-spectrum topical antifungal naftifine compares favorably with a combination high-potency topical steroid-antifungal cream (Lotrisone) in selected fungal infections. Its anti-inflammatory properties may be useful in severe cases of diaper candidiasis.

Seborrheic dermatitis is characterized by salmon-colored patches with greasy yellow scale that begin in the intertriginous areas, especially the diaper area and scalp. Fissuring, maceration, and weeping occasionally develops. Thick, adherent scales on the occiput are referred to as "cradle cap." Although oval red patches may spread to the trunk, proximal extremities, and postauricular areas, affected infants remain healthy and asymptomatic. In dark pigmented children, postinflammatory hypopigmentation is marked but transient.

The cause of seborrheic dermatitis is unknown. However, the yeast *Pityrosporum* has been implicated in adult seborrhea and identified in the scalp of infants with "cradle cap." This organism tends to proliferate in areas where sebaceous glands are most numerous and active, and this probably explains the timing and the distribution of the eruption. Seborrheic dermatitis may clear without treatment by 2 to 3 months of age, but often it persists until 8 to 12 months. Mild keratolytics found in antiseborrheic shampoos (zinc pyrithione, sulfur, and salicylic acid) are helpful in managing "cradle cap." Emollients and low-potency topical steroids will hasten the resolution of cutaneous lesions. Topical antifungals have been approved for treating adult seborrheic dermatitis and may be useful in infants.

Severe multisystem disease may begin with a progressive diaper dermatitis. A seborrheic dermatitis-like eruption is characteristic of *histiocytosis X*. However, the rash tends to become hemorrhagic and erosive, particularly in the diaper area. Scaly, crusted, purpuric plaques also develop on the scalp, trunk, and extremities. Diagnostic skin biopsies demonstrate infiltrates of atypical histiocytes that may involve the liver, lungs, kidneys, and nervous system and result in severe organ dysfunction and death.

Acrodermatitis enteropathica (AEP) classically presents with an erosive diaper dermatitis, diarrhea, and hair loss during the first few months of life. Weeping, crusted, erythematous patches also appear in a periorificial, acral, and intertriginous distribution. Affected infants are irritable, grow poorly, and are prone to infection and septicemia.

AEP is an autosomal recessive disorder of zinc metabolism. Affected infants have either defective or low levels of a zinc-binding protein in the gastrointestinal tract and resultant zinc malabsorption. Breast milk contains a compensatory zinc-binding ligand that facilitates absorption. Consequently, breast-fed infants do not develop symptoms until nursing is discontinued. Zinc is stored in the fetal liver, particularly during the last month of gestation. As a result, affected premature infants who are not breast fed become zinc deficient quickly. Normal infants who require hyperalimentation as well as those with zinc losses from malabsorption states (e.g., cystic fibrosis, chronic infectious diarrhea, short bowel syndrome) will develop an AEP-like rash if they do not receive zinc supplementation. Similar rashes have been reported with biotin deficiency and urea enzyme cycle defects.

AEP responds within several days to high doses of oral or intravenous zinc. Although dietary zinc without supplementation may be adequate in older children with AEP, these patients require close monitoring of growth and development. Some will require lifelong zinc supplements.

VESICULOPUSTULAR DERMATOSES

Vesiculobullous and pustular eruptions present a confusing clinical picture. Specific diagnosis is critical because therapeutic intervention may be lifesaving.

Infections

Viral infections including herpes simplex and varicella-zoster produce characteristic vesiculopustular eruptions. Herpes simplex is a common cause of self-limited oral and cutaneous lesions in toddlers and older children. However, in neonates, there is a high risk of dissemination. Varicella is less common, but if lesions appear during the first week of life, the risk of mortality approaches 30%.

HERPES SIMPLEX

Cutaneous lesions of herpes simplex typically begin at 3 to 10 days of life as 1 to 2 mm, clustered red papules and vesicles that may become pustular, denuded, and hemorrhagic over the following 2 to 3 days. The first lesions commonly develop on the scalp in vertex deliveries and on the feet or buttocks after breech presentation.

Blisters will contain multinucleated giant cells when their contents are prepared on a glass slide with Giemsa or Wright's stain. Viral cultures from blister fluid or denuded areas of skin often demonstrate cytopathic effect within 24 to 36 hours. Early antiviral therapy may decrease the risk and severity of disseminated disease. Skin lesions should be gently cleansed, and excess blister fluid absorbed with a gauze pad to reduce cutaneous spread. Skin lesions may recur for up to 5 years.

VARICELLA

When a mother has varicella within 3 weeks of delivery, her infant has a 25% risk of manifesting congenital chickenpox. Exposure during the first trimester occasionally leads to the development of the neonatal varicella syndrome with linear scars, limb anomalies, ocular defects, and central nervous system involvement.

As in herpes simplex, infants with congenital disease may be well at birth. Infants who develop chickenpox between 3 and 10 days of age are at risk of varicella pneumonitis, encephalitis, and purpura fulminans with widespread bleeding, hypotension, and death. Transplacental antibody protects infants with onset within the first 3 days of life, and disease in infants older than 10 days is rarely severe.

Varicella-zoster immune globulin and parenteral acyclovir may improve outcome and should be considered early in the course of infants at risk for severe disease. As with herpes simplex, lesions contain multinucleated giant cells. These two viral infections can sometimes be differentiated only by culture of the blister contents.

BACTERIAL INFECTIONS

Several common bacterial infections present with vesiculopustular eruptions in infancy. In *bullous impetigo*, slowly enlarging blistering rings surround central umbilicated crusts. Lesions may appear anywhere on the skin surface. However, in young infants, areas prone to trauma, such as the diaper area, circumcision wound, and umbilical stump, are frequent sites of primary infection. Bullous lesions are caused by certain epidermal toxin-producing strains of staphylococcus. Although lesions may remain localized, they are highly infectious and may be inoculated to multiple sites on the patient as well as to caretakers. In newborns and young infants, dissemination of the toxin may result in widespread erythema and blistering typical of *staphylococcal scalded skin syndrome* (SSSS). In this case, gentle pressure on the skin causes the upper epidermis to slide off, leaving a denuded base (Nikolsky's sign).

In bullous impetigo, bacteria are identified in Gram-stained material obtained directly from the rash. In SSSS, it may be impossible to identify a primary cutaneous site of infection. In these children, infection in lungs, bone, meninges, ears, and other noncutaneous sources must be sought.

Because neonates do not localize infection to the epidermis and superficial dermis, any sign of progressive cellulitis or systemic infection should prompt immediate treatment with parenteral antibiotics and supportive care. A nosocomial source should always be suspected. The possibility of skin colonization of personnel should be investigated.

DISSEMINATED CANDIDIASIS

Disseminated candidiasis in the newborn may be confused with bacterial infection. In congenital candidiasis, generalized erythematous papules, vesicles, and pustules are present at or soon after birth. These lesions may slough, leaving large, denuded areas reminiscent of SSSS. The organism is acquired by ascending vaginal or cervical infection. The identification of pseudohyphae and spores from pustules and scales is diagnostic. When infants acquire infection at delivery, the onset of skin lesions may be delayed by 7 to 10 days. Erosive patches with satellite pustules are usually limited to intertriginous areas. Fullterm infants often go on to heal without treatment, although topical antifungals may be helpful. Preterm infants are at high risk for dissemination, and early diagnosis and initiation of parenteral amphotericin may be lifesaving.

MECHANOBULLOUS DISEASES (EPIDERMOLYSIS BULLOSA)

These disorders are a heterogenous group of blistering dermatoses characterized by the development of lesions after trauma to the skin. Epidermolysis bullosa (EB) variants are differentiated by their inheritance pattern, clinical presentation, histopathology, and biochemical markers. Although blisters may appear at birth or in the neonatal period, the onset of lesions in mild, localized forms is often delayed until later childhood or adult life.

EB may be classified into three major types, depending upon the cleavage plane of the blister. In EB simplex, blisters are intraepidermal, and the clinical course is usually mild. In junctional EB, blisters form at the dermal-epidermal junction, usually through the lamina lucida in the basement membrane zone. Although patients may have mild disease comparable to EB simplex, in some children, progressive blistering with involvement of the mucous membranes and gastrointestinal tract leads to inanition, sepsis, and death within the first 2 years of life. Dystrophic EB is characterized by scarring blisters that form in the dermis beneath the basement membrane zone. Blisters may be localized to the hands and feet or widespread with involvement of the dentition, nails, airway, and esophagus.

EB should be considered in infants with recurrent blistering when infection has been excluded. Family history and examination of other family members will aid in clinical diagnosis. A skin biopsy with electron microscopy will provide precise identification of the cleavage plane in the skin. Genetic counseling is important, particularly in severe variants. Prenatal diagnosis is available.

In children without a family history of EB, it may be difficult to determine a prognosis in the newborn period. Infants with dystrophic EB may do very well, but children with junctional disease may pursue a downhill course after a period of stabilization. The appropriate counsel is reassurance. Discussion of prognosis should be postponed pending a period of observation.

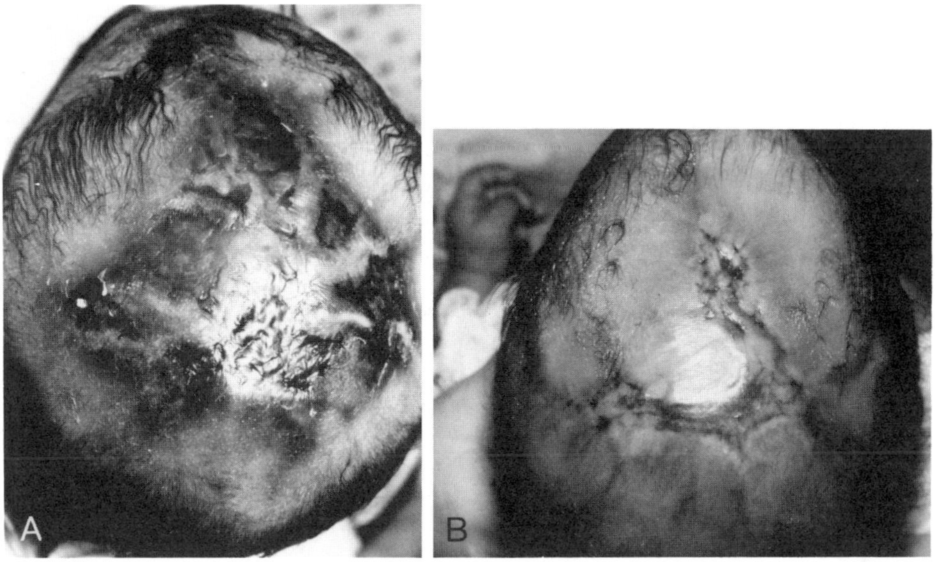

Figure 14.4. A large scalp defect noted at birth (A) healed by 4 months of age (B). The child was otherwise healthy, and the defect was excised with skin expanders at 5 years of age.

Treatment of EB is dependent on severity and is covered in depth in standard reference texts.

APLASIA CUTIS CONGENITA

This is a heterogenous group of disorders whose common feature is congenital absence of the skin. The entity has been recognized for over 150 years, but the cause is unknown. In the classic form, one or several erosions or ulcerations covered with a crust or thin membrane involve the vertex of the scalp (Fig. 14.4). Healing with atrophic, hairless scars occurs over 2 to 6 months, depending on the size and depth of the ulceration. Lesions may extend through the soft tissue into bone. This benign variant is usually inherited as an autosomal dominant trait. Less commonly, the trunk and extremities are involved, and lesions may be associated with limb defects, amniotic band syndrome, epidermolysis bullosa, and chromosomal aberrations.

In uncomplicated aplasia cutis congenita, the defect is amenable to simple excision during later childhood or adult life. Large lesions may require staged excision and the use of tissue expanders. Initially, care must be taken to evaluate the depth of the defect, prevent further tissue damage and infection, and search for associated anomalies. Gentle normal saline compresses, topical antibiotics, and sterile dressings are adequate for most patients. Large defects may respond to occlusive dressings (DuoDERM, Comfeel). Occasionally, early surgery is necessary.

Perinatal trauma to the scalp may result in similar defects noted at birth or within the first month of life. Scalp blood sampling, monitor electrodes, and forceps may produce small ulcers that heal with scarring. Halo scalp ring is a form of localized scalp injury associated with caput succedaneum, which occasionally resolves with a scarring alopecia.

MASTOCYTOSIS

This may first come to clinical attention when cutaneous lesions blister. The disorder typically presents at birth or within the first few months of life. It may present as a solitary mastocytoma, as multiple lesions, or as urticaria pigmentosa. Although the trunk is most commonly involved, these benign mast cell-containing macules, papules, and plaques may involve any cutaneous site as well as the gastrointestinal tract, bone marrow, lungs, kidneys, and nervous system. Skin lesions range from under 1 cm to large, infiltrated plaques that cover the chest or back. Although the overlying epidermis may appear normal at birth, increasing age is associated with progressive, localized hyperpigmentation.

Nonspecific triggers of mast cell degranulation such as rubbing, hot water, vigorous physical activity, and certain medications (e.g., aspirin, anesthetic agents, x-ray contrast material) may produce urtication of cutaneous lesions. Darier's sign is a reliable physical finding in mastocytosis and refers to the hives that form after stroking involved skin. Infants are particularly prone to blister formation, and widespread blistering is associated with fluid and electrolyte losses and increased risk of infection. Other symptoms of histamine toxicity, including chronic diarrhea, gastric ulceration, uncontrolled pruritus, bleeding, and hypotension, may develop.

Pruritus and systemic symptoms are usually controlled with antihistamines. In infants with bullous mastocytosis and/or systemic disease, oral cromolyn sodium 20 to 40 mg/kg/day may be lifesaving. In many children, the number of papules and plaques increases for 1 to 2 years. During childhood, mastocytomas often become less reactive and tan or brown overlying pigmentation fades slowly. Hyperpigmentation, urtication, and systemic symptoms may persist in some individuals.

INCONTINENTIA PIGMENTI (IP)

This is a neurocutaneous syndrome named for the peculiar marble cake swirls of brown pigment that appear on the trunk and occasionally on the extremities in later infancy and early childhood. In the newborn, patches of erythema and blisters are scattered on the trunk, scalp, and extremities. Blisters are typically oriented in lines, swirls, and dermatomal patterns. Although these inflammatory lesions may recur for months, they usually give way to hyperkeratotic warty plaques by several weeks to several months of age. The hyperkeratotic stage is typically followed by increasing pigmentation at 2 to 6 months of age. Occasionally, hyperpigmentation may begin to appear at several weeks of age, and in 10% of infants, it may be the only manifestation at birth. During later childhood, brown streaks often fade to leave atrophic, hypopigmented patches. These subtle scars may be the only manifestation of cutaneous disease in older children and adults.

Histopathology of blisters in the newborn demonstrates characteristic intraepidermal edema and vesicles loaded with eosinophils. When IP is suspected, the child should be evaluated for associated defects, which may involve the central nervous system, heart, eye, skeletal system, and dentition. IP is inherited as an X-linked, dominant disorder and appears to be lethal in males; 97% of affected infants are female. A careful examination of mothers often reveals subtle cutaneous findings.

NEVI

Nevi appear at birth or in the first month of life. They are composed of mature or nearly mature cutaneous elements organized in an abnormal fashion. These hamartomas may be comprised of virtually any epidermal or dermal structure.

Vascular Nevi

Congenital vascular malformations are the most common neoplasms of childhood. Flat, nonpalpable salmon patches and port wine stains are present at birth. Palpable hemangiomas typically appear within the first 2 weeks of life, grow for 6 to 12 months, and resolve spontaneously over the following years.

SALMON PATCHES

Salmon patches occur in 60 to 70% of newborns. Lesions are usually located on the nape of the neck, glabella, forehead, or upper eye lids. Although salmon patches usually fade during the first year of life and tend to be camouflaged by normal pigmentation, they may persist indefinitely, particularly on the neck. The pink patches also darken with crying, breath holding, and physical exertion.

PORT WINE STAINS

Port wine stains (PWS) are present at birth in 0.2 to 0.3% of newborns. Unlike salmon patches, PWS tend to persist unchanged during childhood and to darken in adolescence and adulthood. Small angiomatous papules and underlying soft tissue hypertrophy may also develop.

Although unilateral lesions on the head and neck are most common, any part of the body surface and mucous membranes may be involved. Occasionally, PWSs present in association with extracutaneous defects. Children with involvement of the first division of the trigeminal nerve may have an associated vascular malformation of the ipsilateral meninges and cerebral cortex (Sturge-Weber syndrome). Seizures, mental retardation, hemiplegia, and glaucoma may develop during the first several years of life. The association of cutaneous vascular lesions with limb hypertrophy is typical of Klippel-Trenaunay-Weber syndrome.

Infants with PWSs deserve a thorough physical examination looking for signs of systemic disease. Children with forehead and periorbital involvement require careful neurodevelopmental follow-up, an eye examination to exclude glaucoma, and further neurological studies as indicated.

Rehabilitative cosmetics (e.g., Dermabland, Covermark) provide reasonable, safe, but temporary camouflage of PWSs. Definitive treatment consists of selective photothermolysis using a pulsed, tuneable yellow-dye laser. Treatment in early childhood produces the best outcome with the fewest number of treatments and the least cost (Fig. 14.5).

PALPABLE HEMANGIOMAS

Although rarely present at birth, palpable hemangiomas occur in up to 10% of infants by 4 weeks of age. Lesions typically begin as barely visible telangiectasias or red macules that rapidly grow into 0.5 to 4.0 cm, bright red, compressible tumors or strawberry hemangiomas. Many hemangiomas have a deep dermal or subcutaneous component. Occasionally, lesions lack a superficial component altogether (cavernous hemangiomas).

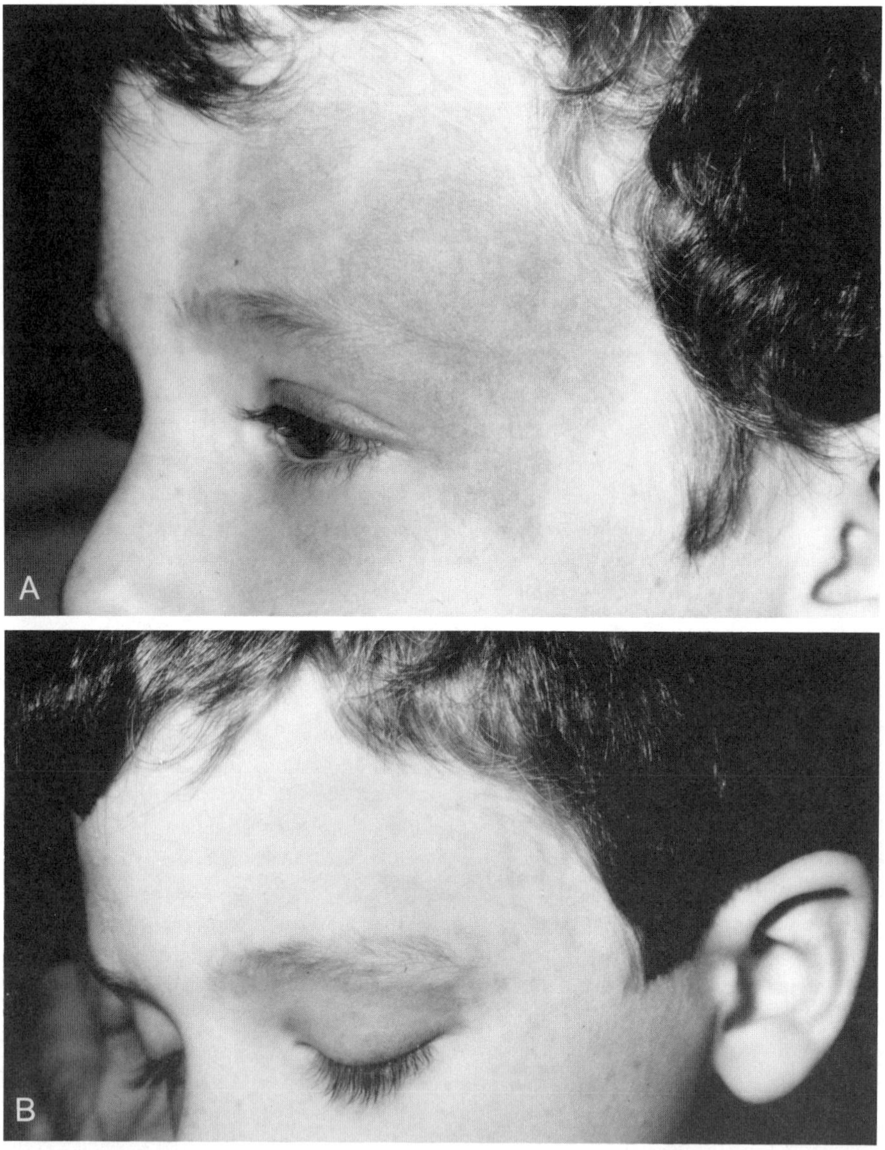

Figure 14.5. A 4-year-old boy with a port wine stain on the left temple (A) demonstrated marked clearing after three pulsed dye laser treatments (B).

Growth of hemangiomas usually stops by 6 to 12 months of age, followed by early signs of involution, such as graying of the lesion (Fig. 14.6). Involution is independent of sex, location, size, number, and depth of the hemangiomas. Although the majority of hemangiomas resolve by 5 to 7 years, persistent lesions continue to improve into adolescence. Scarring, patulous skin, or telangiectasias remain in 30 to 40% of children.

Although hemangiomas are benign tumors and involution is the rule, these lesions may compromise vital functions when they are located near the anus, urethra, airway, and orbit. Large, rapidly-growing lesions in young infants may be associated with high-output

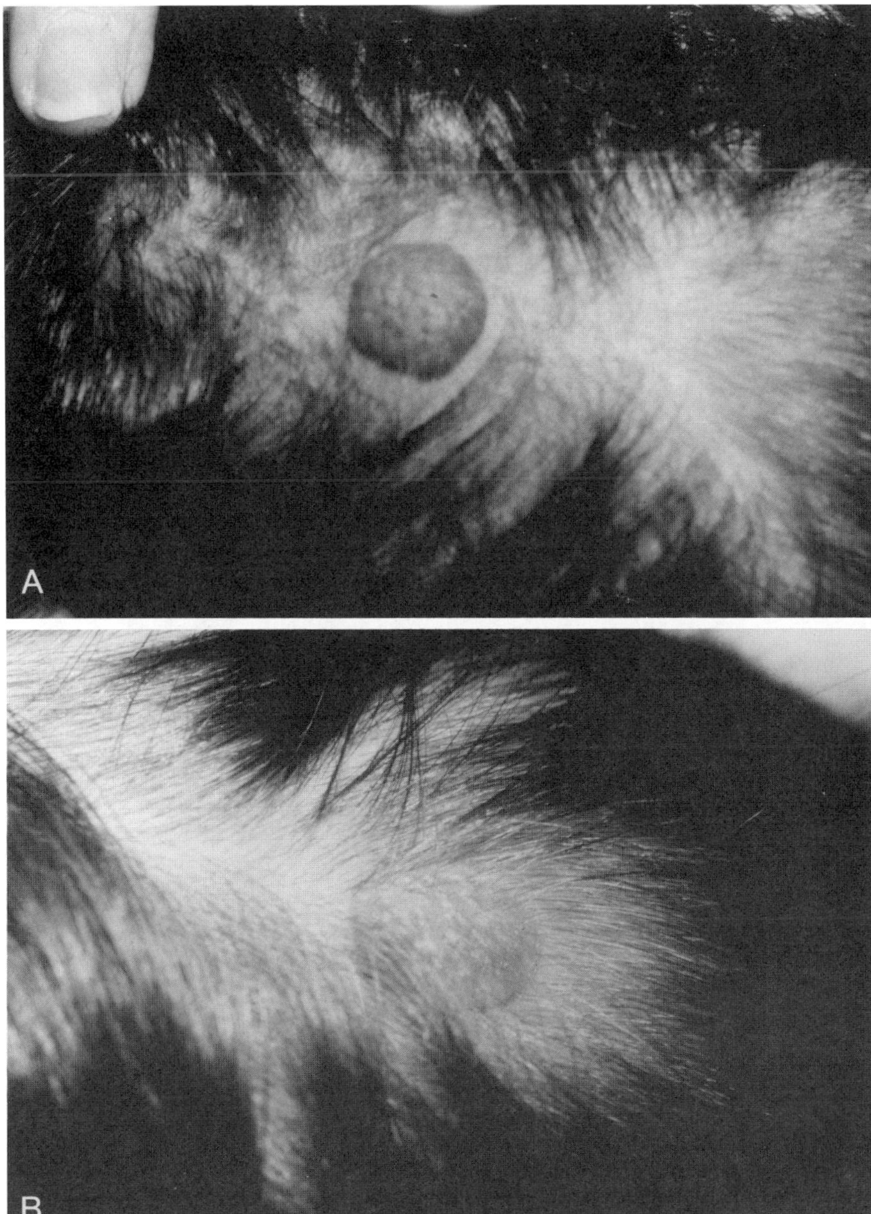

Figure 14.6. A combined strawberry-cavernous hemangioma that appeared on the scalp at 2 weeks of age, peaked in size at 7 months (A), and virtually resolved by 19 months (B).

cardiac failure and bleeding (Kasabach-Merritt syndrome). In these children, treatment with high-dose corticosteroids (prednisone 2 to 4 mg/kg/day) may be lifesaving or prevent complications (e.g., obstructive amblyopia). Midline hemangiomas, particularly in the lumbosacral area, may be associated with underlying vertebral and cord anomalies. Magnetic resonance imaging has proven particularly useful in delineating the extent of these defects.

Hemangiomas in the diaper area are prone to ulceration and infection. Careful hygiene, topical and systemic antibiotics, occlusive dressings, and barrier pastes may be required to prevent cellulitis and scarring.

Although the pulsed dye laser has been approved for palpable hemangiomas, it appears to be particularly useful in treating early, thin lesions and residual telangiectasias later in life. Anecdotal reports indicate that it may also be effective in treating thick, rapidly growing lesions.

Other Nevi

Hamartomatous nevi include a number of congenital lesions containing epidermal and adnexal structures. These nevi can affect hair follicles (nevus pilosis), apocrine and eccrine glands (apocrine and eccrine nevi), fibroblasts (connective tissue nevi), and smooth muscle (smooth muscle and pilar hamartomas).

EPIDERMAL NEVI

Epidermal nevi are a common pediatric finding and must be distinguished from sebaceous nevi. The epidermal nevus presents at birth or during early childhood as a linear group of warty, hyperpigmented papules. Lesions may be small or extend to involve half of the trunk and extremities. Infants with large lesions should be evaluated for associated defects, including seizures, mental retardation, and skeletal and ocular defects (epidermal nevus syndrome). Cutaneous lesions may respond to the application of topical keratolytics such as lactic acid, salicylic acid, and urea. Small lesions may be excised or ablated by carbon dioxide laser.

SEBACEOUS NEVUS OF JADASSOHN

Sebaceous nevus of Jadassohn is characterized by a 1 to 4 cm, linear or round, hairless, yellow, cobblestone-like plaque on the scalp. Although lesions usually involve the head and neck, nevi occasionally appear on the trunk and extremities. Rarely, lesions extend over a large portion of the body surface and are associated with multiple neuroectodermal and mesodermal defects (nevus sebaceous syndrome). Sebaceous nevi are usually removed in later childhood, because of the 15 to 20% risk of benign and malignant growths developing in plaques during adult life. Benign hypertrophy of the sebaceous and apocrine components is common at puberty.

CONGENITAL PIGMENTED NEVI

Congenital pigmented nevi are pigmented plaques, often with dense hair growth, that are noted at birth or during the first few months of life. Pigmented nevi contain nevomelanocytic nevus cells, which are neural crest-derived cells that share with normal skin melanocytes the ability to produce melanin. At birth, the lesions may be light tan with only soft vellus hairs. During infancy, the nevus darkens, and hair may become prominent. Occasionally, darkly pigmented lesions lighten during the first 1 to 2 years of life. Small, dark macules or nodules may also appear within the borders of the nevus.

Giant congenital pigmented nevi may reach over 20 cm in diameter and are associated with a 2 to 15% lifetime risk of melanoma. Early treatment when feasible includes selected surgical excision, particularly of nodular components. Unfortunately, large areas of the nevus may not be amenable to surgical management, and close observation with photographs is required. Regular examinations should include careful palpation of the entire lesion because melanomas may arise deep within the nevus without visible surface changes.

Medium (2 to 10 cm) and small (<2 cm) congenital pigmented nevi may also be associated with a higher risk of malignant change than acquired moles. However, the incidence is unknown, and there are no uniformly accepted guidelines for their management. Small size and high parental anxiety may dictate early surgical excision, but removal of these nevi is usually safely left until later childhood.

DISORDERS OF PIGMENTATION

Although most disorders of pigmentation in infancy and childhood are of cosmetic importance only, some lesions provide clues to the diagnosis of multisystem disease.

Hyperpigmentation

POSTINFLAMMATORY HYPERPIGMENTATION

The most common cause of increased pigmentation is postinflammatory hyperpigmentation (see page 200). This alteration in normal pigmentation follows many inflammatory processes in the skin, such as a diaper dermatitis or traumatic injury. Lesions typically follow the distribution of the resolving disorder. Although epidermal melanocytes appear normal, aberrant delivery of melanin to surrounding keratinocytes results in the deposition of pigment in the dermis. Areas of hyperpigmentation are more marked in darkly pigmented children. No therapy is necessary, and lesions usually fade over several months.

MONGOLIAN SPOTS

These are poorly circumscribed, slate-gray to blue-green, congenital macules. Lesions range from a few millimeters to over 20 cm and are found on the trunk and proximal extremities of 80 to 90% of black infants, 75% of orientals, and 10% of whites. Mongolian spots do not require therapy and usually fade by 3 to 5 years of life. When lesions are clinically confused with a pigmented nevus, a skin biopsy will reveal characteristic melanocytes in the dermis of a mongolian spot.

CAFE AU LAIT SPOTS

Cafe au lait spots are discrete, tan macules that appear at birth or during childhood in 10 to 20% of normal individuals. Lesions vary from the size of freckles to 20 cm or more in diameter and may involve any part of the skin surface. Although most affected children are normal, cafe au lait spots, particularly if six or more lesions over 1.5 cm in diameter are present, may be a marker of classic neurofibromatosis (von Recklinghausen's disease). Lesions are also associated with tuberous sclerosis, Albright's syndrome, leopard syndrome, epidermal nevus syndrome, Bloom's syndrome, ataxia-telangiectasia, and Russell-Silver syndrome.

DIFFUSE HYPERPIGMENTATION

Diffuse hyperpigmentation is rare in infancy and may suggest the presence of an underlying endocrine, hepatic, or nutritional disorder. Hereditary forms of hyperpigmentation may affect cutaneous melanocytes directly.

Hypopigmentation

ASH LEAF MACULES

Hypopigmentation may also occur as a localized or diffuse finding in the skin. Although 0.1% of normal newborns have hypopigmented macules (ash leaf macules), these lesions may be a marker for tuberous sclerosis. These macules appear at birth as 2 mm to 3 cm lesions on the trunk of 70 to 90% of individuals with tuberous sclerosis.

The identification of ash leaf macules may be enhanced in lightly pigmented children by the use of a Wood's light examination. The visible purple light that is emitted by the Wood's light is absorbed by melanin. In a darkened room, subtle areas of depigmentation or hypopigmentation will appear bright violet, whereas normal pigmented skin will absorb most of the light and appear dull purple or black.

Children with hypopigmented macules require close neurodevelopmental observation. Onset of other symptoms of tuberous sclerosis may be delayed for years. Lesions on cosmetically important areas are readily camouflaged by rehabilitative cosmetics such as Dermablend and Covermark.

NEVUS ANEMICUS

Nevus anemicus is often misdiagnosed as an ash leaf macule. This congenital patch, usually located on the trunk, appears pale or mottled compared to surrounding normal skin. However, a Wood's lamp examination demonstrates the presence of normal pigment. A persistent increase in vascular tone seems to account for this phenomenon.

PIEBALDISM (PARTIAL ALBINISM) AND ALBINISM

Piebaldism is a rare autosomal dominant disorder characterized by a white forelock and circumscribed congenital leukoderma. Special variants of piebaldism include Waardenburg's syndrome, in which leukoderma is associated with lateral displacement of the inner canthi and inferior lacrimal ducts, a flattened nasal bridge, and sensorineural deafness; and Wolfe's syndrome, an autosomal recessive disorder associated with multiple neurological deficits.

Albinism is a heterogenous group of inherited disorders manifested by generalized hypopigmentation or depigmentation of the skin, eyes, and hair. It occurs in an autosomal recessive, oculocutaneous form and an X-linked ocular variant.

DISORDERS OF THE HAIR AND NAILS

Although abnormalities of the hair and nails occur as isolated lesions, they may be associated with defects of other ectodermal structures or systemic disease.

In the premature infant, the scalp and forehead may be covered with fine, soft lanugo hair. By full term, most infants have full scalp coverage with normal terminal hair. However, shortly before birth and for up to 4 months after birth, infants undergo a period of brisk shedding when the infantile pattern shifts to a normal adult pattern of hair growth. In light-haired children, the process is often complete before birth, and the hair is sparse at delivery. Shedding is commonly delayed in dark-haired individuals and may occur rapidly during early infancy. Parents should be reassured that this is a normal physiological process.

The normal pattern of hair growth and shaft morphology may be disturbed in a number of hereditary disorders and congenital syndromes.

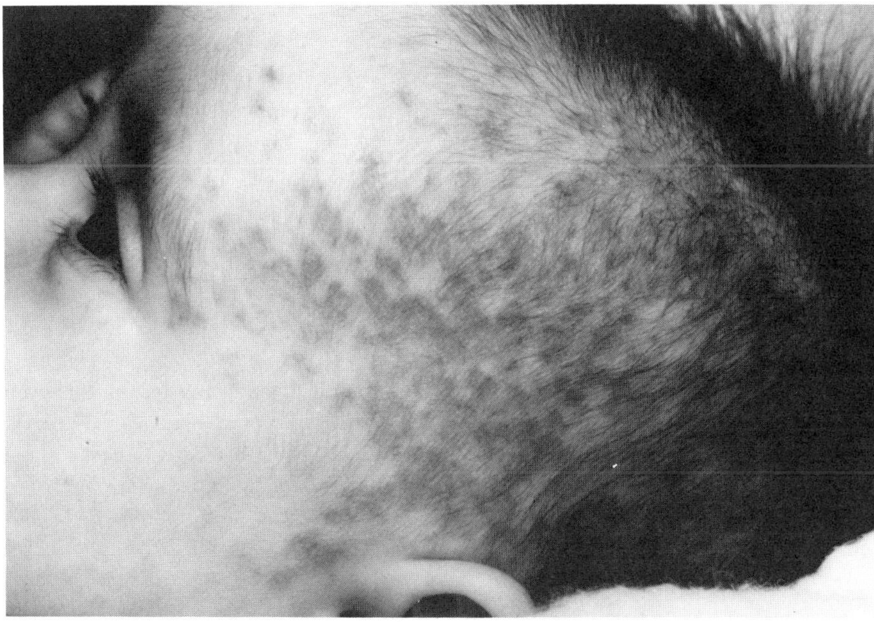

Figure 14.7. Annular erythematous, slightly atrophic plaques spread over the forehead and scalp of a 4-month-old infant with neonatal lupus erythematosus.

Nails are fully formed at birth. Absence, hypoplasia, or dysplasia of the nails may also occur as part of a more widespread cutaneous or systemic disorder.

Sucking blisters on the dorsum of the thumb or index finger are commonly present at birth. They contain clear, sterile fluid and resolve uneventually within several days. Persistent thumb sucking in infancy and early childhood is frequently complicated by chronic candidial and bacterial paronychia. The area at the base of the nail becomes red, edematous, and macerated, and nail dystrophy with rippling and irregular transverse grooving is common. Although the application of topical antibiotics and antifungals may be helpful, lesions usually heal spontaneously in later infancy or childhood when thumb sucking ends.

REACTIVE ERYTHEMAS

Reactive erythema refers to a group of disorders characterized by erythematous macules, plaques, and nodules, which vary in size, shape, and distribution. Unlike specific dermatoses, they represent reaction patterns in the skin triggered by a number of different endogenous and environmental factors. In infants, erythema multiforme, erythema nodosum, urticaria, and vasculitis occur after exposure to various infections and drugs. The management of affected infants, like that of older children and adults, involves identification and elimination of the offending agent and supportive care. Some reactive erythemas are peculiar to infancy.

Neonatal Lupus Erythematosus

Neonatal lupus erythematosus is the most common cause of congenital heart block. Although cutaneous lesions may not appear until several months of age, they are frequently present at birth. Affected infants demonstrate annular, erythematous plaques with a central scale, telangiectasias, atrophy, and hypopigmentation (Fig. 14.7). Lesions typically range from 0.5 to 3.0 cm in diameter and may spread from the scalp and face to the neck, upper trunk, and upper extremities. Although the development of the cutaneous rash does not require sunlight, it may be triggered or exacerbated by sun exposure.

The cause of neonatal lupus is unknown. However, the presence of transplacentally acquired ssA(Ro) and ssB(La) antibodies are thought to play a primary role in pathogenesis. In adults, ssA and ssB antibodies are associated with Sjogren's syndrome and a photosensitive variant of systemic lupus known as subacute cutaneous lupus erythematosus.

In addition to conduction defects and structural cardiac anomalies, affected infants may develop hepatosplenomegaly, anemia, leukopenia, thrombocytopenia, and lymphadenopathy. With the exception of cardiac involvement, neonatal lupus usually resolves spontaneously in 6 to 12 months as transplacentally derived antibody wanes. The use of low- and medium-potency topical steroids on intensely inflamed cutaneous lesions for several weeks may reduce the risk of scarring. Subtle atrophy and pigmentary changes may persist. Rarely, infants will require systemic corticosteroids and supportive care. Parents should be instructed to protect children with sunscreens and avoid direct sun exposure for at least 4 to 6 months. Mothers without clinical signs of lupus also require careful follow-up because they are at increased risk of developing overt disease.

SUGGESTED READINGS

Fitzpatrick TB, Eisen AZ, Wolff K, Freedberg IM, Austen KF. Dermatology in general medicine. New York: McGraw-Hill, 1987.

Hurwitz S. Clinical pediatric dermatology. Philadelphia: Saunders, 1981.

Meneghini CL, Bonifazi E. An atlas of pediatric dermatology. Chicago: Year Book Medical Publishers, 1986.

Rasmussen J. Pediatric dermatology. Pediatr Clin North Am 1983:30(3).

Schachner LA, Hansen RC. Pediatric dermatology. Boston: Churchill Livingstone, 1988.

Weston W. Practical pediatric dermatology. Boston: Little, Brown, 1979.

15

Discharge Planning

Pamela Kimzey Donohue
Christine A. Gleason

An organized, easily implemented, and effective discharge plan is an essential part of the care of the recovering NICU infant. When the discharge process proceeds smoothly, the hospitalization is more likely to be judged successful by parents, hospital staff, and primary care practitioners, even if there were significant medical complications. The reverse is also true. Too often, the impending discharge of the hospitalized NICU infant comes as a surprise to the parents, the primary care pediatrician, and even some of the nursery staff directly responsible for the infant's care. The formation of a multidisciplinary team approach to discharge planning can promote communication and facilitate a timely and well-organized discharge experience for the family members and staff.

THE DISCHARGE TEAM

The family's ability to assume primary care for the infant, the community support services available to the family, and the specialized medical care required by the infant are all concerns that need to be addressed well before the discharge date. A multidisciplinary discharge team can utilize the knowledge and expertise of many disciplines to assess the family's need. The discharge team can be composed of a variety of personnel, depending on the resources of the nursery (Table 15.1). Physicians, nurses, respiratory therapists, social workers, and community health nurses can all play important roles. The core constituents of the discharge planning team are the physician and primary nurse directly responsible for the infant's medical care, the social worker, and the family. The goals of the team are to formulate an organized discharge plan and to implement it effectively.

Physician

It is the role of the physician to anticipate the discharge as early as possible and to notify the other members of the discharge team so the discharge process can be put into effect. Making changes in the infant's medical management for ease of home care should be carefully considered and made a priority. Physicians can help the family establish primary care pediatric follow-up and institute early and ongoing communication with the designated physician to foster continuity of care.

Table 15.1. Multidisciplinary Discharge Team

Core team members
Physician
Primary nurse
Social worker
Family
Primary care follow-up physician
Additional team members
Discharge coordinator
Community health nurse
Respiratory therapist
Follow-up program personnel
Nutrition/lactation consultants
Medical specialists
Billing department representatives

Primary Nurse

The primary nurse can play a key role in coordinating a smooth transition from the hospital environment to home. She or he has intimate knowledge of the infant's past medical history and present care needs. Frequently, the primary nurse has spent more time with the family than any other member of the staff and is best able to anticipate the needs of both the infant and the family in weeks to come. Discharge teaching with the family can be done by the primary nurse.

Social Worker

Ongoing assessment of the family's stability and support systems is imperative in planning for a successful discharge. The social worker working with the family throughout the hospitalization has first-hand knowledge of their coping mechanisms and can lead the team in planning effective discharge strategies. Linking the family with community resources to provide ongoing support and financial assistance, two areas of major concern to most families, can be accomplished by the social worker prior to discharge.

Family

Including the family as part of the discharge team allows them to anticipate the discharge with the nursery staff. Although the discharge date may have been a focus for the family since the date of admission, they may not clearly understand discharge criteria or the process involved in taking a child home safely after a prolonged hospitalization. Participating in planning conferences with medical personnel adds to the family's education about their infant's condition and builds confidence in their own abilities to take over their infant's care.

Discharge Coordinator

With more rapid discharges of more complicated infants, many tertiary care centers have found it helpful to designate one person to be primarily responsible for coordinating the discharge of each child. The discharge coordinator role can be filled from a variety of disciplines. The primary purpose of the coordinator is to gather all the information about the infant and family and assimilate it into a realistic discharge plan. The utilization of the primary nurse for this position seems to be ideal, but staffing constraints often do not permit the primary nurse to take on this kind of responsibility. Employing physician assistants and nurse practitioners in an expanded house officer role that includes supervision of the discharge process is a feasible alternative. In intensive care nurseries with large nursing staffs, a coordinating nurse can also be utilized to gather information and delegate nursing responsibilities.

DISCHARGE PROCESS

Discharging an infant home is a very stressful process for families and is often viewed as another crisis in the hospital course. Anticipating discharge as early as 2 to 3 weeks in advance helps to alleviate some of the anxiety families feel at taking on sole responsibility of the infant for the first time. A predischarge case conference, held well in advance, encourages the team to formulate a plan and a timetable. A cohesive plan minimizes the chance that the family will receive conflicting and therefore confusing information. This consistency becomes particularly important in tertiary care centers and teaching hospitals where staff rotate on a frequent basis.

Medical Criteria for Discharge

Average discharge weight and postconceptional age (PCA) vary considerably among hospital neonatal units. When planning for discharge, it is most useful to think in terms of PCA and the infant achieving behavioral goals rather than attaining a specific weight. Basing the discharge date on a "magical" weight often leads to additional, unnecessary days of hospitalization. There is little disagreement about the following medical criteria for the discharge of NICU infants.

1. Medically stable
2. Able to maintain body temperature in open crib/bassinet
3. Adequate weight gain
4. Nippling all feedings in a reasonable period of time *or* tolerating an alternative feeding plan (e.g., gastrostomy)
5. Parents emotionally and physically ready
6. Primary care physician chosen and involved

Initiating the Discharge Process

Optimally, discharge planning should begin at the time of the infant's NICU admission. It is tempting to use the mother's "due date" to estimate the expected date of discharge, but this date often overestimates the length of hospitalization. It is best to begin by summarizing the aforementioned medical criteria for discharge and informing parents that the infant will be ready to go home when these criteria are met. If a date is necessary, then 34 to 36 weeks postconceptional age (PCA) may be used as an approximation. For premature infants with no major complications, discharge planning can usually begin by 32 weeks PCA. At that time, the discharge team should be convened and notified that discharge is approaching. A general discharge date can be set, but the parents should clearly understand that the date is subject to change if the infant is not yet ready.

Transitions to Home Care

Once a discharge date has been set, every effort should be made to simplify the care the infant will require at home (Table 15.2). Feedings should be changed from premature formula to the more readily available formula (20 kcal/oz) that will be used at home. If the mother plans to breast feed, she should be encouraged to time her visits so that she may breast feed her baby whenever possible. During the last week of hospitalization, the mother should increase her use of the breast pump to 8 times/day, including once at night. This will augment her milk supply. Medications such as diuretics, electrolyte replacements, and methylxanthines should be weaned, if possible. The half-life of these medications should be considered when allowing time to see if the infant really needs them. For example, caffeine has a half-life of 100 hours; therefore, it may be necessary to wait 5 to 7 days to see if apnea/bradycardia recurs. If medications are needed at home, preparations that can be given once or twice a day are preferable to those requiring more frequent administration. The need for an apnea monitor, supplemental oxygen, or other special equipment should be determined (Table 15.3). Any special equipment needed should be ordered well in advance, and equipment should be tested in the hospital. The parents should be given the opportunity to practice using the equipment prior to discharge.

All changes in the infant's management should be made well in advance of the anticipated discharge date. Monitoring the infant's progress in the hospital after changes are made is an important consideration when devising a discharge timeline.

Predischarge Studies

The need for predischarge studies depends on the clinical condition(s) of each individual infant. Commonly ordered studies are listed in Table 15.4. These studies must be ordered in a timely fashion so that appropriate interventions may be implemented and evaluated before the actual discharge date. Obtaining a hematocrit on the morning of

Table 15.2. Transitional Management

Wean from incubator to open crib/bassinet. This usually occurs at 33 to 35 weeks PCA (see chapter 5).
Change premature formula to formula (or breast milk) that will be used at home.
Attempt to wean medications. Consider the half-life of specific medications when formulating a discharge timetable.
For necessary medications, optimize preparations for home administration by considering (a) easy availability, (b) dosage scheduling, (c) patient tolerance.
Determine the need for special equipment at home. Order equipment in time for family teaching to be done with the equipment that will be used at home.

Table 15.3. Home Equipment

Cardiorespiratory monitor
Oxygen therapy equipment
Suction equipment
Gastrostomy replacement tubes
Gavage feeding tubes
Stethoscope
Ostomy care equipment
Wound/skin care equipment

Table 15.4. Commonly Ordered Discharge Studies

Hematocrit and reticulocyte count
Cranial ultrasound
Chest x-ray
Echocardiogram
Eye examination
Metabolic screen (PKU/thyroid)
Hearing screen
Neurodevelopmental evaluation
Special consultant's evaluation

Table 15.5. Discharge Procedure

Discharge family conference (see also Chapter 16)
Parent teaching completed
CPR
Well-child care
Special equipment
Car seat
Special equipment tested in hospital, used by family
Follow-up appointments made and primary care physician contacted
Parents room in with infant after teaching completed
Immunizations given

discharge only to find that a transfusion is indicated not only delays the discharge process but adds to the family's anxiety about their capability to care for the infant at home. Discussing the results with the parents and follow-up pediatrician is critical. If subspecialty follow-up will be needed, obtaining consultation while the infant is still hospitalized facilitates continuity of care. Follow-up physicians are given the opportunity to have a baseline evaluation, and the parents are given the opportunity to ask questions, thus establishing a basic link that helps insure adequate follow-up.

Loose Ends

During the last few days of the hospitalization, a number of tasks need to be completed (Table 15.5). Many of these goals can be realized simultaneously and, with good planning, none of them need delay the discharge. These "loose ends" often are forgotten or given low priority due to time constraints. They are, however, crucial to a successful discharge.

The primary care follow-up pediatrician should be contacted and given a medical update on the infant's condition and how discharge plans are proceeding. Any special follow-up plans and/or recommendations can be discussed at this time. All follow-up appointments with the primary care physician and any specialists should be made well in advance of the discharge date. A final discharge family conference may be held several days before discharge or on the day of discharge. The focus of the discussion should be to summarize the infant's hospital course and problem list, to answer the family's questions, and to correct any misunderstandings. Additionally, family concerns regarding discharge and home care can be addressed, and follow-up appointments, medications, and studies reviewed.

The AAP recommends DPT vaccine at 2 months chronological age. Similar recommendations for *Hemophilus Influenza* vaccine are forthcoming. The vaccine should not be given within 48 hours of discharge (to avoid confusing temperatures, apnea, etc.). Oral polio vaccine should not be given during the hospitalization, but it may be given "on the way out the door."

Discharge Process Summary

Clearly defined discharge criteria provide both the family and staff with a point of reference from which the progress of any child can be judged. As discharge nears, keeping a checklist of goals that need to be accomplished helps keep the staff focused and prevents important elements from "falling through the cracks." Having a physical checklist makes it readily apparent what tasks have not yet been completed (see Appendix).

TRANSFER TO OTHER HOSPITALS

Discharge criteria will vary if an infant is being discharged to a location other than home. If an infant is being transported from a regional referral center back to a community hospital, the capabilities of the receiving hospital must be taken into consideration. Many community hospitals do not have the support services or nursing personnel to care for an infant that a tertiary care center may consider uncomplicated. When transfer is possible, it has been shown to be cost effective and beneficial for families. A pediatric chronic care facility can be utilized for infants requiring prolonged convalescence or for those infants whose families cannot cope with a child with special needs at home. Close consultation between the staffs of the referring and accepting institutions and with the family facilitates a smooth transition.

WORKING WITH FAMILIES

The prolonged hospitalization of a critically ill infant can have a profound effect on family organization. Primary focus on the sick child can lead to disruption of daily routines, feelings of isolation by siblings, and marital discord. The financial burden created by the hospitalization can be overwhelming. By the time of discharge, the family may start to focus on how the infant will fit into their present life style and how they will provide care for an infant who has required such intensive support for such a long time. Concerns about long-term prognosis may increase as worry over survival is lessened.

Early Discharge

Early discharge can be advantageous to families for a number of reasons. Prolonged separation may interfere with parent-infant bonding. For families who live great distances from the hospital, the additional financial burden of travel and lodging may be substantial. Coping with a tertiary care institution, often in an unfamiliar location, adds to the frustration and anxiety. If well-planned and implemented, an early discharge can help preserve the family unit. Parents of infants with relatively uncomplicated courses and shorter lengths of stay may feel just as overwhelmed as parents of more critically ill children. Sensitivity to these differences in perception by the medical staff and the parents can help ease the progression of the discharge process. Parents who visit frequently and communicate with the staff as often as possible become more familiar with their child's responses to daily events. A slow transition of care from nursing staff to parents facilitates the parents' feelings of competence.

Discharge Teaching

Discharge teaching needs to be individualized and goal oriented. Information should be presented to the family in an organized and comprehensive format. The use of both written material and oral presentations is optimal. Comprehensive discharge teaching decreases parental anxiety and increases parental confidence. In addition, it decreases the risk of rehospitalization. Neonatal intensive care graduates are three times as likely to require readmission to the hospital as infants not requiring intensive care.

Although the pattern of illness is the same in NICU graduates and nongraduates, both parental concern and professional anxiety have been shown to contribute to the differences in rates of rehospitalization. Parents need to be given enough information during teaching sessions to enable them to make informed, competent decisions. Educating the family about the signs and symptoms of illness can prepare them for the possibility of readmission and assist them in seeking medical care appropriately.

One of the most valuable teaching tools for the parents is the opportunity for them to room in with the infant in the hospital environment prior to discharge. Ideally, this takes place in a location that provides the parents with the opportunity to assume complete care of their child while being in close proximity to medical staff should back-up be needed.

PRIMARY CARE FOLLOW-UP

Frequently, the discharge of an infant from an intensive care nursery occurs prior to the resolution of the infant's active medical problems. As many as 40% of infants with birth weights <1500 grams require rehospitalization within the first year of life. The peak incidence of readmission occurs between 2 and 4 months of age, and respiratory infections are the leading diagnosis. The postneonatal mortality rate has been shown to be ten times higher in premature NICU graduates than in the general infant population. Given this high-risk population, the importance of firmly established primary care follow-up prior to discharge cannot be over emphasized. For some families, this means helping them locate a pediatrician in their community; for others, it means informing their family pediatrician of the birth of a high-risk infant. Prior to discharge, the family physician can be a valuable resource, providing great support to families and helping the intensive care staff to better understand family dynamics and to be aware of special family problems.

Rapid advancements in neonatal care make it increasingly more difficult for primary care physicians to remain knowledgeable about current treatment modalities for high-risk infants. Physician discomfort in caring for these infants has been cited as one of the factors contributing to the high readmission rate of neonatal intensive care survivors. In 1984, Hurt found that 86% of pediatricians and 12% of family practitioners practicing in an East Coast metropolitan area cared for at least five high-risk infants per year. Nearly 30% of the pediatricians cared for more than 15 NICU graduates per year. Despite the experiences within their own practices, the majority of these physicians felt uncomfortable in dealing with the common problems of this population. When asked about their primary source of information concerning the care of high-risk infants, physicians with ≤ 12 years of experience cited residency training, while those with > 12 years of practice relied on the medical literature. The vast majority of these physicians felt that increased communication with the regional referral center and more training specific to NICU graduates would increase their confidence levels. With 6.8% of all live births resulting in infants with birth weights <2500 grams, more primary care physicians are likely to become involved in the care of high-risk infants.

Regional referral centers can contribute significantly to physician education and facilitate continuity of care by initiating frequent and detailed communication with private pediatricians. Discussing not only past medical history but present treatment rationale and expected outcome should be a part of the discharge process. Providing references aids in education. Reviewing the parents' understanding of their child's condition promotes understanding and trust between the family and the follow-up physician. A phone call to the primary care provider should be made on the day of discharge to provide anthropomorphic data, medication dosages, and dates of prearranged specialized follow-up. A written discharge summary should also be sent, but relying on written communication alone often results in the patient reaching the pediatrician's office before the discharge summary.

SUMMARY

Regionalization of perinatal care, effective back transport, and diagnostic related groups have contributed to decreased length of stay and earlier discharge of infants from neonatal intensive care nurseries. A well-orchestrated discharge process that begins early in the infant's hospitalization is the key to facilitating a smooth transition of both infant and family from the hospital to the home.

SUGGESTED READINGS

Arenson J. Discharge teaching in the NICU: the changing needs of NICU graduates and their families. Neonatal Network 1988; Feb:29–52.

Boynton BR, Boynton CA. Discharge planning for high-risk infants. J Perinatol 1985;5:44–48.

Hurt H. Continuing care of the high-risk infant. Clin Perinatol 1984;11:3–17.

Lang M, Behle MB, Ballard RA. The transition from hospital to home. In: Ballard R, ed. Pediatric care of the ICN graduate. Philadelphia: Saunders, 1988:12–16.

Lewry J, Wailoo MP. Pattern of illness in babies discharged from a special care unit. Arch Dis Child 1985;60:1068–1081.

Lund C, Lefrak L. Discharge planning for infants in the intensive care nursery. Perinatology-Neonatology March/April 1982.

Lynch TM, Jung AL, Bose CL. Neonatal back transport: clinical outcomes. Pediatrics 1988;82:845–851.

McCormick M, Shapiro S, Starfield B. Rehospitalization in the first year of life for high-risk survivors. Pediatrics 1980;66:991.

Wegman ME. Annual summary of vital statistics—1987. Pediatrics 1988;82:817–827.

16

The Family's Perspective

Phoebe Rostov

The birth of an infant is an event that is most often associated with celebration. For most families, the 9 months of pregnancy bring change and preparation. The physical changes of the "mother-to-be" trigger contemplation of the mothering role and how it impacts on her sense of self. Fathers-to-be are similarly challenged. Siblings watch their mother's body change and grow; they struggle with complex thoughts as they imagine being the big brother or sister and wonder in what other ways their family will change. In addition, financial issues arise, often leading to job or career decisions.

Adjustments are gradual and subtle; nurseries are painted, furniture is bought or borrowed, books on pregnancy are read, childbirth classes are scheduled, books are read to siblings, and grandparents make plans to be available after the baby's birth. Pediatricians are interviewed, decisions to breast or bottle feed are made, and the prenatal visits with sonograms (baby's first picture) and the sound of the growing infant's heartbeat (received with a sigh of relief and quiet excitement) take place. These make the reality of the new baby sharper each day. Unless the pregnancy is identified as high-risk, problems like premature birth are not discussed. Women fight back fears of having an unhealthy baby. Questions bravely asked of physicians about potential medical problems or discussions with family and friends about "What if my baby has something wrong?" are appropriately met with reassurance.

THE UNEXPECTED

When a pregnancy ends prematurely or if a fullterm infant has medical or surgical problems, expectations are abruptly shattered. In each case, the parents and family respond in a unique way, influenced by the special circumstances of their situation, including the obstetrical history, prior infant losses, the special meaning of this particular infant, previous emotional trauma, the mode of family functioning, individual coping styles, the age of the parents, and socioeconomic factors.

However, the sense of loss is common to all in this situation. They feel the loss, not only of the imagined and hoped-for healthy infant, but also of the roles of mother, father, sibling, and grandparent of that imaginary infant. The new roles for which they have prepared, the conflicts and emotions with which they have struggled, and the solutions they have chosen suddenly do not fit the new situation.

It is only when the loss is acknowledged and grieving for the healthy infant has begun that family members can begin all over again, learning about new realities, setting new expectations, and preparing for the new baby under an entirely new set of circumstances.

"Do I Send Out Birth Announcements or Not?"

It is essential that health professionals understand the stresses encountered by parents during their infant's hospitalization and after discharge. The overriding issues are: (a) the premature birth or the medical condition necessitating hospitalization; (b) the intensive care hospitalization itself; and (c) the discharge from the hospital. These situations result in individual and family crises that disturb or destroy psychological equilibrium.

Health professionals can assist by providing information and emotional support. If the parents' adaptation is successful, a sense of balance is regained, and the infant can be integrated into the family. Like the medical course, the progression from stress to crisis to adaptation to resolution is not smooth. Parents experience a wide range of emotions, moving in and out of stability as one stress is overcome only to be replaced by another.

FOSTERING THE PARENT/INFANT RELATIONSHIP

Hospitalization of a newborn infant necessitates the separation of the infant from the parents. Whether an infant is "down the hall," in a regional center hundreds of miles away, or simply on the other side of an incubator wall, the natural development of parenting behavior is thwarted. The parent still wants to function as caretaker and nurturer, but he or she is prevented from doing so by the circumstances of the hospitalization and by the anxiety that inevitably follows.

It becomes the responsibility of the intensive care nursery staff, through policies and procedures as well as through daily interactions with families, to facilitate parental involvement by specifically addressing issues related to privacy, separation, and parental roles.

Privacy

If medical conditions permit, privacy affords parents the opportunity to make emotional connections with their infant. Parents require privacy in order to touch their infant, to examine him or her from head to toe, and to observe and assimilate the entire situation. They need privacy for their fears and privacy for their hopes.

A screen around the infant's incubator or warming bed can create a private space by shutting out the overwhelming NICU environment and decreasing feelings of self-consciousness. Privacy provides the chance for parents to risk interacting with their infant, whether by singing a song or talking about the day's events, whether with a touch, a kiss, or a long, loving, worried gaze.

The staff must balance the family's need for information and support with their need for privacy. Parents need enough information to help them feel safe with their infant. Yet, it is important to make sure that, with the best intention of orienting parents to the unit and to the medical condition of their infant, they are not, in fact, being overwhelmed with information. Sometimes an introduction to the infant by nursing staff, reassurance that medical staff is close by, a promise to check in at frequent intervals, and a chair by the "screened" bedside are all that the new parent needs.

Separation

NICU policies should be designed to minimize the inevitable separation between infant and parents.

LIBERAL VISITING HOURS

Ideally, the intensive care nursery should allow visiting 24 hrs/day. Parents' schedules vary, travel time to the hospital can be lengthy, and the parental need to visit may occur at anytime.

Psychologically, it is crucial that parents always know that their infant belongs to them and is accessible at all times. Understandable and unnecessary frustration, sadness, and confusion can surface when visiting hours restrict parent/child contact. Parents may justifiably ask, "Whose baby is this, mine or the hospital's?"

PHONE CALLS

Once again, it is important that parents be able to contact the nursery at any time to check on their infant and to maintain a sense of connection when physical visitation is not possible.

It is recommended that phone calls be restricted to parents only. At first, parents may oppose such a policy. They may request that other relatives and friends be allowed phone contact, not realizing that information given to persons other than parents can result in unnecessary misunderstandings and confusion. Furthermore, limiting phone contact to parents permits frequent updates while minimizing the time that the staff is away from the infant. In addition, such a policy can be viewed as an early opportunity for the staff to support parents in their unique relationship with their infant by giving the parents the opportunity to make decisions about what information should be shared and with whom.

It is important for the staff to be aware that phoning the unit for information can be an emotionally charged task for parents. As one parent described:

> . . . do you know how many times I stared at the telephone this morning and just couldn't pick it up to call? What if Robbie had a bad night? I just don't think I could've handled hearing that over the phone. I would call every hour if I could know ahead of time that I would hear good news. . . . Do you know what else? Every time I call and talk to the nurse caring for Robbie, I feel so far away from him that I have to choke back the tears. When I try to stay busy when I can't visit, it's easier. Calling reminds me how much I miss being with him. . .

It is not unusual for parents to call the unit and not be sure what they want to know. They just want to feel connected with their infant and be reassured. Nurses or other staff members receiving calls from parents can assist by structuring the telephone call. Specific questions can be suggested when parents are oriented to the unit.

In addition to medical information, comments that allow a parent to visualize their infant over the telephone can have a positive impact. Months after the conversation took place, a parent recalled the following answer she received from her son's primary nurse after asking how he was doing:

> . . . you would think that Brian knows that his mom is on the phone. He just turned his head this way. His cheeks are getting plump, and his eyes look so big this morning. He is really alert today. Would you like me to turn on his music box for him after we're finished talking?

ACCOMMODATIONS

For parents who do not live near the hospital, overnight accommodations and a place for parents to rest after traveling from home can encourage more frequent visitations as well as longer stays. A nursery staff member, such as a social worker, should be available to discuss options with parents and facilitate obtaining accommodations.

VISITING POLICY

Siblings, friends, and family outside of the immediate family should be allowed to accompany parents at their discretion. The opportunity to introduce their hospitalized infant to friends and family and to observe reactions and respond to questions gives parents the chance to anticipate reactions from others after the infant is discharged. Through such interactions, parents can become comfortable with their child's unique beginnings. Furthermore, visitation by close friends offers an additional opportunity for support.

If possible, siblings should be encouraged to visit. Visitation can help the sibling adjust to the different, more complicated, and confusing family while at the same time helping parents with the task of integrating the new infant into their existing family.

Parental Roles

Throughout the pregnancy, parents have been anticipating the needs of the new infant and have visualized themselves as providing closeness, comfort, and attention to their infant's primary, daily needs. From a psychological perspective, the primary task of parents who are coming to terms with the hospitalization of their newborn is the redefinition of their parental roles and responsibilities. Parental involvement is initially very limited, and in order to begin to establish a meaningful relationship with their infant, parents must identify and perform alternate parenting tasks. Otherwise, their lack of involvement tends to increase anxiety and guilt and leads to a sense of detachment and incompetence.

Ms. H. called daily regarding the medical status of her 26-week infant, who was on a respirator. Initially, she visited every other day. During visits, she would sit by the bedside, staring at the monitor, reviewing her son's daily log, or talking with the nurses. When she was encouraged to touch her infant, Ms. H. refused, replying, "You know what he needs now. I'll wait until he's a little bigger and off that machine." Visits began decreasing, and Ms. H. appeared more withdrawn when at the bedside. The social worker spoke with her during a visit, and Ms. H. began crying, stating, "I don't even feel like he's my baby. I sit and watch and can't do anything for him. The nurses are more comfortable with my own baby than I am."

Parents require a great deal of assistance in identifying ways that they can be involved. Again, parents need to acknowledge and mourn the fact that they are unable to take responsibility for direct caretaking and are unable to hold, cuddle, and comfort their infant as they had envisioned. However, it is essential that new responsibilities are undertaken immediately and not put off until the infant is "healthy."

SOURCE OF INFORMATION

Roles to be defined and encouraged include those of decision-maker, information gatherer, advocate, and observer. Parents will be viewing their child from a unique perspective, and their perceptions should be sought and defined as important information that only parents can offer. The importance of functioning in this role is revealed in the following example:

> Jessica had been in the nursery for about 3 weeks. I was not handling my visitor status well and was beginning to feel more and more insignificant because the nurses seemed to know best what to do for her and I felt I had nothing to offer.
>
> I was really taken aback when the new attending physician walked up to me at Jessica's incubator and introduced herself. When I asked the doctor how my baby was doing, she looked at me with a smile and asked, 'How does she seem to you?'
>
> The doctor then spent time obtaining information from me regarding Jessica's history and my impressions of her medical course. After that discussion, I felt different. I felt that I did know my daughter and that, in a way, I was an expert too.

If the parents are included in the treatment team, it will be a normal course of action to obtain information from them, to include them in discussions, and to acknowledge and respect their position as decision-makers.

PROVIDER OF CONTINUITY

Parents are in a unique position to offer continuity from hospital to home. The staff should emphasize this fact early in the hospitalization by creating an environment that encourages parents to establish certain routines that will be continued at home. For example, parents can bring in toys, mobiles, and music boxes that can be placed in the incubator and later transferred to the home nursery. Clothes, blankets, and toys do not need to be left in the "empty nursery" at home awaiting the infant's arrival. Instead, they can be a part of the infant's world in the hospital.

ACUTE PHASE OF HOSPITALIZATION

Emotionally, most parents find themselves in a "state of shock" after the delivery of an infant who requires admission to the NICU. Frequently, they describe themselves as feeling numb or disassociated from the events around them. This initial shock can be viewed as functional because it enables parents to make contact with an environment that might otherwise be too painful or overwhelming.

Disappointment and Helplessness

After the initial contact with the infant and the nursery, numbness subsides and is replaced by a sense of loss of the imagined healthy infant along with fear for the survival of the real and critically ill infant. It is during this time that parents experience a pervasive sense of helplessness. They are haunted by questions regarding the reasons for the infant's medical problems. They suffer a never-ending review of each moment of the pregnancy and experience feelings of self-blame and guilt. They also experience a challenging of their religious beliefs and sense of fairness.

Parents require support and information throughout the initial hospitalization. The medical team must present the reality of the medical status and the prognosis both to give the parents a realistic picture as well as to establish trust. However, at the same time, parents need support and reassurance as they begin to form a relationship with their child. The parent is at the start of a tightrope walk, maintaining a delicate balance between reality on one side and optimism on the other.

Guilt

Attempts to reassure parents that their infant's problems are in no way related to anything they did or did not do rarely interrupt questions and ruminations. When a child is born with medical problems, the mother experiences a sense of failure at not having been able to protect her infant and keep him or her healthy. Fortunately, the intensity of self-blame and guilt and the preoccupation with causal factors usually subside as the parent is able to function in a newly defined parenting role.

The mother who has been compliant with medical care and advice throughout the pregnancy and adapted her lifestyle accordingly asks "Why me?" For the mother who has not been compliant or who has engaged in such activities as drug or alcohol usage, the birth of the sick infant may be the first time that the reality of her behavior becomes clear. Although denial of the linkage between her behavior and its impact on the infant may continue, feelings of guilt and self-blame are often intense. In either case, this is an opportune time for intervention by a mental health practitioner.

Stress and Accommodation

During the acute phase of hospitalization, parents are faced with the task of incorporating the demands of parenting a hospitalized infant into the existing family structure. Individual emotional problems or problems in the couple's relationship with one another may come to the surface. The consequences of these problems are magnified by the tendency of parents to become socially isolated. They view their situation as private and unique and narrow their support network.

Throughout the initial period of hospitalization, parents finds themselves on an emotional roller coaster whose ups and downs are determined by advances or setbacks in their infant's condition. Fortunately, with ongoing information and support, most parents are able to make the necessary adjustments to regain a sense of equilibrium and maintain an effective level of functioning.

ONGOING HOSPITALIZATION

When infants do well and parents observe their progress and are increasingly able to participate in their care, feelings of relief and competence surface. Parents often describe the existence of a special parent/infant relationship.

> . . . It's as if we have already survived something together. I used to watch Ryan in his isolette and feel both his and my helplessness. It was hard to watch him without worrying. Now I see him and I think, 'What a miracle. What a gift.' I have had the chance to watch and touch and love my baby when most babies his age aren't born yet. . . .

Surprisingly, the shift from the initial acute phase of illness to the ongoing hospitalization can also be unsettling. Once again, adjustments are required. Just when parents have organized and solidified their new routines, the situation shifts. At the advice of their friends and the staff, parents have finally given themselves permission to visit at the hospital less frequently in order to recuperate and focus their attention on home and family needs. Now, they find themselves again pulled to the hospital.

Parent as Caretaker

The hospitalization should be a period of gradual weaning of caretaking responsibilities from nurse to parent. Instruction, encouragement, and placement of the parents in their parental role should become central ingredients in parent/staff interactions. Parents benefit from opportunities to be in charge of their infant and to practice being the sole caretaker as early as possible. Although this can be approximated within the nursery setting, it is not until parents are truly alone with their infant that they can begin to feel competent. Walks down the hallway, feeding in a separate room, or just some private, parent/child "play time" in a separate room off of the nursery can help to allay anxieties and result in increased feelings of comfort and competence.

FIRSTS

In an effort to preserve some of the special moments that would normally occur between parents and the newborn infant, "firsts" should be saved for parents whenever possible. This means, for example, first nipple feeding, dressing in infant clothes for the first time, and first bath.

Return to the Community Hospital

After the acute phase of illness has resolved and the infant is in the "feeding and growing" period of hospitalization, infants hospitalized at a regional neonatal center may have the opportunity to be transported back to their community hospital for the remainder of their hospitalization. Although the fact that an infant is medically stable enough to be transported to and cared for in a community hospital should be reassuring, parents frequently experience increased anxiety when the issue of back transport is raised.

Parents become dependent on the medical staff that has treated their infant since birth. Survival is attributed to that medical team, and ongoing recovery is gladly entrusted to that hospital's NICU staff. Activities that can facilitate a smooth transition to another hospital include informing parents of the communication between the NICU staff and the physicians at the other hospital, a parental tour of the community hospital's nursery, an orientation to the new facility, including names of staff who will be caring for the infant, and a review of hospital policies. The more consistent the policies, particularly regarding visitation and handling, the easier for parents to make the adjustment. When parents and infant arrive at the new hospital, it is an opportune time for the medical staff to demonstrate their knowledge of the infant's history, to recall information obtained from specific members of the medical team from the sending hospital, and to approach the parents as experts regarding their own infant.

DISCHARGE

"When will my infant be able to come home?" is among the first questions asked by parents of an infant admitted to a neonatal intensive care unit. This question is repeatedly asked and addressed throughout the hospitalization, and it is sometimes a surprise to both parents and the staff when the announcement of a discharge date is met with mixed emotions and a lack of preparation, emotionally and physically, on the part of the parents.

The Date

Why do parents find themselves unprepared emotionally and physically at the time of their infant's discharge? Although they anticipate discharge from the time of admission, parents constantly fear that their infant will not recover and may never come home. Until a specific date is offered by the physician, the frequently asked question, "*When* can my baby come home?" is actually a substitute for the frightening and therefore unspoken real question, "*Will* my baby come home?" Parents cannot think of their infant coming home without facing the anxiety-provoking possibility that it may not happen. For this reason, parents often have not directly faced the issues surrounding their infant's discharge.

Old Insecurities

Both parents and the staff are caught off-guard when the reaction to the news of discharge is not exclusively one of relief and excitement. What occurs instead is a resurfacing of the feelings and concerns of the initial phase of the hospitalization. A sense of helplessness recurs and brings with it anxiety and changes in behavior. Parents become irritable; the frequency of visits and phone calls may decrease; and jealousy of the relationship between the staff and the infant may reappear.

Parents make adjustments in order to cope with the grief and daily stresses of relating to a critically ill newborn. Such adjustments are commonly confused with the broader and more complex task of becoming parents of an infant whose life just happened to begin in a neonatal intensive care unit. It is with the reality of impending discharge that parents are confronted with making the stressful transition from NICU visitor to home caretaker.

Parents see their hospital-based competence deteriorating into home-based insecurities.

> . . . When I was told that Jenny would be able to come home in time for Christmas, I almost collapsed. The doctors and nurses seemed so excited about delivering the news, I began to wonder what was wrong with me. The guilt at knowing that a part of me wished she could stay longer was unbearable . . . but I was scared and unprepared. I wanted Christmas to be so special for Michael (older sibling); he has felt so pushed aside. It was going to take so much to prepare for the holiday without her discharge. I know I should be excited, and everyone knows that I have waited for this day for 5 months, but I don't know how I'll ever be ready. . .

In an attempt to help parents feel comfortable and ready to have their infant discharged from the intensive care unit, there is sometimes a tendency on the part of the medical staff to minimize the infant's medical course and to normalize his or her health to a degree that is not accurate. Statements such as, "Taking Jonathan home now is like taking home any other newborn," typically do not reassure a parent. Instead, they serve to negate Jonathan's early birth, surgery for a patent ductus, difficult weaning from a ventilator, discharge with a monitor, and all the strength, love, and stamina it took for his parents to weather such a medical course for their first born. It is best to review the hospital course, the critical times as well as the progress, in order to give the parents a chance to integrate the information in a different way now that discharge is a reality.

NEW REALITIES

Discharge creates a whole new set of problems that, if not anticipated, can be disorienting to parents and exasperating to caretakers.

Postpartum Depression

Some women experience a delayed postpartum depression after being home with their infants. This can be intensified if the mother does not anticipate how overwhelming the isolation and child-care demands of that initial period at home can be. The postpartum depression feeds on itself. Self-disappointment increases when mothers experience anything other than ecstasy at their infant's survival and homecoming.

Interpersonal Adjustments

Any birth requires that a couple make emotional room for a third person. Special difficulties are presented with the birth of a preterm infant because the preparation period was cut short. Many parents are just beginning to feel settled with the shift in their life-style and the emotional demands of coping with their infant's hospitalization when they are faced with another major adjustment related to their infant's discharge home. Feelings of fear related to the homecoming and a revived sense of grief are sometimes expressed as anger toward one another.

Siblings

Siblings are faced with their own concerns. Even in the best of situations, the birth of a sibling is a time of emotional upheaval. When it is an early birth, siblings have not been prepared for the separation from their parents and for the intensity of their parents' feelings. Parents are physically absent and emotionally preoccupied. The sibling must adjust during the infant's hospitalization, only to be confronted with new adjustments at the time of homecoming. It is no wonder then that the "not so new" addition to the family is greeted with mixed emotions.

Financial Consequences

The financial consequences of long-term neonatal hospitalization are great. Even couples with insurance can find that their percentage of the bill is overwhelming. In situations where both members of a couple had been working prior to delivery, the loss of one income increases financial stress. This can lead to conflicts related to returning to work as opposed to staying at home. Infants who require special home-care equipment and/or medical care present ongoing financial demands.

Isolation

As mentioned above, one of the most frequently experienced stresses is that of isolation. Parents often do not realize how socially dependent they had become on the support group that was always available during hospital visits. In addition, medical precautions can lead to the restriction of visitors and the limitation of outings. Alternative caretakers are difficult to find. This means that parents have decreased opportunities for socialization and decreased time with one another. Social isolation is heightened for the parents of infants with problems requiring specialized care.

When parents do participate in social activities with their infants, they are confronted with the reactions of others. Comments on size, developmental achievements, equipment, etc. require a parent to recount and relive their infant's history. This can be painful and intimidating.

Fatigue

Finally, mention should be made of the stress related to physical fatigue. Parents have not had time to recuperate from the physical and emotional exhaustion incurred while their infant was hospitalized before they are faced with the demands of normal and perhaps specialized infant care needs. Most premature infants at the time of discharge are slow and/or frequent feeders. A frequent postdischarge cry from parents is "Where's the night shift?" After observing the hospital environment where cares were scheduled, feedings measured, and changes and observations recorded, parents are often reluctant to use common sense. The price is exhaustion.

Intervention

What can health care professionals do to help families manage more effectively and thereby minimize crises when they occur at discharge? During the hospitalization, the following interventions have proven to be helpful:

1. By providing continuity of staff, external stability is provided for the family;
2. A staff member trained to address the family's psychological needs should be available. An experienced social worker is critical to this effort;
3. Siblings need to be included in the hospital experience. Parents need to be educated regarding how to prepare their children, address their questions, anticipate reactions, and have their involvement with the new sibling be as positive as possible;
4. Family members and friends who will provide support and future caretakers should be identified early and included in visits and discharge teaching. It is useful when pediatric follow-up is identified as early as possible and the future pediatrician is included in communications regarding an infant's medical status;
5. When discharge is anticipated, it is important for parents to be notified as early as possible and to be included in the planning. Offering parents opportunities for private time with their infants, including overnight stays, prior to discharge allows parents to make a more gradual transition toward becoming the primary caretaker;
6. Providing reading material and facilitating communication with "graduate" parents is a way of minimizing potential isolation and normalizing experiences that will be encountered once at home.

SUGGESTED READINGS

Affleck G, Tennen H, Rowe J, Roscher B, Walker L. Effects of formal support on mothers' adaptation to the hospital-to-home transition of high-risk infants: the benefits and costs of helping. Child Dev 1989;60:488–501.

Arenson J. Discharge teaching in the NICU: the changing needs of NICU graduates and their families. Neonatal Network 1988;6:29–30, 47–52.

Barbero GJ. Children with recurrent hospitalizations: a problem of disabled children, parents, and physicians. Develop Behav Pediatr 1984;5:319–324.
Brown LP, York R, Jacobsen B, Gennaro S, Brooten D. Very low birth-weight infants: parental visiting and telephoning during initial infant hospitalization. Nurs Res 1989;38:233–236.
Consolvo CA. Siblings in the NICU. Neonatal Network 1987;5:7–12.
Daga SR, Shinde SB. Mothers' participation in neonatal intensive care and its impact. J Trop Pediatr 1987;33:274–277.
Dillard RG, Auerbach KG, Showalter AH. A parents' program in the intensive care nursery: its relationship to maternal attitudes and expectations. Soc Work Health Care 1980;5:245–251.
Giacoia GP, Rutledge D, West K. Factors affecting visitation of sick newborns. Clin Pediatr 1985;24:259–262.
Giblin PT, Roland ML, Waller JB Jr, Ager JW. Correlates of parenting on a neonatal intensive care unit: maternal characteristics and family resources. J Genet Psychol 1988;149:505–514.
Hayward EA, Janes-Kelley S, Sikora M. Rooming-in: a preventative health care measure in the neonatal intensive care unit. Neonatal Network 1988;7:29–34.
Lind RF, Pruitt RL, Greenfeld D. Previously infertile couples and the newborn intensive care unit. Health and Social Work 1989;14:127–133.
Mahan CK, Kreuger JC, Schreiner RL. The family and neonatal intensive care. Social Work Health Care 1982;7:67–78.
Mohan VM, Karen S. Maternal involvement in the care of high risk infants in a sick newborn nursery—a prospective study. Indian Pediatr 1986;23:121–125.
Noble DN, Hamilton AK. Families under stress: perinatal social work. Health and Social Work 1981;6:28–35.
Paludetto R, Faggiano-Perfetto M, Asprea AM, DeCurtis M, Margara-Paludetto P. Reactions of sixty parents allowed unrestricted contact with infants in a neonatal intensive care unit. Early Hum Dev 1981;5:401–409.
Perrault C, Collinge J, Outerbridge EW. Family support in the neonatal intensive care unit. Dimens Health Serv 1979;56:16–18.
Philipp C. Parental perceptions of children who were hospitalized in neonatal intensive care units. Child Psychiatry Hum Dev 1983;14:76–86.
Rushton CH. Promoting normal growth and development in the hospital environment. Neonatal Network 1986;4:35–41.
Salitros PH. Transitional infant care: a bridge to home for high-risk infants. Neonatal Network 1986;4:35–41.
Satariano HJ, Briggs NJ, O'Neal C. Discharged from neonatal intensive care: how satisfied are the parents? Pediatr Nurs 1987;13:352–353.
Solnit A, Stark N. Mourning and the birth of a defective child. Psychoanal Study Child 1961;16:523–537.
Taylor PS. Promoting parental care of high-risk babies. Aust Nurs J 1986;15:31–33.
Tennen H, Affleck G, Gershman K. Self-blame among parents of infants with perinatal complications: the role of self-protective motives. J Pers Soc Psychol 1986;50:690–696.
Troy P, Wilkinson-Faulk D, Smith AB, Alexander DA. Siblings visiting in the NICU. Am J Nurs 1988;88:68–70.
Valentin LD. The problems of grief and separation in the special care baby unit. Nurs Times 1981;4:1942–1944.
Vas Dias S. Psychotherapy in special care baby units. Nurs Times 1987;83:50–52.
Whetsell MV, Larrabee ME. Using guilt constructively in the NICU to affirm parental coping. Neonatal Network 1988;6:21–27.
Zeanah CH, Canger CI, Jones JD. Clinical approaches to traumatized parents: psychotherapy in the intensive care nursery. Child Psychiatry Hum Dev 1984;14:158–169.
Zeskind PS, Sacino R. Effects of maternal visitation to preterm infants in the neonatal intensive care unit. Child Develop 1984;55:1887–1893.

Appendices

A. Laboratory Values

	Age 1 week			Age 3 weeks			Age 5 weeks			Age 7 weeks		
Constituent	Mean	SD	Range	Mean	SD	Range	Mean	SD	Range	Mean	SD	Range
Na (mEq/L)	139.6	±3.2	133–146	136.3	±2.9	129–142	136.8	±2.5	133–148	137.2	±1.8	133–142
K (mEq/L)	5.6	±0.5	4.6–6.7	5.8	±0.6	4.5–7.1	5.5	±0.6	4.5–6.6	5.7	±0.5	4.6–7.1
Cl (mEq/L)	108.2	±3.7	100–117	108.3	±3.9	102–116	107.0	±3.5	100–115	107.0	±3.3	101–115
CO_2 (mM/L)	20.3	±2.8	13.8–27.1	18.4	±3.5	12.4–26.2	20.4	±3.4	12.5–26.1	20.6	±3.1	13.7–26.9
Ca (mg/dl)	9.2	±1.1	6.1–11.6	9.6	±0.5	8.1–11.0	9.4	±0.5	8.6–10.5	9.5	±0.7	8.6–10.8
P (mg/dl)	7.6	±1.1	5.4–10.9	7.5	±0.7	6.2–8.7	7.0	±0.6	5.6–7.9	6.8	±0.8	4.2–8.2
BUN (mg/dl)	9.3	±5.2	3.1–25.5	13.3	±7.8	2.1–31.4	13.3	±7.1	2.0–26.5	13.4	±6.7	2.5–30.5

Appendix A.1. Serum electrolyte values in preterm infants (Birth Weight 1500 to 1750 grams). (Reprinted from Klaus MH, Fanaroff AA. Care of the high risk neonate. 3rd ed. Philadelphia: Saunders, 1986. Adapted from Thomas J, Reichelderfer T. Premature infants: analysis of serum during the first seven weeks. Clin Chem 1968;14:272. Used with permission of the American Association of Clinical Chemistry.)

	Term	Preterm
WBC count (cells/mm^3)		
No. of infants	87	30
Mean	8.2	9.0
Median	5	6
SD	7.1	8.2
Range	0–32	0–29
± 2 SD	0–22.4	0–25.4
Percentage polymorphonuclear cells	61.3%	57.2%
Protein (mg/dl)		
No. of infants	35	17
Mean	90	115
Range	20–170	65–150
Glucose (mg/dl)		
No. of infants	51	23
Mean	52	50
Range	34–119	24–63
CSF/blood glucose (%)		
No. of infants	51	23
Mean	81	74
Range	44–248	55–105

Appendix A.2. Cerebrospinal fluid examination in high-risk neonates without meningitis. (Reprinted with permission from Sarff L, Platt L, McCracken G. Cerebrospinal fluid evaluation in neonates: comparison of high-risk infants with and without meningitis. J Pediatr 1976;88:473.)

B. Growth Parameters

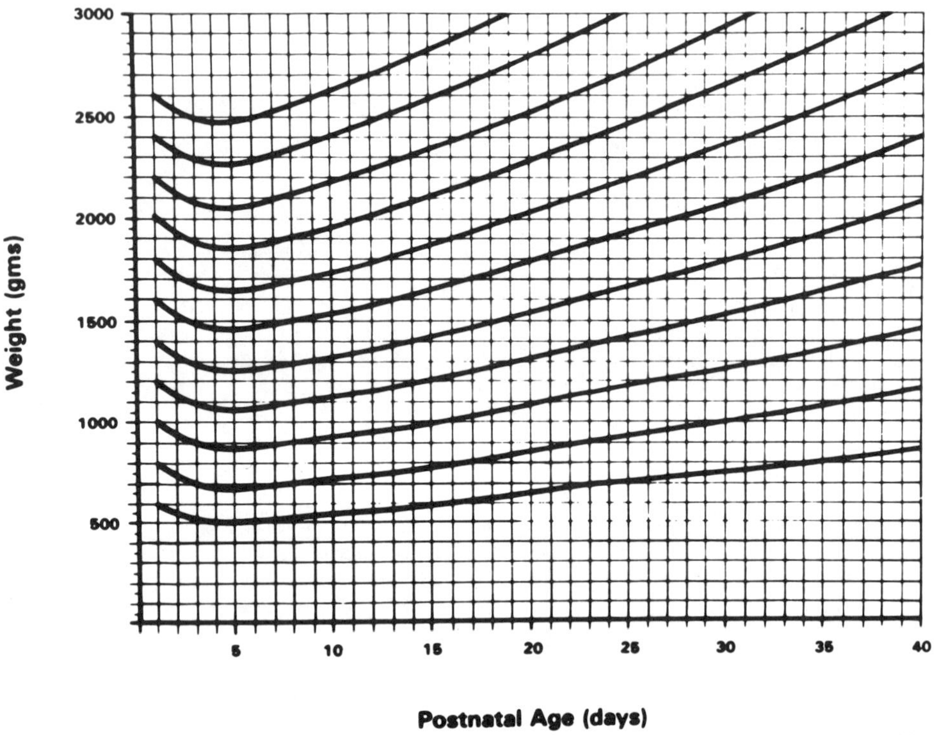

Appendix B.1. Postnatal growth grid (growth curves for 1000 gram birth weight groups). (Reprinted from Shaffer SG, Quimiro CL, Anderson JV, Hall RJ. Postnatal weight changes in low birth weight infants. Pediatrics 1987;79:702–705. Reproduced by permission of Pediatrics.)

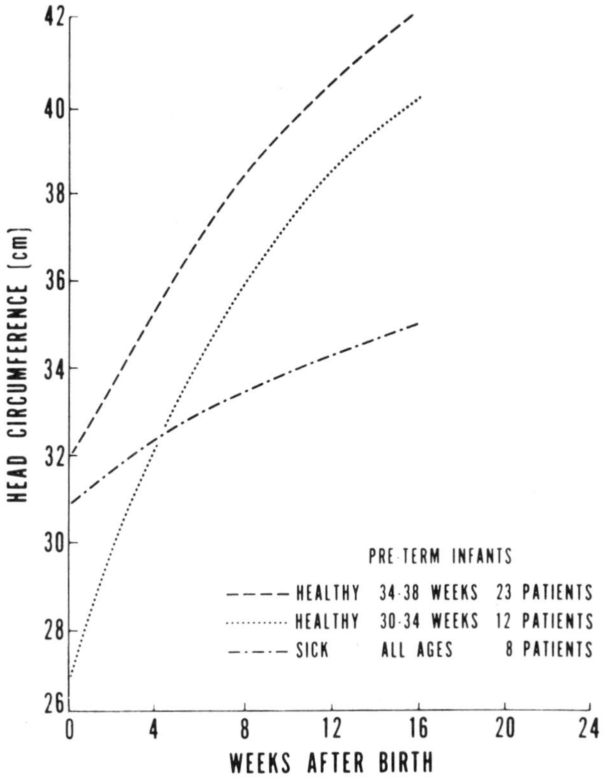

Appendix B.2. Head circumference growth chart. (Reprinted with permission from Sher PK, Brown SB. A longitudinal study of head growth in pre-term infants. I. Normal rates of head growth. Develop Med Child Neurol 1975;17:705–710.)

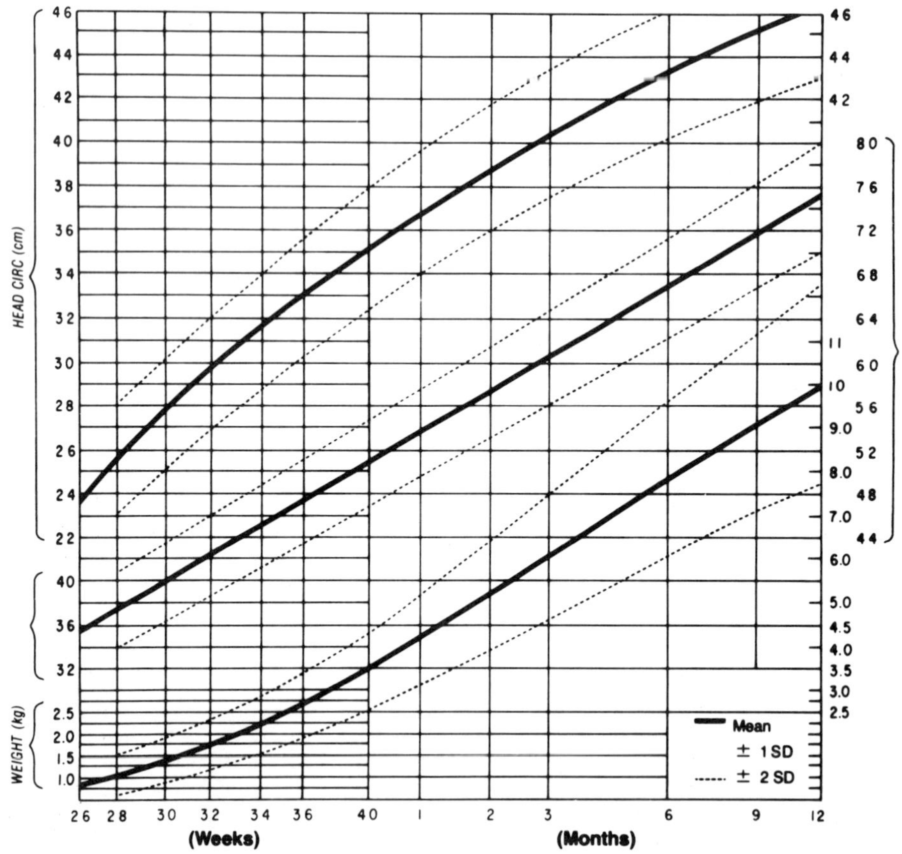

Appendix B.3. Growth record for infants birth to 1 year, sexes combined. (Used and reprinted with permission of Ross Laboratories, Columbus, OH 43216, © 1987 Ross Laboratories. Adapted and used with permission from Babson SG, Benda GI. Growth graphs for the clinical assessment of infants of varying gestational age. J Pediatr 1976;89:814.)

POUNDS	OUNCES 0	1	2	3	4	5	6	7	8	9	10	11	12	13	14	OUNCES 15
0	—	28	57	85	113	142	170	198	227	255	283	312	340	369	397	425
1	454	482	510	539	567	595	624	652	680	709	737	765	794	822	850	879
2	907	936	964	992	1021	1049	1077	1106	1134	1162	1191	1219	1247	1276	1304	1332
3	1361	1389	1417	1446	1474	1503	1531	1559	1588	1616	1644	1673	1701	1729	1758	1786
4	1814	1843	1871	1899	1928	1956	1984	2013	2041	2070	2098	2126	2155	2183	2211	2240
5	2268	2296	2325	2353	2381	2410	2438	2466	2495	2523	2551	2580	2608	2637	2665	2693
6	2722	2750	2778	2807	2835	2863	2892	2920	2948	2977	3005	3033	3062	3090	3118	3147
7	3175	3203	3232	3260	3289	3317	3345	3374	3402	3430	3459	3487	3515	3544	3572	3600
8	3629	3657	3685	3714	3742	3770	3799	3827	3856	3884	3912	3941	3969	3997	4026	4054
9	4082	4111	4139	4167	4196	4224	4252	4281	4309	4337	4366	4394	4423	4451	4479	4508
10	4536	4564	4593	4621	4649	4678	4706	4734	4763	4791	4819	4848	4876	4904	4933	4961
11	4990	5018	5046	5075	5103	5131	5160	5188	5216	5245	5273	5301	5330	5358	5386	5415
12	5443	5471	5500	5528	5557	5585	5613	5642	5670	5698	5727	5755	5783	5812	5840	5868
13	5897	5925	5953	5982	6010	6038	6067	6095	6123	6152	6180	6209	6237	6265	6294	6322
14	6350	6379	6407	6435	6464	6492	6520	6549	6577	6605	6634	6662	6690	6719	6747	6776
15	6804	6832	6860	6889	6917	6945	6973	7002	7030	7059	7087	7115	7144	7172	7201	7228
16	7257	7286	7313	7342	7371	7399	7427	7456	7484	7512	7541	7569	7597	7626	7654	7682
17	7711	7739	7768	7796	7824	7853	7881	7909	7938	7966	7994	8023	8051	8079	8108	8136
18	8165	8192	8221	8249	8278	8306	8335	8363	8391	8420	8448	8476	8504	8533	8561	8590
19	8618	8646	8675	8703	8731	8760	8788	8816	8845	8873	8902	8930	8958	8987	9015	9043
20	9072	9100	9128	9157	9185	9213	9242	9270	9298	9327	9355	9383	9412	9440	9469	9497
21	9525	9554	9582	9610	9639	9667	9695	9724	9752	9780	9809	9837	9865	9894	9922	9950
22	9979	10007	10036	10064	10092	10120	10149	10177	10206	10234	10262	10291	10319	10347	10376	10404

Appendix B.4. Conversion of pounds and ounces to grams.

C. Miscellaneous

Age	< 1.0 kg	1.0–1.5 kg	1.5–2.5 kg	> 2.5 kg
Birth	33 ± 15	39 ± 18	42 ± 20	49 ± 19
1 week	41 ± 15	47 ± 18	50 ± 20	60 ± 19
2 weeks	45 ± 15	50 ± 18	53 ± 20	64 ± 19
4 weeks	48 ± 15	53 ± 18	56 ± 20	68 ± 19

Appendix C.1. Normal mean arterial pressure in the newborn. Values given as mean +95% confidence limits for single measurements. (Reprinted with permission from Stork EK, Carlo WA, Kleigman RM, et al. Pediatr Res 1984;18:321A.)

Weeks	1	2	3	4	5	6	7	8	9	10
< 1500 gm	0.40	0.30	0.25	0.25	0.25	0.25	0.25	0.25	0.35	0.45
28–32 weeks	(0.05)	(0.04)	(0.03)	(0.03)	(0.03)	(0.03)	(0.03)	(0.03)	(0.04)	(0.05)
1500–2000 gm	0.45	0.40	0.40	0.45	0.45	0.45	0.50	0.50	0.60	0.70
32–36 weeks	(0.05)	(0.05)	(0.05)	(0.05)	(0.05)	(0.05)	(0.05)	(0.05)	(0.06)	(0.06)
2000–2500 gm	0.50	0.45	0.50	0.60	0.70	0.75	0.75	0.75	0.75	0.80
36–40 weeks	(0.05)	(0.05)	(0.05)	(0.06)	(0.06)	(0.06)	(0.60)	(0.60)	(0.60)	(0.70)
>2500 gm	0.55	0.55	0.55	0.60	0.75	0.80	0.85	0.85	0.85	0.85
Term	(0.60)	(0.60)	(0.60)	(0.60)	(0.70)	(0.70)	(0.80)	(0.80)	(0.80)	(0.80)

Appendix C.2. Serum Vitamin E (mg/dl) (Mean ± [1 SD]). (Reprinted with permission from Klaus MH, Fanaroff AA. Care of the high-risk neonate. 3rd ed. Philadephia: Saunders, 1986.)

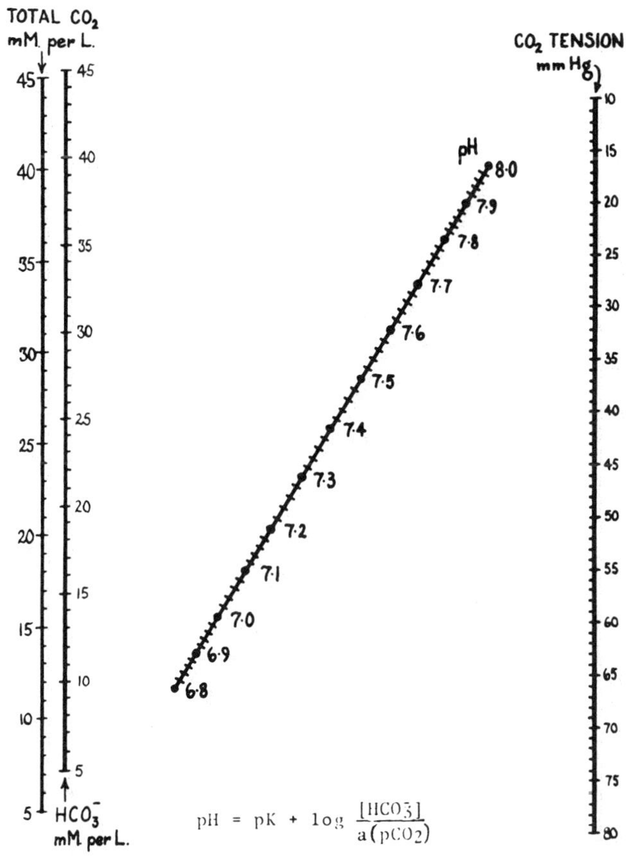

$$pH = pK + \log \frac{[HCO_3^-]}{a(pCO_2)}$$

where pK = 6.10 and a = 0.0301

Appendix C.3. Henderson-Hasselbalch Nomogram. Line chart for graphic calculation of serum or plasma values by the Henderson-Hasselbalch equation. A straight line through given points on any two scales cuts the other two scales at points indicating simultaneously occurring values. (From Cole CH. The Harriet Lane handbook. 10th ed. Chicago: Year Book Medical Publishers, 1984. Adapted from McLean FC. Application of the law of chemical equilibrium (law of mass action) to biological problems. Physiological Reviews 1983;18:495. Used with permission of the American Physiological Society.)

NAME ______________________ DOB ______ GA ______ BWT __________

1. Discharge criteria: A) Medically stable
   B) Gaining weight
   C) Nippling all feeds
   D) Temperature stable in bassinet
   E) Family ready

   Anticipate discharge 2–3 weeks in advance. Discharge as early as 34 weeks postconceptional age (PCA) for infants without major problems, therefore begin discharge planning as early as 32 weeks.

   Calendar date for 32 weeks PCA: __________

2. Anticipating Discharge:
   1. ___ Primary care pediatrician Name ______________________
   2. ___ 20 kcal/oz formula with Fe started
   3. ___ Nipple feeds started ___ nippling all ___
   4. ___ Weaned to bassinet
   5. ___ Medication changes made for optimal home management: started ___ completed ___
   6. ___Caffeine/theophylline discontinued. Date discontinued: ______________
   7. ___Family notified and involved in discharge plan

3. Predischarge studies:
   ___ Echocardiogram ordered ___ done ___
   ___ CXR ordered ___ done ___
   ___ Head sonogram ordered ___ done ___
   ___ Neurodevelopmental exam ordered ___ done ___
   ___ BAERS scheduled ___ done ___
   ___ Hct/reticulocyte count ordered ___ done ___
   ___ Head circumference measured
   ___ ROP exam scheduled ___ done ___
   ___ Metabolic screens done ___

4. Discharge needs:
   ___ Discharge family conference
   ___ Medication prescriptions written
   ___ Special equipment ordered
   ___ Follow-up appointments made
   ___ Primary care physician contacted
   ___ Neurodevelopmental exam arranged (Follow-up as recommended)
   ___ ROP exam scheduled (Follow-up as recommended)
   ___ Speech and Hearing appointment made (Follow-up as recommended)
   ___ Other specialty appointments made
   ___ DPT ordered ___ done ___ (2 months of age—do not give within 48 hrs of discharge).
   ___ OPV ordered ___ done ___ (2 months of age—given at time of discharge).
   ___ Hib (Recommendations forthcoming)

Appendix C.4. Medical discharge checklist. Division of Neonatology, The Johns Hopkins Hospital, 1990.

Index

Page numbers in *italics* denote figures; those followed by "t" denote tables.

Abdomen
  distention, in feeding tolerance, 28
  wall defects, surgical management, 189–190
Abruptio placenta, in developmental disabilities, 151–152
Acidosis, respiratory, in chronic lung disease, 109
Acne, neonatal, 204
Acquired immunodeficiency syndrome (*see* Human immunodeficiency virus infection)
Acrocyanosis, 202
Acrodermatitis enteropathica, 206
Acropustulosis of infancy, 203
Acyclovir
  in herpes simplex virus infection, 95–96
  in varicella, 207
Adenine arabinoside, in herpes simplex virus infection, 95
β-Agonists, in chronic lung disease, 117t, 119
AIDS (*see* Human immunodeficiency virus infection)
Airway obstruction, apnea and, 36, 40
Albinism, 216
Albuterol, in chronic lung disease, 117t, 119
Aldactone (spironolactone), in chronic lung disease, 116–118, 117t
Allergic contact dermatitis, 205
Alupent (metaproterenol), in chronic lung disease, 117t, 119
Amino acids, requirements, 6
Aminophylline, in apnea, 43
Ammonia, excess blood levels, apnea in, 41
Ampicillin, in streptococcal infection, 86
Amylase activity, 11
Anemia, 49–60
  apnea and, 39
  clinical course, 49, *50*
  erythropoietin in, 49–52, *51*
  hematocrit in, 52–53
  management, 54–59, *54–55*, 57t–58t, *58*, 113
  nutritional deficiencies in, 54–57, *54–55*
  pathophysiology, 49–53, *51*
  signs and symptoms, 53, 53t
  transfusion therapy in, 57–59, 57t–58t, *58*
Anesthesia
  apnea and, 190
  thyroid function effects, 172
Angioplasty, in left heart disease, 72
Antihistamines, in mastocytosis, 210
Anus, imperforate, colostomy in, 192
Aorta, coarctation, 70–72
Aortic valve defects, 70–72
Apgar score, developmental disability risk and, 153
Aplasia cutis congenita, 209, *209*
Apnea
  central, 36, 40
  clinical presentation, 37–41, 38t, 40t, 42t
  definition, 33–34
  diagnosis, 41, 42t
  hematocrit and, 53
  in chronic lung disease, 105, 110
  incidence, 34–35, *34*
  mixed, 36
  monitoring, 45–46, 46t
  obstructive, 36
  of prematurity, definition, 33
  pathogenesis, 35–37, *35*, *37*, 40
  pathological, 33, *34*
  pathological conditions with, 39–41, 40t, 42t
  postanesthetic, 190
  treatment, 41–44, 42t–44t
  vs. gestational age, 34, *34*
Apparent life-threatening event, home monitoring for, 45–46, 46t
Arrhythmias, cardiac, 74–76
Arterial blood gases (*see* Blood gases, arterial)

Arterial hemoglobin oxygen saturation, in chronic lung disease, 109–110, *110*, 114–115
Arterial pressure, vs. postnatal age, 243
Ash leaf macules, 216
Asphyxia, hearing loss and, 180
Aspiration, in feeding, 112–113
Asymmetry, in neurodevelopmental examination, 138t, 139
Atrial beats, premature, 74–75
Auditory brainstem response, in hearing screening, 180–184, *181*, *183*
Auditory stimulation, as developmental intervention, 143–144

Bacteria, colonization of newborn, 85–86
Bacterial meningitis, 86, 180
Balloon angioplasty, in left heart disease, 72
Barotrauma, chronic lung disease and, 104–105, *104*
Basal metabolic rate, preterm infant, 5–6
Bathing, skin irritation in, 198
Behavioral abnormalities, in neurodevelopmental examination, 140
Benzyl alcohol, respiratory effects, 44
Betamethasone, thyroid function effects, 172
Bilirubin level, hearing loss and, 179–180
Blindness, 134
  in retinopathy of prematurity, 125, 129, 131
Blisters, 206–210
  sucking, 217
Blood
  loss, anemia in, 52–53
  pH, in chronic lung disease, 108–109
  sampling, heel stick nodules from, 201, *201*
Blood gases, arterial, measurement
  in cardiovascular disorders, 65
  in chronic lung disease, 108–109, 108t, 115
Blood pressure, vs. age, 62, 243
Blood urea nitrogen, serum levels, 239
Body composition, fetus, 2–4, 2t, *3*
  vs. preterm infant, 6, *7*
Body temperature, regulation (*see* Thermoregulation)
Bradycardia, 74
  hematocrit and, 53
  in apnea, 34, 45–46, 46t
  in chronic lung disease, 105, 110
  in patent ductus arteriosus, 41
Brain
  atrophy, developmental disabilities and, 156
  calcification in, developmental disabilities and, 156
  hemorrhage
    developmental disabilities and, 155–157
    in fullterm newborn, 158
  imaging, developmental disabilities and, 155–158, 156t
  infarction, in fullterm newborn, 158
Brainstem immaturity, apnea and, 35, *35*
Breast milk
  antithyroid drugs in, 172
  calcium in, 14
  carbohydrates in, 11
  discharge planning and, 222
  fortification, 14, 15t, 21, 27–28
  HIV transmission in, 91–92
  immune factors in, 20–21, 21t
  lipids in, 9–10
  preterm
    protein content, *7*, 8
    vs. term, 21, 22t
  protein in, *7*, 8, 21, 22t
  sodium in, 12
  term vs. preterm, 21, 22t
  vitamins in, 19
  vs. formula, 20–21, 21t–22t
  weight gain and, 6, *7*
  zinc in, 17, 206
Breathaire (terbutaline), in chronic lung disease, 117t
Breathing
  cessation (*see* Apnea)
  in hypercapnia, 37, *37*
  in hypoxia, 37, *37*
  modulators, 35, *35*
Bronchodilators, in chronic lung disease, 117t, 118–119
Bronchopulmonary dysplasia, 103 (*see also* Chronic lung disease)
Bronkosol (isoetharine), in chronic lung disease, 117t, 119
Bullous impetigo, 207
BUN (blood urea nitrogen), serum levels, 239
Burns, 200, *200*

Cafe au lait spots, 215
Caffeine, in apnea, 42–43, 43t
Calcification, intracranial, developmental disabilities and, 156
Calcium
  absorption, 13
  deficiency, 13, 15–16

excretion, 14
in fetal body composition, *3*
in formulas, 14
in milk, 14
in parenteral nutrition, 15, 16t
requirements, 13–16, *14*, 15t
serum levels, 239 (*see also* Hypocalcemia)
Caloric requirements (*see* Energy, requirements)
Candidiasis, 205–206
disseminated, 208
Carbohydrate
in breast milk, immunological function, 21t
requirements, 10–11
storage, 10–11
supplementation in formula, 28
Carbon dioxide (*see also* Hypercapnia)
Henderson-Hasselbalch nomogram for, 245
measurement in chronic lung disease, 108–109
serum levels, 239
Cardiac catheterization, in ventricular septal defect, 70
Cardiovascular disorders
arrhythmias, 74–76
blood gas measurement in, 65
chest radiography in, 65
chromosomal, 65–66, 65t
cor pulmonale, 76–77, 109, 116
cyanotic congenital, 72–74, 72t
echocardiography in (*see* Echocardiography)
electrocardiography (*see* Electrocardiography)
evaluation in, 61–65
functional murmurs, 66–67
heart block, 76
history, 61–62
in chronic lung disease, 107
left heart disease, 70–72
patent ductus arteriosus (*see* Patent ductus arteriosus)
physical examination in, 62–64
premature beats, 74–75
pulmonary artery stenosis, 66
pulmonary flow murmur, 67
pulmonary venous anomalies, 73
single ventricle without pulmonary stenosis, 73–74
sinus rhythm, 74
supraventricular tachycardia, 75–76
tetralogy of Fallot, 72–73
truncus arteriosus, 73
ventricular septal defect, 68–70
Cardiovascular shunt (*see also* Patent ductus arteriosus)
apnea in, 41
transfusion therapy in, 59
ventricular septal defect, 68–70
Catheterization
arterial
scars resulting from, 199–200, *199*
tissue necrosis in, 200
cardiac, in ventricular septal defect, 70
central venous, infections from, 87
Cavernous hemangioma, 211–214, *213*
Central apnea, 36, 40
Central nervous system (See also Brain)
disorders, apnea and, 40
HIV infection, 92
syphilis manifestations in, 97–98
Central venous catheter, infections from, 87
Cerebral palsy, 133–134, 134t
brain hemorrhage and, 157
Cerebrospinal fluid constituents, 239
Checklist, for discharge planning, 224, 246
Chemical burns, 200, *200*
Chemoreflex, laryngeal, in apnea, 38–39
Chickenpox, congenital, 207
Chlamydial infection, 96–97
Chloride
requirements, 12
serum levels, 239
Chlorothiazide
in chronic lung disease, 116, 117t, 118
in patent ductus arteriosus, 68
Chromosomal disease
cardiovascular, 65–66, 65t
developmental disability risk and, 155
Chronic lung disease, 103–124
assessment, 105–111, 106t, 108t, *110*
bronchodilators in, 118–119
clinical evaluation, 105–108, 106t
complications, 111t
definitions, 103–104
discharge planning, 120–122, 120t–121t
diuretics in, 116–118, 117t
fluid management in, 115–116
history, 105, 106t
laboratory studies, 108–111, 108t, *110*
management, 111–119, 111t–112t, 114t, 117t
goals in, 103, 103t
monitoring in, 110
nutrition in, 111–113, 112t
outcome, 122–123
oxygen therapy in, 113–115, 114t

Chronic lung disease—*continued*
pathogenesis, 104–105, *104*
steroid therapy in, 119
Cleft lip/palate, hearing loss in, 179
Clonus, sustained, in neurodevelopmental examination, 138t, 139
Clothing, thermoregulation and, 82t
Cold stress, 198
Color, skin
harlequin changes, 202–203
in cardiovascular disorders, 62
Color Doppler echocardiography, 64
Colostomy, 192–193
Computed tomography, developmental disabilities and, 136, 155–158, 156t
Conduction abnormalities, 74–76
Congenital heart disorders (*see under* Cardiovascular disorders)
Congenital infections (*see under* Infections)
Congestive heart failure
in chronic lung disease, 116
in patent ductus arteriosus, 68
in ventricular septal defect, 70
Conjunctivitis, chlamydial, 96–97
Constipation, in feeding tolerance, 28
Contact dermatitis, 205
Continuous murmur, 63
Continuous positive airway pressure, in apnea, 43–44
Conversion, metric-pounds, 243
Copper requirements, 16–17
Cor pulmonale, 76–77
in chronic lung disease, 109, 116
Cortical atrophy, developmental disabilities and, 156
Corticosteroids
in chronic lung disease, 119
in hemangioma, 213
Cradle cap (seborrheic dermatitis), 206
Cranial imaging studies, in developmental disabilities, 136
Cranial neuropathy, in neurodevelopmental examination, 138t, 139
Craniofacial malformation, hearing loss in, 179
Crib-O-Gram, in hearing screening, 182
Cromolyn sodium
in chronic lung disease, 119
in mastocytosis, 210
Cryotherapy, in retinopathy of prematurity, 131
Cutis marmorata, 202
Cyanosis
in apnea, 34
in cardiovascular disorders, 62
in congenital heart disease, 72–74, 72t
in skin disorders, 202
Cysteine, requirements, 6
Cystic fibrosis, enterostomy in, 192
Cytomegalovirus infection
hearing loss and, 179
transfusion-acquired, 59, 89
vertically transmitted, 89–90

Dapsone, in acropustulosis of infancy, 203
Darier's sign, in mastocytosis, 210
Deafness (*see* Hearing loss)
Demographic factors, in developmental disabilities, 150, 151t
Depression, postpartum, 235
Dermatitis, 205–206
Dermatology (*see* Skin)
Development (*see also* Developmental disabilities; Growth; Neurodevelopmental outcome)
language, 143–144
hearing loss and (*see* Hearing loss)
thyroid gland, 162–163
Developmental disabilities
abnormal behavior in, 140
assessment, 135
asymmetries in, 139
auditory stimulation in, 143–144
causes, 149–150
cerebral palsy, 133–134, 134t, 157
common patterns in, 138–140, 138t
community resources and, 145–146
cranial neuropathy in, 139
daily care scheduling, 141
definition, 133
discharge planning, 144–145, 145t
emotional interventions, 140
examination in, 136–140, 137t–138t
hyperreflexia in, 139
hypertonia in, 138–139, 138t
hypotonia in, 138, 138t
interventions in, 140–144, 146t
mental retardation, 134, 169–170
minimal cerebral dysfunction, 135
monitoring, 135–140, 137t–138t
neck extensor hypertonia in, 138–139, 138t
nonnutritive sucking benefits, 141–142
oromotor abnormalities in, 139
parent counseling, 144–146, 145t
positioning techniques, 142–143
risk factors for, 144–145, 149–160

cranial imaging and, 155–158, 156t
degrees, 152–159, 153t–154t, 156t
demographic, 150, 151t
examination in, 136–140, 137t–138t
neonatal, 151t, 152
neurodevelopmental examination and, 136–140, 137t–138t, 158–159
obstetrical, 151–152, 151t
prenatal, 150–151, 151t
vs. causation, 149–150
with highly increased risk, 153t, 155
with mildly increased risk, 152–153, 153t
with moderate increased risk, 153–154, 153t–154t
sensory evaluation in, 139–140
sensory impairment, 134–135 (*see also* Hearing loss; Retinopathy of prematurity)
social interventions, 140
stimulation techniques, 143–144
types, 133, 134t
visual stimulation in, 144
Dexamethasone
in chronic lung disease, 119
in hyperthyroidism, 173
Diaper dermatitis, 205–206
Diarrhea, in rotavirus infection, 88
Digoxin
in cor pulmonale, 77
in left heart disease, 71
in supraventricular tachycardia, 76
in ventricular septal defect, 70
Diphtheria-tetanus-pertussis immunization, 98
Discharge planning, 219–226
checklist for, 224, 246
coordinator for, 220–221
date designation, 234
developmental disabilities and, 144–145, 145t
equipment needs, 222, 222t
family conference in, 223
family considerations in, 224–225
family role in, 233–234
for chronic lung disease, 120–122, 120t–121t
for early discharge, 224–225
for enteral feeding, 29
for follow-up care, 225–226
for thermoregulation, 81–82
for transfer to other hospital, 224
for transitions to home care, 222, 222t
immunization in, 223–224
initiation, 221
insecurities developing in, 234
loose ends in, 223–224, 223t
medical criteria for, 221
predischarge studies, 222–223, 223t
process, 221–224, 222t–223t
teaching, 225
team for, 219–221, 220t
Diuretics
in chronic lung disease, 116–118, 117t
in left heart disease, 71
in patent ductus arteriosus, 68
in pulmonary edema, 116
in ventricular septal defect, 70
Diuril (chlorothiazide)
in chronic lung disease, 116, 117t, 118
in patent ductus arteriosus, 68
Dobutamine, in left heart disease, 71
Dopamine, in left heart disease, 71
Doppler echocardiography, 64–65
Down's syndrome, cardiovascular disorders in, 65, 65t
Doxapram, in apnea, 44
Drugs
abuse
apnea in, 40
developmental disability risk and, 150–151, 151t
HIV infection and, 91
hypothyroidism induced by, 168
thyroid function effects, 172
topical, skin absorption, 197–198
Ductus arteriosus, patent (*see* Patent ductus arteriosus)

Early diastolic murmur, 63
Early systolic murmur, 63
Echocardiography, 64–65
in arrhythmias, 75–76
in chronic lung disease, 108t, 109, 115
in cor pulmonale, 77
in left heart disease, 71
in patent ductus arteriosus, 67–68
in ventricular septal defect, 69
Edema, pulmonary
in chronic lung disease, 115–116
in left heart disease, 71
Electrocardiography, 64
in arrhythmias, 75–76
in chronic lung disease, 108t, 109, 115
in cor pulmonale, 77
in patent ductus arteriosus, 68

Electrolyte values, serum, 239
Emotional interventions, developmental, 140–141
Encephalitis, herpes, 95–96
Encephalomalacia, developmental disabilities and, 158
Encephalopathy, hypoxic-ischemic, 154, 154t
Energy
  requirements
    components, 5–6, *7*
    fetal, 3–4, *4–5*
    in chronic lung disease, 111–112
    in enterostomy, 193
    postnatal, 4–6, 5t, *7*
    preterm infant, 4–6, 5t, *7*
  storage in fetus, 3–4, *4–5*
Enfamil Human Milk Fortifier, composition, 15t
Enteral feeding (*see under* Feeding)
Enteric infections, viral, 88
Enterostomy, 192–193
Epidermal nevi, 214
Epidermolysis bullosa, 208–209
Equipment
  for home care, 222, 222t
  for oxygen therapy, 121
Erythema, reactive, 217–218, *217*
Erythema toxicum neonatorum, 203
Erythromycin, in chlamydial infection, 96–97
Erythropoietin, in postnatal anemia, 49–52, *51*
Esophageal atresia, 187–188
  gastrostomy in, 191
Euthyroid sick syndrome (low T_3 syndrome), 171
Extensor hypertonia, in neurodevelopmental examination, 138–139, 138t
Eye
  chlamydial infection, 96–97
  retinopathy in (*see* Retinopathy of prematurity)
  stimulation, as developmental intervention, 144

Family, 227–237
  accommodation to situation, 232
  birth announcements by, 228
  counseling on developmental disability, 144–146, 145t
  disappointment, 231
  fatigue, 236
  financial impacts on, 235
  guilt feelings, 232
  hearing loss history in, 179
  helplessness feelings, 231
  impact of unexpected problems on, 227–228
  in acute phase of hospitalization, 231–232
  in discharge planning, 220, 223–225, 233–234
  insecurities, 234
  interpersonal adjustments in, 235
  interventions for, 236
  isolation, 235–236
  lodging accommodations for, 230
  parental roles during hospitalization, 140, 230–231
  participation as caretaker, 233
  phone call policy, 229
  postpartum depression and, 235
  privacy for, 228
  reaction to ongoing hospitalization, 232–233
  relationship with infant, 228–231
  return to community hospital and, 233
  separation from infant, policies concerning, 228–230
  sibling problems in, 235
  stress in, 232
  visiting policy for, 229–230
Fat necrosis, subcutaneous, 204–205
Father (*see* Family)
Fatigue, caretaker, after discharge, 236
Fatty acids
  essential, 8–9
  in formulas, 9–10, 10t
Feeding, enteral (*see also* Breast milk; Formulas)
  advancing, 25–27
  apnea and, 38–39
  aspiration in, 112–113
  breast milk vs. formula, 20–21, 21t–22t
  concentration, 27–28, 112
  discharge planning and, 29, 222
  factors affecting, 19
  frequency, 27
  gastric residuals in, 28
  gavage, 22–25, 24t–25t
    apnea and, 38
    gastrostomy for, 25, 112, 141–142, 191–192
    in chronic lung disease, 112
    nonnutritive sucking in, 141–142
  in enterostomy, 193–194
  in esophageal atresia, 187–188
  initiation, 20
  methods for, 22–25, 24t–25t

necrotizing enterocolitis and, 20, 25–26
nonnutritive sucking in, 141–142
osmolality, 26
regulation, 4
tolerance
in chronic lung disease, 105, 112–113
monitoring, 28–29, 28t
transpyloric, 23
Fever, 80–81, 81t
Fistula, tracheoesophageal, 187–188
Fluid and electrolyte balance
in chronic lung disease, 115–116
in enterostomy, 193
Folate deficiency, in anemia, 56–57
Follow-up care, after discharge, 225–226
Formulas
calcium in, 14, 15t
carbohydrates in, 11
concentration, 27–28, 112
high-calorie, 70
in chronic lung disease, 112
in enterostomy, 193–194
in ventricular septal defect, 70
lipids in, 9–10, 10t
preterm, 10t, 22
protein content, 7–8, 8t
sodium in, 12–13
vitamins in, 18t
vs. breast milk, 20–21, 21t–22t
weight gain and, 6, *7*
zinc in, 17
Fortification, breast milk, 14, 15t, 21, 27–28
Fungal infections, 205–206, 208
Furosemide
in chronic lung disease, 117–118, 117t
in left heart disease, 71
in patent ductus arteriosus, 68

Galactose absorption, 11
"Gasping syndrome," 44
Gastric residual, between feedings, 28
Gastroesophageal reflux
after esophageal atresia correction, 188
apnea and, 39
continuous gavage feeding in, 25
in chronic lung disease, 112–113
Gastrointestinal system, viral infections, 88
Gastroschisis, surgical management, 189–190
Gastrostomy
complications, 191–192
for gavage feeding, 25, 112, 141–142, 191–192
in abdominal wall defect, 189
in chronic lung disease, 112
indications, 191
Gavage feeding, 22–25, 24t–25t
apnea and, 38
gastrostomy for, 25, 112, 141–142, 191–192
in chronic lung disease, 112
nonnutritive sucking in, 141–142
Genioglossus muscle activity, in sleep, 36
Genital herpes virus infection, 94–96
Gentamicin, in streptococcal infection, 86
Giant congenital pigmented nevi, 214–215
Glucoamylase activity, 11
Glucose
absorption, 11
in cerebrospinal fluid, 239
Glycerides, 9, 9t
Graft-versus-host disease, in transfusion therapy, 59
Gram-negative organisms, in nosocomial infections, 86–87
Grams, conversion to pounds/ounces, 243
Graves' disease, maternal, neonatal hyperthyroidism in, 172–173
Growth
as nutritional assessment, 29
assessment, 135–136
fetal, 2–3, *2–3*, 2t
head circumference, 136, 241–242
in chronic lung disease, 111–112, 112t
intrauterine retardation, 152
postnatal, *2–3*, 240, 242

Hair disorders, 216
Handicapped infant (*see* Developmental disabilities)
Handling techniques, as developmental interventions, 142–143
Harlequin skin color change, 202–203
Head circumference growth
chart for, 241–242
developmental disabilities and, 136
Hearing loss, 135, 177–186
incidence, 177
interventions, 178
risk factors, 178–180, 178t
screening for, 140
importance, 177
methodology, 180–182, *181*
programs, 182–185, *183*, 185t
rationale, 177–178
timing, 182

Heart block, congenital, 76
Heart disorders (*see* Cardiovascular disorders)
Heart rate, 74
  in cardiovascular disorders, 62
Heart sounds, in cardiovascular disorders, 63
Heat regulation (*see* Thermoregulation)
Heel stick nodules, 201, *201*
Hemangioma, 211–214, *213*
Hematocrit
  in anemia, 53, 53t
    transfusion indications and, 57–59, 57t–58t, *58*
  in chronic lung disease, 111
  variations in, 49, *50*
Hemoglobin, fetal, oxygen affinity, 50
Hemoglobin oxygen saturation, in chronic lung disease, 109–110, *110*, 114–115
Hemorrhage, brain
  developmental disabilities and, 155–157
  in fullterm newborn, 158
Henderson-Hasselbalch nomogram, 245
Hepatitis B, 93–94
  immunization, 94
  transfusion-acquired, 89
Hepatitis C, transfusion-acquired, 89
Hering-Breuer reflex, continuous positive airway pressure and, 43
Hernia
  incisional, in enterostomy, 193
  inguinal
    in abdominal wall defect, 189
    in chronic lung disease, 107
    surgical management, 190
Herpes simplex virus infection, 94–96, 207
Hirschsprung's disease, colostomy in, 192
Histiocytosis X, skin manifestations, 206
HIV infection (*see* Human immunodeficiency virus infection)
Holosystolic murmur, 63
Home monitoring, apnea, 45–46, 46t
Hood, for oxygen therapy, 113–114
Hormones, thyroid (*see* Thyroid gland)
Human immunodeficiency virus infection, 91–93
  transfusion-acquired, 89
Hyaline membrane disease, 103
Hydrocephalus
  developmental disabilities and, 157
  monitoring for, 136
  surgical management, 194–195
Hyperammonemia, apnea in, 41
Hyperbilirubinemia, hearing loss and, 179–180
Hypercapnia
  in chronic lung disease, 109
  ventilatory response to, 37, *37*
Hyperpigmentation disorders, 215
Hyperreflexia, in neurodevelopmental examination, 138t, 139
Hypertension, pulmonary
  in chronic lung disease, 107, 109
  in ventricular septal defect, 70
Hyperthermia, 80–81, 198
  apnea and, 39
Hyperthyroidism, neonatal, 172–173
Hyperthyrotropinemia, transient, 171
Hypertonia, neck extensor, in neurodevelopmental examination, 138–139, 138t
Hypocalcemia, 15–16
  apnea in, 41
  in chronic lung disease, 111
Hypochloremia, in chronic lung disease, 110
Hypoglycemia
  apnea in, 41
  developmental disability risk and, 152–153
Hypokalemia, in chronic lung disease, 110
Hyponatremia, 12
  apnea in, 41
  in chronic lung disease, 110
Hypophosphatemia, 15–16
  in chronic lung disease, 111
Hypopigmentation disorders, 216
Hypopituitarism, thyroid dysfunction in, 170
Hypoplastic left heart syndrome, 70–72
Hypothermia, 80–81
  apnea and, 39
Hypothyroidism
  central, 170
  clinical signs, 167
  maternal, 171
  permanent, 168–170
  primary, 167–170
  secondary (central), 167
  tertiary (central), 167
  transient, 167–168
Hypothyroxinemia
  in hypothyroidism, 166t, 167–170
  in thyroxine-binding globulin deficiency, 166t, 170
  transient, 166–167, 166t
Hypotonia, in neurodevelopmental examination, 138, 138t
Hypoxia/hypoxemia
  erythropoietin response to, 50, 52

hearing loss and, 180
symptoms, 114–115, 114t
ventilatory response to, 37, *37*
Hypoxic-ischemic encephalopathy, 154, 154t

Ileostomy, 192–193
Imaging, cranial, developmental disability risk and, 155–158, 156t
Immune factors, in breast milk, 20–21, 21t
Immunization, 223–224
diphtheria-tetanus-pertussis, 98
hepatitis B, 94
polio, 99, 224
Immunoglobulin A, in breast milk, 21t
Impetigo, bullous, 207–208
Incontinentia pigmenti, 210
Incubator, 80–81, 81t–82t, 222, 222t
Indomethacin, in patent ductus arteriosus, 68
Infarction, brain, in fullterm newborn, 158
Infections, 85–102 (*see also specific infection*)
apnea and, 41
catheter-related, 87
congenital
developmental disability risk and, 153
hearing loss and, 179
enteric, 88
Gram-negative, 86–87
immunization for, 98–99
nosocomial, 85–89
opportunistic, in HIV infection, 92
respiratory, 87–88
skin, 207–208
streptococcal, 86
transfusion-acquired, 89
vertically transmitted (congenital), 89–98
Influenza, 88
Inguinal hernia
in abdominal wall defect, 189
in chronic lung disease, 107
surgical management, 190
Inotropic drugs, in left heart disease, 71
Intercostal muscular activity, in sleep, 36
Intestinal dysfunction
in abdominal wall defect, 189
in enterostomy, 193
in necrotizing enterocolitis therapy, 194
Intrauterine growth retardation, 152
Intraventricular hemorrhage, developmental disabilities and, 155–157
Iodine
absorption through skin, 197
deficiency, hypothyroidism in, 167
excess, hypothyroidism in, 167–168
placental transfer, hypothyroidism in, 168
requirements, 17
Iron, in nutrition, 54–55, *54–55*
Irritability, in neurodevelopmental examination, 140
Isoetharine, in chronic lung disease, 117t, 119

Jadassohn, sebaceous nevus of, 214
Jaundice, mechanism, 52
Jejunostomy, 192–193
Jitteriness, in neurodevelopmental examination, 140

Kasabach-Merritt syndrome, 213

Labyrinthine primitive reflex, 142
Lactase activity, 11
Lactoferrin, in breast milk, 21t
Lactose, in milk, 11
Language development, 143–144
hearing loss and (*see* Hearing loss)
stimulation, as developmental intervention, 143–144
Laryngeal chemoreflex, in apnea, 38–39
Laser surgery, in hemangioma, 214
Lasix (*see* Furosemide)
Left heart disease, 70–72
Length, vs. postnatal age, 242
Lethargy, in neurodevelopmental examination, 140
Leukoderma, 216
Leukomalacia, periventricular, developmental disabilities and, 155, 157–158
Light intensity, in retinopathy of prematurity, 130
Lipase, in breast milk, 10
Lipid
absorption, 9–10
classes, 8, 9t
dietary, 9–10, 10t
energy storage in, 3–4, *4–5*
fatty acids, 8–10, 10t
functions, 8, 9t
glycerides, 9, 9t
in fetal body composition, 2t
in formulas, 9–10, 10t
phospholipids, 9, 9t
sterols, 9, 9t
supplementation in formula, 28
Liver morphology
in abdominal wall defect, 189
in chronic lung disease, 107

Low T_3 syndrome, 171
Lugol's solution, in hyperthyroidism, 173
Lung disorders (*see also* Chronic lung disease)
  cor pulmonale in, 76–77, 109, 116
Lupus erythematosus, neonatal, 217–218, *217*
Lymphocytes, in breast milk, 21t
Lymphocytic interstitial pneumonitis, in HIV infection, 92
Lysozyme, in breast milk, 21t

Magnetic resonance imaging, developmental disabilities and, 136, 155–158, 156t
Malaria, transfusion-acquired, 89
Maltase activity, 11
Mastocytosis, 210
Mechanical ventilation, in apnea, 44
Mechanobullous diseases, 208–210
Medications (*see* Drugs)
Melanosis, transient neonatal pustular, 203
Meningitis
  hearing loss and, 180
  streptococcal, 86
Mental retardation, 134
  developmental disability risk and, 155
  in hypothyroidism, 169–170
Metabolic disorders, apnea in, 41
Metabolism, preterm infant, 5–6
Metaproterenol (Metaprel), in chronic lung disease, 117t, 119
Methimazole, neonatal thyroid effects, 172
Methylxanthines, in apnea, 42–43, 42t–44t
Metric system, conversion to pounds/ounces, 243
Microcephaly, 155
Milia, 204
Miliaria, 204
Minimal cerebral dysfunction, 135
Mitral valve obstruction, congenital, 70–72
Moles (*see* Nevi)
Mongolian spots, 215
Monitoring
  apnea, 45–46, 46t
  developmental disabilities, 135–140, 137t–138t
  chronic lung disease, 110
  equipment for, 222
  feeding tolerance, 28–29, 28t
  oxygen therapy, 114–115, 114t, 122
Mother (*see* Family)
Murmurs, in cardiovascular disorders, 63–64, 66–67

Nail disorders, 216–217
Nasal cannula, for oxygen therapy, 113
Nasogastric tube feeding, 23, 24t, 112
Neck extensor hypertonia, in neurodevelopmental examination, 138–139, 138t
Neck position, apnea and, 39
Necrosis
  fat, subcutaneous, 204–205
  from arterial catheters, 200
Necrotizing enterocolitis
  apnea in, 41
  enterostomy in, 192
  feeding advancement and, 25–26
  feeding initiation and, 20
  medical management, 194
  surgical management, 192
Neonatal factors, in developmental disabilities, 152
Neurodevelopmental examination, 136–140, 137t–138t, 158–159
Neurodevelopmental outcome (*see also* Developmental disabilities)
  chronic lung disease and, 123
  hearing loss effect on, 177–178
Neutral thermal environment, 79
Nevi
  epidermal, 214
  hemangioma, 211–214, *213*
  pigmented, 214–215
  port wine stains, 211, *212*
  salmon patches, 211
  sebaceous, of Jadassohn, 214
Nevus anemicus, 216
Nifedipine, in cor pulmonale, 77
Nikolsky's sign, in scalded skin syndrome, 207
Nodules, heel stick, 201, *201*
Nonnutritive sucking, as developmental intervention, 141–142
Nosocomial infections, 85–89
  bacterial, 85–87
  viral, 87–89
Nutrition, 1–31
  calcium, 13–16, *14*, 15t–16t
  carbohydrate, 10–11, 21t, 28
  copper, 16–17
  deficiencies (*see also specific substance*)
    in anemia, 54–57, *54–55*
  energy requirements and
    fetal, 2t, 3–4, *4–5*
    in chronic lung disease, 111–112
    preterm infant, 4–6, 5t, *7*

enteral feeding in (*see* Feeding, enteral)
enterostomy and, 193–194
for fetal growth reproduction, 2–3, *2–3*, 3t
in chronic lung disease, 111–113, 112t
lipid, 8–10, 9t–10t, 28
minerals, 11–17, 12t, *14*, 15t–16t
objectives, 1
parenteral
calcium in, 15, 16t
in enterostomy, 193
phosphorus in, 15, 16t
soft tissue damage in, 200, *200*
vitamin D in, 15
phosphorus, 13–16, *14*, 15t–16t
potassium, 12t, 13
protein, 6–8, 8t
sodium chloride, 11–13, 12t
trace elements, 16–17
vitamins (*see* Vitamins)
water, 11–13
zinc, 16–17

Obstetrical factors, in developmental disabilities, 151–152, 151t
Obstructive apnea, 36
Omphalocele, surgical management, 189–190
Opportunistic infections, in HIV infection, 92
Oral polio vaccine, 224
Oromotor abnormalities, in neurodevelopmental examination, 138t, 139
Oromotor stimulation, as developmental intervention, 141–142
Osmolality, in enteral feeding, 26
Otoscopy, in hearing screening, 184
Ounces, conversion to grams, 243
Oximetry, pulse (*see* Pulse oximetry)
Oxygen
deficiency (*see* Asphyxia; Hypoxia/hypoxemia)
measurement, in chronic lung disease, 108–109
toxicity, chronic lung disease and, 104–105, *104*
Oxygen saturation, in chronic lung disease, 109–110, *110*, 114–115
Oxygen therapy
delivery systems, 113–114
discharge planning, 120–122, 120t–121t
equipment for, 121
in apnea, 44
in chronic lung disease, 104, 113–115, 114t, 120–122, 120t–121t
in left heart disease, 71
monitoring, 114–115, 114t, 122
retinopathy of prematurity and, 113, 125–127, *127*

Pacifiers, as developmental intervention, 141–142
Panhypopituitarism, hypothyroidism in, 170
Pansystolic murmur, 63
Papile grading system, brain hemorrhage, 157
Parenteral nutrition (*see under* Nutrition)
Parents (*see* Family)
Patent ductus arteriosus, 67–68
apnea in, 41
in chronic lung disease, 107
in pulmonary atresia, 72–73
left heart disease and, 70–72
Pathological apnea, 33, *34*
Penicillin, in streptococcal infection, 86
Penicillin G, in syphilis, 98
Periodic breathing, 33–34
Periventricular hemorrhage, developmental disabilities and, 155–157
Periventricular leukomalacia, developmental disabilities and, 155, 157–158
Pertussis, immunization, 98
pH
blood, in chronic lung disease, 108–109
Henderson-Hasselbalch nomogram for, 245
Phenobarbital, thyroid function effects, 172
Phenytoin, thyroid function effects, 172
Phlebectasia, congenital, 202
Phone calls, policy for, 229
Phospholipids, 9, 9t
Phosphorus
absorption, 13
deficiency, 13, 15–16
excretion, 14
in fetal body composition, *3*
in formulas, 14, 15t
in milk, 14
in parenteral nutrition, 15, 16t
requirements, 13–16, *14*, 15t
serum levels, 239
Piebaldism, 216
Pigmentation disorders, 210, 215–216 (*see also* Nevi)
Pigmented nevi, congenital, 214–215
Pituitary gland dysfunction, hypothyroidism in, 170
Pneumocystis carinii pneumonia, in HIV infection, 92

Pneumography, in apnea, 45
Pneumonia, 88
  in HIV infection, 92
Pneumonitis
  chlamydial, 96–97
  herpes, 95–96
  in cytomegalovirus infection, 90
  lymphocytic interstitial, in HIV infection, 92
Polio vaccine, 99, 224
Polycose carbohydrate supplement, 28
Polycythemia
  as fetal adaptation, 50, 52
  developmental disability risk and, 153
Polysomnography
  in apnea, 45
  in chronic lung disease, 110
Porencephaly, developmental disabilities and, 156
Port wine stains, 211, *212*
Positioning
  apnea and, 39
  as developmental intervention, 142–143
Postpartum depression, 235
Potassium
  deficiency, 110
  requirements, 12t, 13
  serum levels, 239
Pounds, conversion to grams, 243
Precordial activity, in cardiovascular disorders, 63
Prednisone, in hemangioma, 213
Premature beats, 74–75
Prenatal factors, in developmental disabilities, 150–151, 151t
Prickly heat (miliaria), 204
Privacy, for family, 228
Propranolol
  in hyperthyroidism, 173
  in supraventricular tachycardia, 76
Propylthiouracil, neonatal thyroid effects, 172
Prostaglandins, in left heart disease, 71
Protein
  absorption, 6
  energy storage in, 3–4, *4*
  in breast milk, 21, 21t–22t
  in cerebrospinal fluid, 239
  in fetal body composition, 2t, *3*, 7
  requirements, 6–8, 8t
Proventil (albuterol), in chronic lung disease, 117t, 119
Pulmonary artery stenosis, murmurs in, 66
Pulmonary atresia, with tetralogy of Fallot, 72–73
Pulmonary edema
  in chronic lung disease, 115–116
  in left heart disease, 71
Pulmonary flow murmur, 67
Pulmonary function, in chronic lung disease. 107, 108t, 109
Pulmonary hypertension
  in chronic lung disease, 107, 109
  in ventricular septal defect, 70
Pulmonary veins, anomalous insertion, 73
Pulse oximetry
  in cardiovascular disorders, 65
  in chronic lung disease, 108t, 109, *110*, 115
  in oxygen therapy monitoring, 114–115
Pulsed Doppler echocardiography, 64–65
Pulses, in cardiovascular disorders, 63
Pustular skin disorders, benign, 203–204

Quality-of-life issues (*see* Developmental disabilities)

Radiography
  in cardiovascular disorders, 65
  in chronic lung disease, 108, 108t, 115
  in patent ductus arteriosus, 68
Radioimmunoassay, thyroid hormones, 162
Rash, diaper, 205–206
Reactive erythema, 217–218, *217*
Reflux, gastroesophageal (*see* Gastroesophageal reflux)
Resin T_3 uptake test, 162, 166t, 170
Respiratory acidosis, in chronic lung disease, 109
Respiratory distress (*see also* Chronic lung disease)
  in esophageal atresia, 187
  in patent ductus arteriosus, 68
  thyroxine deficiency and, 172
Respiratory infections, viral, 87–88
Respiratory muscles, activity in sleep, apnea and, 36
Respiratory rate, in cardiovascular disorders, 62
Respiratory syncytial virus infection, 88
Reticulocyte response, transfusion therapy and, 58, *58*
Retinopathy of prematurity, 125–132
  classification, 127–129, *128*, *130*
  clinical presentation, 127–129, *128*, *130*
  diagnosis, 129, *130*

historical view, 125
management, 129–131
oxygen therapy and, 113
pathophysiology, 113, 125–127, *126–127*
regression, 128–129
screening for, 140
Retrolental fibroplasia (*see* Retinopathy of prematurity)
Reverse triiodothyronine, 161–163, 165, 171
Ribavirin, in respiratory infections, 88
Rickets, 111–112
Right ventricular preejection period, in chronic lung disease, 109
Right ventricular systolic time interval, in chronic lung disease, 109
Ritodrine, thyroid function effects, 172
Rotavirus infections, 88
Rubella syndrome, congenital, hearing loss and, 179

Salmon patches, 211
Salt, requirements, 11–13, 12t
SaO_2 (oxygen saturation), in chronic lung disease, 109–110, *110*, 114–115
Sarnat staging system, for hypoxic-ischemic encephalopathy, 154, 154t
Scalded skin syndrome, 207–208
Scaly skin disorders, 205–206
Scars, 199–200, *199–200*
Scheduling daily care, as developmental intervention, 141
Screening
for hearing loss (*see under* Hearing loss)
for retinopathy of prematurity, 140
for thyroid hormones, 165–166
Sebaceous gland hyperplasia, 203
Sebaceous nevus of Jadassohn, 214
Seborrheic dermatitis, 206
Seizures, developmental disability risk and, 152, 154
Selenium requirements, 17
Sensory impairment, 134–135 (*see also* Hearing loss; Visual impairment)
in neurodevelopmental examination, 138t, 139–140
Sensory stimulation, as developmental intervention, 143–144
Sepsis
apnea and, 41
nosocomial, 86–87
Septal defect, ventricular, 68–70
Shivering, heat production in, 80
Short bowel syndrome, continuous gavage feeding in, 25
Shunt
cardiovascular (*see* Cardiovascular shunt; Patent ductus arteriosus)
in hydrocephalus, 195
Siblings
emotional concerns, 235
visiting policy, 230
Sinus rhythm, 74
Skin
barrier properties, 197–198
care, in enterostomy, 192–193
evaluation, 201–202
function, 197, 198t
structure, 197, 198t
thermoregulatory function, 198
topical agents use on, 197–198
Skin disorders
acne, 204
acrocyanosis, 202
acrodermatitis enteropathica, 206
acropustulosis of infancy, 203
albinism, 216
allergic contact dermatitis, 205
aplasia cutis congenita, 209, *209*
ash leaf macules, 216
burns, 200, *200*
cafe au lait spots, 215
candidiasis, 205–206
catheter damage, *199*, 200
chemical burns, 200, *200*
cradle cap (seborrheic dermatitis), 206
cutis marmorata, 202
diagnosis, 204
diaper dermatitis, 205–206
epidermal nevi, 214
epidermolysis bullosa, 208–209
erythema toxicum neonatorum, 203
fat necrosis, 204–205
harlequin color change, 202–203
heel stick nodules, 201, *201*
hemangioma, 211–214, *213*
herpes simplex infection, 207
histiocytosis X, 206
hyperpigmentation, 215–216
hypopigmentation, 216
in herpes simplex virus infection, 95
in syphilis, 97–98
incontinentia pigmenti, 210
infections, 207–208
mastocytosis, 210

Skin disorders—*continued*
mechanobullous, 208–210
melanosis, 203
milia, 204
miliaria, 204
Mongolian spots, 215
nevi, 210–215, *212–213*
nevus anemicus, 216
piebaldism, 216
pigmentation abnormalities, 215–216
pigmented nevi, 214–215
port wine stains, 211, *212*
prickly heat, 204
pustular, 203–204
reactive erythemas, 217–218, *217*
salmon patches, 211
scaly, 205–206
sebaceous gland hyperplasia, 203
sebaceous nevus of Jadassohn, 214
seborrheic dermatitis, 206
staphylococcal scalded syndrome, 207–208
surgical scars, 199, *199*
thermal burns, 200
transient vascular phenomena, 202–203
varicella, 207
vesiculopustular, 206–210, *209*
Sleep
apnea in, 36
patterns, developmental effects, 141
polysomnography in, 45, 110
respiratory muscular activity in, 36
Social interventions, developmental, 140–141
Social worker, in discharge planning, 220
Sodium
disorders (*see* Hyponatremia)
serum levels, 239
Sodium chloride, requirements, 11–13, 12t
Speech development, 143–144
hearing loss and (*see* Hearing loss)
Spironolactone, in chronic lung disease, 116–118, 117t
Staphylococcal scalded skin syndrome, 207–208
Steroids
in chronic lung disease, 119
thyroid function effects, 172
Sterols, 9, 9t
Stimulation, sensory, as developmental intervention, 141–144
Strawberry hemangioma, 211–214, *213*
Streptococcal infections, nosocomial, 86
Stress, in family, 232
Subarachnoid hemorrhage, developmental disabilities and, 158
Sucking
apnea and, 38
blisters from, 217
nonnutritive, as developmental intervention, 141–142
Sudden infant death syndrome, home monitoring for, 45–46, 46t
Supraventricular tachycardia, 75–76
Surfactant deficiency, in chronic lung disease, 104, *104*
Surgical management, 187–196
abdominal wall defects, 189–190
colostomy, 192–194
esophageal atresia, 187–188
gastroschisis, 189–190
gastrostomy, 191–192
hydrocephalus, 194–195
ileostomy, 192–194
inguinal hernia, 190
omphalocele, 189–190
scarring in, 199–200, *199*
undescended testes, 190
Syphilis, 97–98, 179
Systolic ejection murmur, 63

T_3 (*see* Triiodothyronine)
T_4 (*see* Thyroxine)
T_3 RU (resin T_3 uptake) test, 162, 166t, 170
Tachycardia, 74
in chronic lung disease, 106
supraventricular, 75–76
Tachypnea
in cardiovascular disorders, 62
in chronic lung disease, 106
Taurine, requirements, 6
TBG (*see* Thyroxine-binding globulin)
Teaching, before discharge, 225
Temperature regulation (*see* Thermoregulation)
Teratogenesis, in developmental disabilities, 150–151, 151t
Terbutaline, in chronic lung disease, 117t
Testis, undescended, surgical management, 190
Tetanus, immunization, 98
Tetracycline, in chlamydial infection, 96
Tetralogy of Fallot, with pulmonary atresia, 72–73
Theophylline
in apnea, 42–43, 42t–44t
in chronic lung disease, 117t, 118–119

toxicity, 44t
Thermal burns, 200
Thermal stress, apnea and, 39
Thermogenesis, 80
diet-induced, 6
Thermoregulation, 79–83
discharge advice for, 81–82
energy requirements and, 6
goals, 79
homeostatic mechanisms in, 80
incubator in, 80–81, 81t–82t, 222, 222t
physical principles in, 79, 80t
skin function in, 198
types of instability, 80–81, 81t
Thumb sucking blisters, 217
Thyroid gland, 161–175
aplasia, 168–169
development, 162–163
disorders
hyperthyroidism, 172–173
hyperthyrotropinemia, 171
hypothyroidism
maternal, 171
neonatal, 167–170
hypothyroxinemia, 166–170, 166t
low T_3 syndrome, 171
medication-induced, 172
respiratory distress syndrome and, 172
screening for, 165–166
thyroxine-binding globulin deficiency, 170
thyroxine-binding globulin excess, 173
function, premature vs. fullterm infant, 163, 163t, *164*, 165, 165t
hormones, 161–162
hypoplasia, 168–169
Thyroid-stimulating hormone
deficiency, 171
function, 161
in hyperthyroidism, 172
in hyperthyrotropinemia, 171
in hypothyroidism, 166t, 167–170
in hypothyroxinemia, 166–167, 166t
in low T_3 syndrome, 171
in premature vs. fullterm infant, 163, 163t, *164*
in thyroid development, 162
in thyroxine-binding globulin deficiency, 166t, 170
laboratory testing for, 162
medication effects on, 172
screening for, 165–166
Thyrotoxicosis, neonatal, 172–173
Thyrotropin (*see* Thyroid-stimulating hormone)
Thyrotropin-releasing hormone, 161–162, 166–167
Thyroxine
binding, 161–162
deficiency, 166 172, 166t
excess, 171–173
in premature vs. fullterm infant, 163, 163t, *164*, 165t
in thyroid development, 162–163
laboratory evaluation, 162
replacement therapy with, 169, 171
screening program for, 165–166
synthesis, 161
Thyroxine-binding globulin, 161–162
deficiency, 170
excess, 173
in low T_3 syndrome, 171
in premature vs. fullterm infant, 163, 163t, 165
in thyroid development, 162–163
laboratory evaluation, 162
medication effects on, 172
Tonic labyrinthine primitive reflex, 142
Topical agents, skin absorption, 197–198
Touching, as developmental intervention, 143
Toxoplasmosis, hearing loss and, 179
Trace elements, requirements, 16–17
Tracheoesophageal fistula, 187–188
Tracheomalacia, 187–188
Transfusion therapy
complications, 59
in anemia, 57–59, 57t–58t, *58*
infections from, 89
soft tissue damage in, 200
TRH (thyrotropin-releasing hormone), 161–162, 166–167
Triiodothyronine
deficiency, 171
in hyperthyroidism, 172–173
in premature vs. fullterm infant, 163, 163t
in thyroid development, 162–163
laboratory evaluation, 162
medication effects on, 172
respiratory distress syndrome and, 172
reverse, 161–163, 165, 171
synthesis, 161
Trisomy 13, cardiovascular disorders in, 66
Trisomy 18, cardiovascular disorders in, 66
Trisomy 21 (Down's syndrome), cardiovascular disorders in, 65, 65t
Trophamine, minerals in, 15, 16t

Truncus arteriosus, 73
TSH (*see* Thyroid-stimulating hormone)
Tube feeding (*see* Gavage feeding)
Turner's syndrome, cardiovascular disorders in, 66
Two-dimensional echocardiography, 64–65
Tyrosine, requirements, 6

Ultrasonography, developmental disabilities and, 136, 155–158, 156t
Umbilical artery catheterization, tissue necrosis in, 200

Vagal stimulus, in supraventricular tachycardia, 76
Valvotomy, in left heart disease, 72
Varicella, congenital, 207
Vascularization, retina, 126–127, *126–127*
Ventilation
  in hypercapnia, 37, *37*
  in hypoxia, 37, *37*
Ventolin (albuterol), in chronic lung disease, 117t, 119
Ventricle (brain)
  dilation, developmental disabilities and, 157
  shunting, in hydrocephalus, 195
Ventricle (heart)
  premature beats associated with, 75
  septal defect, 68–70
  single, without pulmonary stenosis, 73–74
Verapamil, in supraventricular tachycardia, 76
Vernix caseosa, 198
Vesiculopustular dermatoses, 206–208
Viral infections (*see also specific virus*)
  enteric, 88
  nosocomial, 87–89
  respiratory, 87–88
  transfusion-acquired, 89
Visiting policy, 229–230
Visual impairment, 134–135
  in retinopathy of prematurity, 125, 128–129, 131
Visual stimulation, as developmental intervention, 144
Vitamin(s)
  deficiencies, in enterostomy, 193–194
  requirements, 17–19, 18t
  supplements, 18–19
Vitamin D
  in parenteral nutrition, 15
  requirements, 15
Vitamin E
  in retinopathy of prematurity, 129–130
  requirements, 56
  serum levels, vs. age, 244

Waardenburg's syndrome, 216
Water
  in fetal body composition, 2t
  requirements, 12
Weaning, from incubator, 81, 81t–82t, 222, 222t
Weight
  birth, hearing loss and, 179
  fetal, vs. gestational age, 2–3, *2–3*, 2t
  vs. blood pressure, 243
  vs. energy requirements, 6, *7*
  vs. mineral content, 14–15, *14*
  vs. postnatal age, 240, 242
Whooping cough, immunization, 98
Wolfe's syndrome, 216
Wolff-Parkinson-White syndrome, 75–76
Wood's light examination, 216

Zidovudine, in HIV infection, 91, 93
Zinc
  deficiency, 206
  requirements, 16–17